SURGERY - PROCEDURES, COMPLICATIONS, AND RESULTS

A SURGEON'S PERSPECTIVE ON DIALYSIS PATIENTS

SURGERY - PROCEDURES, COMPLICATIONS, AND RESULTS

Additional books and e-books in this series can be found on Nova's website under the Series tab.

SURGERY - PROCEDURES, COMPLICATIONS, AND RESULTS

A SURGEON'S PERSPECTIVE ON DIALYSIS PATIENTS

MARIA FRANKOVIČOVÁ
EDITOR

nova
Medicine & Health
New York

Library of Congress Cataloging-in-Publication Data

Names: Frankovicova, Maria, editor.
Title: Surgeon's perspective on dialysis patient / Maria Frankovicova, University Pavol Jozef Safarik, Professor of Surgery; Chief of Department of Vascular Surgery, East Slovak Institute of Cardiovascular Diseases, Medical Faculty of Safarik University, Kosice, Slovakia, editor.
Identifiers: LCCN 2021006052 (print) | LCCN 2021006053 (ebook) | ISBN 9781536192629 (hardcover) | ISBN 9781536193145 (adobe pdf)
Subjects: LCSH: Hemodialysis--Patients.
Classification: LCC RC901.7.H45 S87 2021 (print) | LCC RC901.7.H45 (ebook) | DDC 617.4/61059--dc23
LC record available at https://lccn.loc.gov/2021006052
LC ebook record available at https://lccn.loc.gov/2021006053

Published by Nova Science Publishers, Inc. † New York

CONTENTS

PREFACE

Every year a large number of chronic patients undergo dialysis at dialysis departments in the Slovak Republic. Each one of them is connected to the artificial kidney 100 to 160 times. The most valuable property of these patients is a quality and long-term functioning arteriovenous fistula since it is one of the essential conditions for successful dialysis. The surgeon who creates arteriovenous access must thoroughly examine the patient before the operation, properly evaluate the vascular system and choose the most favorable way of the vascular access for long-term hemodialysis. Patients with chronic renal failure have impaired hemostasis, several of them have diabetes and their vascular system is affected by atherosclerosis. Determination of the operational plan and optimal vascular access is strictly individual and depends not only on the vascular system of the patient but also on the general condition, age and prognosis of the disease. A quality arteriovenous fistula should conform to the requirements of the simplest and the shortest operation as possible, using local anesthesia. Underestimation of any fact can result in the creation of many non-functional AV fistulas. AV fistulas operations for the purpose of long-term hemodialysis are an integral part and one of the most problematic issues of Vascular Surgery. There are more and more patients who are in the long-term hemodialysis program. The average age of patients is increasing. All these factors have resulted in the need to create more and more AV fistulas because their usability is limited. The correct operational tactics, individual approach to the patient and precise surgical technique of the vascular surgeon contributes to the improvement of the quality of life of sick patients, of whom only a small percentage is so lucky that the disease is cured by successful kidney transplantation.

Chapter 1 - The basic prerequisite to successful long-term hemodialysis treatment is the possibility of repeated connection of the patients ‘circulation to the extracorporeal circulation of the hemodialysis machine. This requires a simple and reliable vascular access that provides a sufficient blood volume for the hemodialysis machine. In the chapter the authors present vascular accesses with their advantages and disadvantages, they also describe the history of arteriovenous fistula development.

Chapter 2 - In this chapter the authors describe the anatomy of the arteries and veins of the upper limb. The authors present the most frequently used veins of the forearm and arm to create AV shunt: at the forearm v. cephalica, v. mediana cubiti in the cubital fossa. In the arm area v. basilica, that is very often the last option to create the vascular access for long term dialysis program, with failure or closure of AV shunts formed in the areas of the forearm and cubital fossa.

Chapter 3 - Chronic kidney disease (formerly also chronic renal insufficiency) is irreversible impairment of renal functions. It is defined as abnormalities of kidney structure and function that are present for more than 3 months. The disease should be classified based on the cause, a category determined by glomerular filtration, and albuminuria. The prevalence of chronic kidney disease has been rising at a rapid pace over the last decades, gaining epidemic proportions and has become one of the major public health problems. The worldwide prevalence varies from country to country, with a prevalence of 10-13%.

Chapter 4 - In this chapter the authors present the most frequently created vascular accesses: Subcutaneous arteriovenous fistula, Fistula in fossa Tabatiere, Distal radiocephalic fistula, Radiobasilic AVF with transposition, Radiobasilic AVF with transposition, Distal ulnar-basilic fistula, Proximal radiocephalic fistula, Fistula in fossa cubitalis, brachiobasilic AVF with transposition and other options.

Chapter 5 - The purpose is to create an AV fistula that can be easily cannulated and withstand repeated punctures. The first fistula is introduced in the limb as distally as possible. Doppler ultrasonography **is** a simple examination that will help us map the arteriovenous system on the limbs. AV fistulae are created in super aseptic operating rooms where reconstructive vascular operations are performed.

Chapter 6 - Chronic kidney disease is characterized by a gradual loss of kidney function. The most common causes of kidney malfunction are diabetes mellitus, high blood pressure and glomerulonephritis. Chronic renal disease may not be apparent until a kidney function is significantly decreased. Treatment is focused on the treatment of underlying causes to slow progression of kidney dysfunction. Once kidney functions are significantly impaired and progress to end stage kidney failure, patient may need dialysis. There are different types of dialysis, between them hemodialysis with three primary methods to gain access to the blood for hemodialysis. This chapter deals with problems with maturation of native arteriovenous access and arteriovenous grafts and possibilities to prevents these complications. In this chapter the authors also deal with treatments options.

Chapter 7 - Health care of patients with vascular access for hemodialysis requires the collaboration of a nephrologist, a vascular surgeon, an interventional radiologist, and an angiologist. The vascular access is reported to be one of the six factors determining morbidity and, indirectly, the mortality of dialysis patients. Surgery of arteriovenous connections for the needs of long-term hemodialysis is an integral yet at the same time part one of the most problematic parts of vascular surgery. The principle of care for hemodialysis access is to maintain good function as long as possible with a minimum of complications and interventions.

Chapter 8 - Long-term central venous access means the introduction of a catheter into the lumen of a vein. Central vein cannulation is also vital in acute life-saving conditions. The permanent catheter is inserted into the superior or inferior vena cava. The most commonly used access paths are subclavian vein, internal jugular vein, external jugular vein. Access path via the femoral vein is associated with a higher incidence of complications.

Chapter 9 - Patients with chronic kidney disease, where kidney functions are significantly impaired and progress to end stage kidney failure, may require dialysis. There are different types of dialysis, one of which is hemodialysis. There are three primary methods of establishing vascular access for hemodialysis purposes. Clinical monitoring of AV fistulas, outside and during hemodialysis, can detect AV fistula dysfunction in a timely manner and thus can timely prepare SAVF formation. Any patient with a dysfunctional or non-functional native AV fistula, or with an AV fistula using a prosthesis, is a candidate for SAVF. AV shunt should be monitored at least once a month during hemodialysis and in patients with AV failure SAVF should be considered as the first option for any patient in whom AV fistula has failed.

Chapter 10 - The essence of PD (peritoneal dialysis) is the exchange of substances between the peritoneal dialysis solution inserted into the peritoneal cavity. The exchange takes place by transport through the peritoneum. PD requires a multidisciplinary approach: a nephrologist, nurses, a surgeon, a dietitian, a social worker, and a pharmacologist, with the patient's connection to the transplant center.

Chapter 11 - The number of patients who need a long-term hemodialysis is constantly increasing. The most frequent complications of arteriovenous fistula type subcutaneous vascular accesses include infections, thromboses, and complications due to low blood flow. Complications can include skin necrosis or defects. Skin defects can be most often covered by a flap, a skin transplant or a skin substitute. The flaps are classified according to several criteria as local and distant flaps. The Limberg flap is one of the most commonly used flaps used to cover defects after removal of necrosis in complications of hemodialysis accesses. For definitive cover of the skin, the authors can also use an autograft, for temporary cover using skin substitutes of various origin. Skin substitutes can be divided into biologic, synthetic, biosynthetic, and combined. Reconstruction of tissue defects is needed in case of an extensive defect or a loss of organ function.

Chapter 12 - Kidney transplantation is the treatment method that, from a medical point of view, most comprehensively replaces the function of the organ in the event of its irreversible failure. The first human kidney was unsuccessfully transplanted by Voronoy in Ukraine in 1933. The first kidney transplantation in former Czechoslovakia was performed in Hradec Králové in 1961. In general, organ transplants (Tx) require the technique of vascular anastomosis or surgical connection of vessels, which would allow flow from one vessel to another. Without such a connection, there is no hope of success.

Chapter 13 - Modern cardiology can be classified into two lines, namely invasive and non-invasive. Invasive (using blood) examination methods are used when a non-invasive examination procedure (such as non-invasive imaging tests) determines a diagnosis for which conservative treatment is not sufficient, or when, according to the latest recommendations by the European Society of Cardiology, it is necessary to choose an invasive cardiology procedure. Invasive examination methods are performed through various vascular accesses (for example, in selective coronarography access through the femoral artery or the radial artery is used). In this case, a collision of cardiology, angiology, and vascular surgery occurs at the site of puncture, which may be complemented by various complications. Associated patient diagnoses, such as renal failure at various stages, including the need for dialysis or type 2 diabetes mellitus at the stage of chronic complications, may also be a complication itself. In the next chapter, the authors will mention two main examination methods, namely selective coronarography and CT angiography, however, invasive cardiology offers many more predominantly arrhythmology-related invasive examinations (invasive electrophysiological examinations, ablations of supraventricular tachycardias, atrial fibrillation ablation using cryo energy and the radiofrequency energy). All these examinations are performed through vascular accesses.

Chapter 14 - The authors present five interesting case reports from their department concerning vascular accesses and their complications.

Chapter 15 - In this part of the publication, the author wants to draw attention to possible complications in dialysis patients from the point of view of a thoracic surgeon. It deals with the possible consequences of the cannulation of large veins, pleural tap, inflammatory complications in the pleural cavity. In individual subchapters he deals with pneumothorax, hemothorax, pleural effusion, thoracic empyema, and fibrothorax. He describes their clinical symptoms, diagnostic possibilities, and the treatment itself.

Chapter 16 - Chronic renal failure, dialysis and renal transplantation are associated with wide range of cutaneous manifestations. Uremia has very important impact on occurrence of dermatological symptoms and skin lesions. Cutaneous changes can be nonspecific – mainly pruritus, disorders of skin appendages, dry skin, dyschromia, or specific – calcinosis, perforating dermatoses, bullous dermatoses. Immunosuppressants have strong impact on occurrence of skin infections and skin cancer. Comorbidities associated with chronic renal failure, more often diabetes, obesity, immunosuppressive therapy and dialysis have also influence on management, diagnosis and treatment of cutaneous disorders.

INTRODUCTION

M. Frankovičová

The prolongation of lives and working capabilities in patients suffering from the final stage of chronic kidney disease (CKD) is possible either through kidney transplantation or systematic hemodialysis. Due to the fact that kidney transplantation remains only hope for many of the patients even today, hemodialysis tends to be the permanent solution of their health condition.

The main requirement of a long-term hemodialysis treatment is the possibility of connecting the patient's blood circulation with the artificial kidney's flow.

Proper vascular access means a high-quality and a well-developed arteriovenous connection, the so-called AV fistula, or a catheter leading into the patient's vascular system, which enables connecting the patient to the hemodialysis apparatus repetitively. Satisfactory development and long-term function of the fistula depend on the patient's vessel condition, the lumen of limb arteries and veins, the technical success of the arteriovenous fistula's creation, and the proper post-surgery and post-dialysis treatment.

The establishment of adequate vascular access with patients within the long-term hemodialysis program is often considered the so-called Achilles heel in the field of vascular surgery. This statement seems to be quite accurate, as even despite a well-developed and respected scheme of steps in individual cases, some patients need to go through repetitive surgeries, corrections, or modifications. Even the best vascular access may disappear with time. It is very important for the surgeon to have the exact plan in mind and to have sufficient experience in the field of vascular surgery.

As we have invested 35 years into creating vascular access of the so-called arteriovenous connections, we have decided to write a surgical aid for surgeons and doctors who deal with or would like to deal with the creation of arteriovenous connections in patients within the long-term hemodialysis program. This paper has been written to be easy to follow so that it would effectively help doctors to familiarize themselves with the given subject matter, and so that a surgeon reading this work would not need to spend enormous time self-studying, as previous generations needed to.

The history of vascular access creation at the Department of Surgery in Košice dates back to times when it was led by prof. MUDr. Emil Matejíček, DrSc, who was dealing with this subject matter mainly in his experiments and later on in his practice as well. The first publication about arteriovenous connections was written by prof. MUDr. Július Vajó, DrSc, who considerably contributed to the development of surgical techniques used to create high-quality vascular access in patients dialyzed at dialysis departments in Košice. The vascular team also consisted of MUDr. Eduard Milichovský and doc. MUDr. Igor Kundrát, CSc. In cooperation with prof. MUDr. Miroslav Mydlík, DrSc, MUDr. Róbert Roland and prof. MUDr. Ľudmila Podracká, CSc, several papers were published, and as a result, they enriched the knowledge about the subject matter and informed about new findings and experience. In the 90s, the team of vascular collaborators at the 1st Department of Surgery in Košice led by prof. MUDr. Juraj Bober, CSc. was joined by the following names: MUDr. František Arendárčik, MUDr. Mária Kubíková, MUDr. Jana Blažejová, MUDr. Peter Zavacký, MUDr. Norbert Torma and MUDr. Štefánia Hudáková. These doctors were performing surgeries of patients within the long-term hemodialysis program. Upon the delimitation of the Department of Vascular Surgery and the establishment of the Department of Vascular Surgery within VÚSCH, a.s., the vascular team was expanded with further names of professionals: MUDr. Marián Tomečko, PhD, MPH, MUDr. Vladimír Sihotský, PhD, MUDr. Martina Zavacká, PhD, MPH, MUDr. Andrej Smola, MUDr. Jana Pobehová, PhD, MUDr. Tatiana Granda, MUDr. Pavel Staško, PhD, MHA, MUDr. Ivan Žurkovský, MUDr. Ivan Kopolovets, MUDr. Peter Berek, PhD (the current superintendent at the Department of Vascular Surgery), MUDr. Michal Virág and MUDr. Lukáš Vaško. The number of surgeries has increased within the last 20 years and has reached four-digit numbers. This is influenced by the fact that mainly in recent years we have solved complicated vascular access of the so-called complicated patients who went through repetitive surgeries at different surgery departments within the eastern region of Slovakia. The results of our efforts have been presented at numerous professional scientific congresses, seminars, and internships not only in our country but also abroad.

This book is the source of theoretical as well as practical information for the pre-gradual, post-gradual training of surgeons, vascular surgeons, students of medicines, nephrologists, internists, and doctors of other disciplines within medicine. This book was translated by PaedDr. Peter Protivňak.

In: Surgeon´s Perspective on Dialysis Patient ISBN: 978-1-53619-262-9
Editor: Maria Frankovicova

Chapter 1

VASCULAR ACCESS

M. Frankovičová**, MD
Department of Vascular Surgery,
East Slovak Institute of Cardiovascular Diseases,
Faculty of Medicine,
Pavol Jozef Šafárik University in Košice,
Košice, Slovakia

ABSTRACT

The basic prerequisite to successful long-term hemodialysis treatment is the possibility of repeated connection of the patients 'circulation to the extracorporeal circulation of the hemodialysis machine. This requires a simple and reliable vascular access that provides a sufficient blood volume for the hemodialysis machine.

In the chapter we present vascular accesses with their advantages and disadvantages, we also describe the history of arteriovenous fistula development.

Keywords: vascular access, arteriovenous fistula, history

---

* Corresponding Author's E-mail: mfrankovicova@vusch.sk.

Establishing vascular access in patients enrolled in a long-term dialysis program is the task of the vascular surgeon.

Failure of vascular access is a major cause of hemodialysis morbidity and the most important factor influencing the financial cost of hemodialysis.

One of the basic conditions of long-term hemodialysis treatment is the possibility of repeated connection of the circulatory system of patients to the extracorporeal circulation of the dialysis machine. This requires a simple and reliable vascular access that provides a sufficient blood volume for the hemodialysis machine, which is also available for repeated cannulations (250 - 300) per year and meets the criteria of being the most distant location possible to maintain more proximal sites for the eventual future vascular accesses. In general, the vascular access must provide an extracorporeal flow of at least 250 - 300ml/min without recirculation of previously dialyzed blood into the circulation. By connecting the vein with the artery, we change the hemodynamic conditions, which gradually lead to the vascular reconstruction of the vein and its arterialization. Arterialization of the venous wall will enable the repeated punctures needed to connect the patient to the hemodialysis machine. Although the creation of an arteriovenous fistula belongs to the group of simpler vascular procedures, the issue of indication, operation, and resolution of complications is demanding and requires an experienced vascular surgeon and a comprehensive multidisciplinary approach.

This includes specialists in areas such as vascular surgery, nephrology, interventional radiology, and internal medicine, which are in daily contact with dialysis patients.

The overall increase in the dialysis population is associated with a sharp increase in the number of complications associated with establishing vascular access. Despite improved conditions for ensuring vascular access and subsequent monitoring of patients in the hemodialysis program as well as improved technologies for detecting complications, 18% of patients still die in the terminal stage of renal failure due to the loss of vascular access. The selection of suitable arteries and veins to ensure vascular access is primarily a matter of the erudition of the vascular surgeon.

The technique of surgery is a major problem area of establishing a properly functioning fistula. The cause of the failure may be technically incorrect adaptation of the vessel walls, incorrectly chosen method of anastomosis, rotation of the venous segment, bending of the venous arm of the fistula, insufficient hydrodilation, or pressure on the drainage arm. Other causes may be intraoperative and postoperative complications such as bleeding, thrombosis, infection, and neuropathy. The most common cause of dysfunction and subsequent vascular access failure is the thrombosis of the arteriovenous fistula. In approximately 80% of cases, the arteriovenous fistula (AVF) thrombosis is caused by a vascular obstruction or venous stenosis.

Along with the development of aortic surgery at the end of the 19th and the beginning of the 20th century, papers focused on techniques of peripheral arterial reconstruction also appeared. In 1906, Guthrie and Carrel presented the results of an extensive experimental study dealing with, among other things, direct suturing of a damaged arterial wall, transplantation of blood vessels, organs, and limbs. Independently, Carrel in France and Alfred Exner in Austria were working on the technique of vascular anastomosis. Alexis Carrel was more successful and was awarded the Nobel Prize in Physiology and Medicine in 1912 as the first surgeon ever. Alexis Carrel is considered to be the father of vascular surgery and his vascular suture is basically used to this day. However, we can talk about the real development of vascular surgery only after the Second World War. In addition to the rapid development of surgical techniques, the development of anesthesia, the use of antibiotics, progress in the administration of blood transfusions, the clinical utility of heparin, but also the development of diagnostics, especially angiography, all contributed to its progress. The concept of an arteriovenous fistula for hemodialysis was developed by Brescia, Cimino, and Appell. The first arteriovenous fistula was performed in 1965 by Appell, as a side to side anastomosis between the radial artery and the cephalic vein on the forearm.

The first modern hemodialysis treatment was performed by Willem Kolff on March 17, 1943, in a small hospital in Kampen, Netherlands. He initially used needles for venipuncture to obtain blood by puncturing the femoral artery and then returning it through a cannulated vein. Later, he surgically dissected the radial artery, but this was accompanied by severe bleeding during heparinization (Kolff 1965).

In 1949, Nils Alwall unsuccessfully tried to use rubber tubing and glass cannulas to connect an artery with a vein. Based on this idea, later in 1960, Quinton, Dillard and Scribner (Seattle USA) developed the external Scribner shunt (Quinton 1960), which consisted of thin-walled Teflon cannulas, one of which was inserted into the radial artery and the other one into the cephalic vein on the distal forearm. The outer parts were connected by a Teflon hose, which was later replaced by a flexible silicone tube (Konner 2005).

Because of this external shunt, it was no longer necessary to create new access before each HD. It is therefore rightly considered a milestone in the surgery of vascular access for long-term hemodialysis treatment (Figure 1).

In 1969, MUDr. J. Vajó implanted the first external arteriovenous fistula according to Scribner in Košice.

In the following period, there were several publications describing many complications. Problems such as bleeding, uncontrollable infection, and skin necrosis arose around the insertion and fixation of the cannulas.

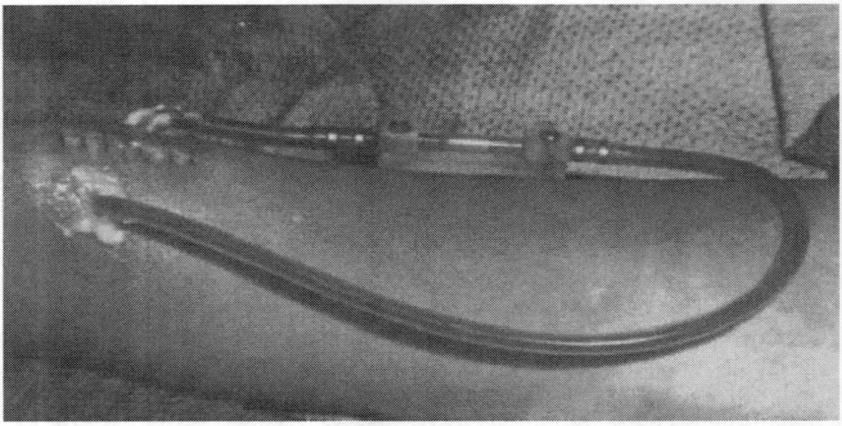

Figure 1. Quinton-Scribner shunt [https://www.researchgate.net/figure/281733078_fig4_Fig-55-QuintonScribner-shunt].

In 1960, prof. E. Matejíček (the Surgical Clinic in Košice) who had dealt with the aforementioned issues for a number of years, published an experimental paper on the consequences of hemodynamic changes after AV fistulas in the “Vnitřní lékařství Journal” (Journal of Internal Medicine).

In 1961, Shaldon (London, UK) introduced the percutaneous insertion of a catheter into the femoral artery and vein (Shaldon 1961). He later preferred veno-venous catheterization for less extensive bleeding complications than after the removal of the catheter from the artery (Konner 2005).

The first arteriovenous fistula was created on February 19, 1965, by the surgeon Dr. Appel. It was a radiocephalic AVF with a side-to-side anastomosis (Figure 2). The results of their team were published by Brescia, Cimino, Appel, and Hurwich in 1966 in the now legendary work "Chronic hemodialysis using venipuncture and a surgically created arteriovenous fistula" (Brescia 1966).

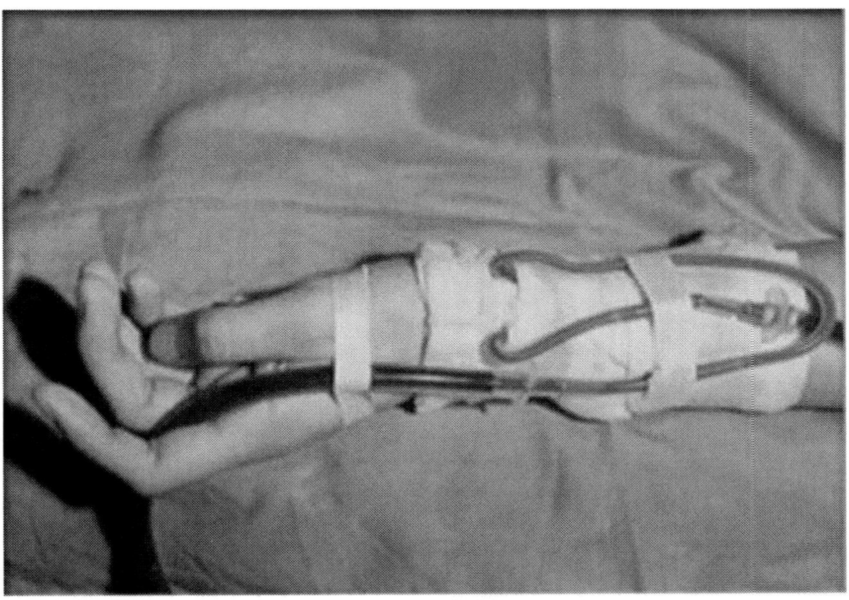

Figure 2. Implanted Scribner's shunt in a 53-year-old patient F.F. in 1970 at the Surgical Clinic in Košice (from the archive of Prof. MUDr. J. Vajó, DrSc.).

This fistula is, to this day, considered to be *the most optimal form* of creating high-quality vascular access for patients enrolled in a long-term dialysis program.

Radiocephalic fistula is the standard by which all other methods of vascular access are assessed. Currently, the arteriovenous fistula of the forearm is used as the primary connection to the hemodialysis machine. However, in some patients, the use of these fistulas is out of the question and therefore other possibilities for creating good vascular access are used. In Košice, hemodialysis treatment began to be used in 1966 at the department of internal medicine.

In 1968, Lars Rohl (Heidelberg, Germany) described an end-to-side anastomosis between the cephalic vein and the radial artery. The benefit of this type of anastomosis was the use of the cephalic vein, which is located laterally and is not suitable for side-to-side anastomosis (Rohl 1968). The end-to-side anastomosis is still the gold standard in the surgery of vascular accesses (Brescia, Cimino, Rohl). In 1970, the internal AV fistulas according to Cimino and Brescia started to be used in Košice for vascular access intended for hemodialysis. The first internal AV fistula for hemodialysis on the left forearm was created by prof. E. Matejíček on May 8, 1970. The creation of internal AV fistulas at the surgical department in Košice was provided by MUDr. Milichovsky, MUDr. Vajó and MUDr. Frankovičová. The first transcutaneous cannulation of the subclavian vein was performed by MUDr. Vajó in December 1972 at FN Košice.

The brachiocephalic AVF was first described by Cascardo (Cascardo 1970). Until 1970, this approach was used in the treatment of 15 patients suffering from chronic kidney disease.

In 1977, Gracz described the cubital AVF between the perforating vein and the proximal radial artery (or brachial artery) (Gracz 1977) (Figure 3).

In 1979 Althaus et al. described the AV fistula between the brachial artery and the transposed basilic vein. In the Czechoslovak literature, prof. J. Breza, the head of the Department of Urology in Bratislava, dealt with this topic and published the results of this novel way of creating vascular access in 1985 in our literature. Prof. M. Frankovičová et al. described the advantages and disadvantages of this vascular access in 2001.

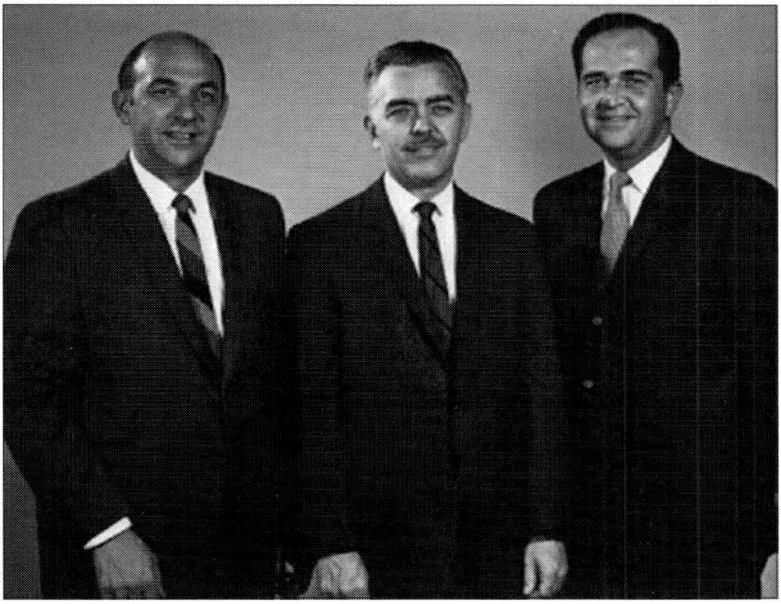

Figure 3. Pioneers of AVF surgery - Brescia, M. J., Cimino, J. E., Appel, K. (Devender Singh, A tribute to the inventor of arteriovenous fistula for hemodialysis: James E. Cimino. 2019).

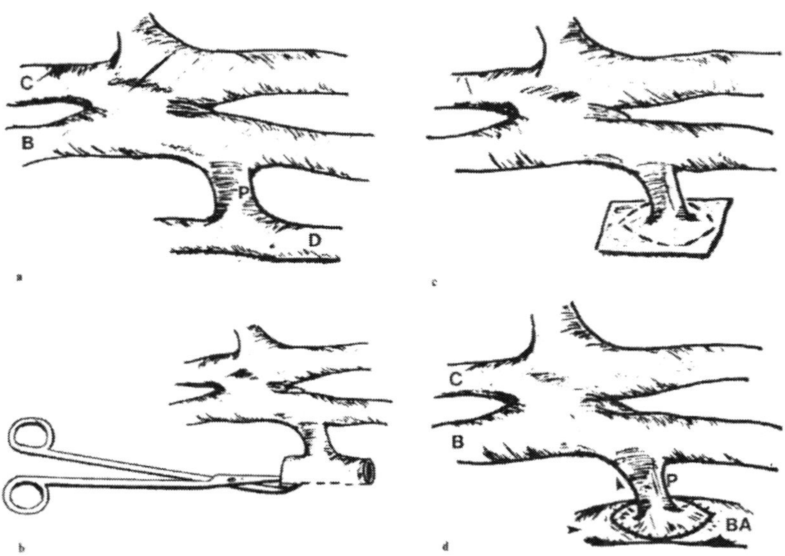

Figure 4. Diagram of the original cubital AVF according to Gracz (Gracz 1977).

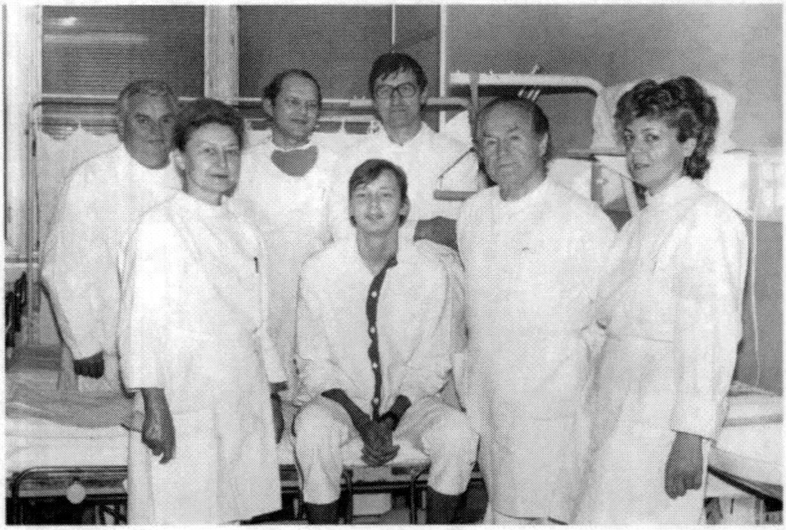

Figure 5. The first kidney transplantation at the surgical department in Košice (Surgical team: Prof. Matejíček, MUDr. Klimešová, MUDr. Frankovičová, coordinator: MUDr. Szabo-Nacko, anesthesiologist: MUDr. Gramová, nephrologist: MUDr. Roland, the patient J. B. in the center).

Kestlerová and Bachleda have published alternative ways of creating high-quality vascular access in Czech and Slovak literature.

In Košice, the first Perm-Cath for hemodialysis was implanted on March 13, 1991, through the internal jugular vein onto a 34-year-old patient by Prof. MUDr. J. Vajó. The issue was also dealt with by prof. MUDr. J. Radoňak. The issues of vascular accesses were later addressed by prof. MUDr. Mária Frankovičová, PhD., whose habilitation thesis on vascular accesses was defended in 1996, and in 2000 a monograph on surgical arteriovenous fistulae was published in Bratislava by HERBA publishing. A team of authors led by prof. MUDr. M. Frankovičová, PhD. wrote a professional publication about the advantages and disadvantages of AV fistulas in the anatomical snuffbox.

In 1995 Berkoben and Schwab emphasized in their paper "Maintenance of permanent hemodialysis vascular access patency" that the most important thing for hemodialysis success is cooperation of the vascular surgeon, nephrologist, and dialysis worker. They underline the importance of the crucial role of the vascular surgeon and the appropriate anatomical and functional conditions on the patient's blood vessels.

The number of patients treated with regular dialysis treatment as of 31st December 2014 in Slovakia was 4022, which is 26 patients less than in 2012, but this also represents an increase of 36% compared to the year 2000. 471 patients were included in the waiting list for transplantation. 115 patients underwent kidney transplantation and 183,591 hemodialyses were performed. Diabetic nephropathy is the most common diagnosis leading to kidney failure. As many as 35% of all dialysis patients suffer from this complication of diabetes, and the statistical occurrence is on the rise. This is followed by kidney inflammation, which leads about 16% of the patients to the need for dialysis. The third most common diagnosis leading to dialysis is nephrosclerosis, which is observed in about 10 - 12% of cases. Last year, 661 patients involved in long-term hemodialysis died, i.e., 16% of all treated. The most common cause of death is cardiovascular disease, which kills up to 61% of patients. Statistics show an increasing trend in cases of cancer and kidney infections, by 15 - 16% for each of the complications.

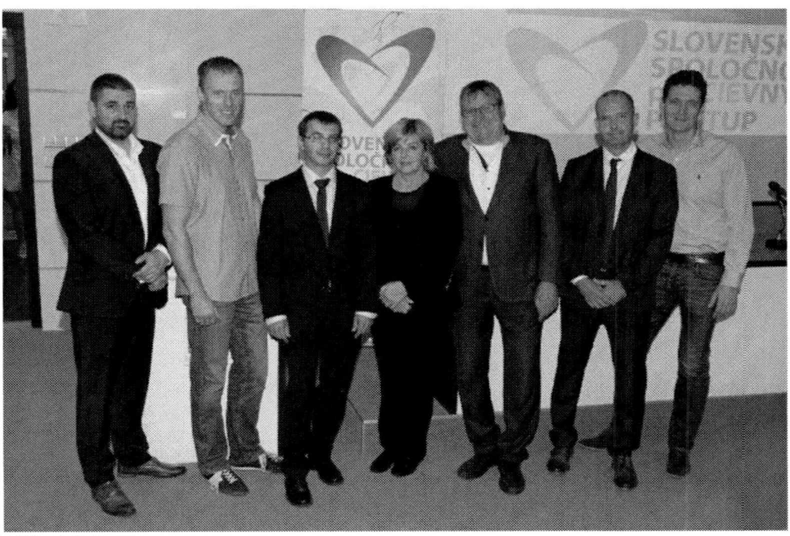

Figure 6. Members of the Committee of the Slovak Society for Vascular Access (Košice 2018).

The vascular surgeons of the city of Košice dealing with the issue of vascular access for long-term hemodialysis have increased their efforts by creating the Slovak Society for Vascular Access, founded in January 2017.

The creation of a high-quality AV fistula can only be achieved by an extensive evaluation of numerous criteria: the patient's vascular condition, his condition, the number and quality of previous vascular treatments, and localization of AV fistulas. At present, MUDr. Necpal, MUDr. Širila and MUDr. Staško improved preoperative mapping and thus evaluated the selection of the most suitable vessels to create first-rate vascular access. To quote MUDr. Roubal, the indication of the order of fistulas is an art that influences the surgical results and those depend to a large extent on the experience of the *vascular surgeon performing the operation*.

REFERENCES

Althaus, P., Schonberger, B., Simmel, F., Hansen, Ch. 1979. "Subkutane Arteriovenose Anastomosen zur Hemodialyse". *Tsch. Gesundheitwesen,* 3:139 - 143. [Subcutaneous Arteriovenous Anastomoses for Hemodialysis. *Tsch. Healthcare*]

Bachleda, P., Utíkal, P., Zadrazil, J. 1993. "Indications for Arteriovenous Fistula for Hemodialysis". *Acta Univ. Palacki Olomouc Fac. Med.,* 135:69 - 70.

Baláž, P., Rokošný, S., Klein, D., Adamec, M. 2008. "Aneurysmorhaphy is an Easy Technique for Arteriovenous Fistula Salvage". *J. Vasc. Surg.,* 9:81 - 84.

Bourquelot, P., Rawa, M., Van Laere, O. 2012. "Long-Term Results of Femoral Vein Transposition for Autogenous Arteriovenous Hemodialysis Access. *J. Vasc. Surg.,* 56:440 - 445.

Breza, J., Rezníček, J., Zvara, V. 1985. "Príprava Krvného Riečišťa pre Hemodialýzu Vytvorením Fistuly Medzi a. Brachialis a do Podkožia Ramena Transponovanou v. Basilica." *Rozhl. Chir.,* 64:11. [Preparation of the bloodstream for hemodialysis by creating a fistula between the brachial artery and the subcutaneous shoulder transposed using the basilic vein. *Rozhl. Chir.*, 64:11].

Brescia, M. J., Cimino, J. E., Hurwich, B. J. and Appel, K. 1966. "Chronic Hemodialysis Using Venipuncture and a Surgically Created Arteriovenous Fistula: NEJM". *New England Journal of Medicine,* doi: 10.1056/NEJM196611172752002.

Cascardo, S., Acchailoo, S. A., Bevin, E. G. 1970. "Proximal Arteriovenous Fistulas for Hemodialysis when Radial Arteries are Unavailable". *Proc. Eur. Dial. Transi.,* 27:42.

Costa, B. N., Rivera, C. F., Rodriguez, M. C., Romero, T. H., Muniz, A. L., Hermida, T. F., Lista, F. S., Diaz, P. I., Hernandez, A. A. 2017. "Angiosarcoma Developing in an Arteriovenous Fistula after Kidney Transplantation". *Case Rep. Transplant.,* 2017: 2426859.

Frankovičová, M., Arendárčik, F., Blažejová, J., Kubíková, M., Martinček, M., Harbuľák, P. Samek, Peter, Roland, R. 1993. "Problems of a Good Vascular Access in Patients in Hemodialysis Program" *Paper presented at the 27. Czecho-Slovak Surgical Congress with international participation*, Banska Bystrica, Slovakia, September 9 - 11.

Frankovičová, M., Bober, J., Arendárčik, F., Kubíková, M., Martinček, M., Lacková, V., Kriegerová, K., Samek, P. 1995. "Rekonštrukčné Cievne Výkony v Našom Klinickom Materiáli", *Slovenský lekár: Časopis Rodinnej Medicíny a Slovenskej Lekárskej Komory,* 2:16 - 17. ["Reconstructive vascular procedures in our clinical material", *Slovak Physician: Journal of Family Medicine and the Slovak Medical Chamber,* 2: 16 - 17].

Frankovičová, M. 1994. "Cievny Štep v Rekonštrukčnej Chirurgii" *Foia Facultatis Medicae Universitas Šafarikiana Cassoviensis*, 51:171 - 175 ["Vascular Graft in Reconstructive Surgery" *Foia Facultatis Medicae Universitas Safarikiana Cassoviensis*, 51: 171 - 175].

Frankovičová, M., Kubíková, M., Arendárčik, F., Martinček, M., Sabol, F., Roland, R., Grejtovská, B. 1997. "Úskalia Vytvárania Tepnovo-Žilových Spojení pre Potreby Dlhodobej Hemodialýzy". *Prakticka flebologie,* 3 - 4:153. ["Pitfalls of creating arterial-venous connections for the needs of long-term hemodialysis". *Practical phlebology,* 3 - 4: 153].

Frankovičová, M. 2000. *Chirurgia Tepnožilových Spojení pre Potreby Dlhodobej Hemodialýzy*. Bratislava: Herba. [*Surgery of arterio-venous junctions for the needs of long-term hemodialysis treatment*].

Frankovičová, M., Roland, R., Vajó, J., Blažejová, J. 1985. "Príspevok k Novému Operačnému Prístupu pre Vytvorenie Tepennožilovej Spojky u Chorých v Dlhodobom Hemodialyzačnom Programe", *Rozhl. Chir.,* 64, 10:663 - 665. [Contribution to a new surgical approach for the formation of an arterial vein junction in patients in a long-term hemodialysis program, *Rozhl. Chir.,* 64,10: 663 - 665].

Frankovičová, M., Kubíková, M., Arendárčik, F., Torma, N., Hudáková, Š., Roland, R., Podracká, Ľ., Bober, J. 2001. "Výhody a Nevýhody Brachobazilických A-V Skratov u Dospelých a u Detí." *Lekársky obzor.,* 7 - 8:251 - 252. [Advantages and Disadvantages of Brachobasilic A-V Shorts in Adults and Children.]

Gracz, K. C., Ing, T. S., Soung, L. S., Armbruster, K. F., Seim, S. K., Merkel, F. K. 1977. "Proximal Forearm Fistula for Maintenance Hemodialysis". *Kidney Int.,* 1:71 - 75.

Hudáková, Š., Frankovičová, M., Kubíková, M., Torma, N. 2000. "Vascular Access for Chronic Hemodialysis – Results and Analysis of Complications." *Przeglad lekarski,* 57, 6:112.

Kestlerová, M., Týblová, M., Kočandrle, V. 1981. "Arteriovenous Fistulae for Hemodialysis Using Vein Allotransplants". *Rozh. Chir.,* 60,5:313 - 318.

Kolff, W. J. 1965. "First Clinical Experience with the Artificial Kidney". *Ann. Int. Med.,* 62: 608 - 619.

Konner, K. 2005. "History of Vascular Access for Haemodialysis". *Nephrol. Dial. Transplant.,* 20:2629 - 2635.

Kubíková, M., Frankovičová, M., Arendárčik, F., Roland, R., Grejtovská, B., Martinček, M., Sabol, F., Šudák, M., Vojtaník, P., Medviďová, J. 1997. "Arteriovenózne Fistuly pre Potreby Dlhodobej Hemodialýzy". *Prakticka flebologie,* 3 - 4(VI):154 ["Arteriovenous fistulas for long-term hemodialysis". *Practical Phlebology*, 3 - 4 (VI): 154].

Quinton, W., Dillard, D., Scribner, B. H. 1960. "Cannulation of Blood Vessels for Prolonged Hemodialysis". *Amer. Trans. Amer. Soc. Artef. Intern. Organs,* 6, 10 - 11:104 – 113.

Rohl, L., Franz, H. E., Mohring, K. 1968. "Direct Arteriovenous Fistula for Hemodialysis". *Scand. J. Urol. Nephrol.,* 2:191 - 195.

In: Surgeon´s Perspective on Dialysis Patient ISBN: 978-1-53619-262-9
Editor: Maria Frankovicova

Chapter 2

ARTERIES AND VEINS OF UPPER LIMBS

L. Vaško[1,*], MD and M. Virág[1], MD
[1]Department of Vascular Surgery,
East Slovak Institute of Cardiovascular Diseases,
Faculty of Medicine, Pavol Jozef Šafárik University in Košice,
Košice, Slovakia

ABSTRACT

In this chapter we describe the anatomy of the arteries and veins of the upper limb. We present the most frequently used veins of the forearm and arm to create AV shunt: at the forearm v. cephalica, v. mediana cubiti in the cubital fossa. In the arm area v. basilica, that is very often the last option to create the vascular access for long term dialysis program, with failure or closure of AV shunts formed in the areas of the forearm and cubital fossa.

Keywords: arteries of the upper limb, veins of the upper limb

* Corresponding Author's E-mail: mudr.lukas.vasko@gmail.com.

Arteries of the Upper Limb (Arteriae Membri Superioris)

Their aim is to supply the upper limb with oxygenated blood. They are the branches of the subclavian artery - a. subclavia. By its branching, the subclavian artery provides nutrition for the upper part of the torso, part of the neck, and the entire upper limb. In the human body, the subclavian arteries are bilateral: the left one (a. subclavia sinistra), which protrudes directly from the aortic arch (arcus aortae), and the right one (a. subclavia dextra), which arises from the brachiocephalic trunk (truncus brachiocephalicus).

After a short course in the chest, a. subclavia passes through the superior thoracic aperture (apertura thoracica superior) above the cupula pleurae and the first rib (costa prima), then continues below the clavicle (clavicula), continuing as the axillary artery (a. axillaris).

Axillary artery further extends through the axillary fossa (fossa axillaris) up to the surgical neck of the humerus (collum chirurgicum humeri), or the lower edge of m. pectoralis major, where it passes to the brachial artery (a. brachialis). It is crossed by the pectoralis minor (m. pectoralis minor), which is located in front of it (ventrally). Therefore, we divide the course of the artery into three sections, considering its position towards the muscle:

The first section – artery is positioned medially (closer to the middle part) from the pectoralis minor muscle

The second section – artery is positioned behind the pectoralis minor muscle

The third section – artery is positioned laterally from the pectoralis minor muscle

The axillary artery is in the first section enclosed in the fibrous sheath, together with the vein (v. axillaris) and network of nerves - brachial plexus (plexus brachialis). It creates small branches connecting to the subscapularis muscle (m. subscapularis) – rr. subscapulares and superior thoracic artery for the first two intercostal spaces – a. thoracica superior.

There are two branches coming out of the second section of a. axillaris. It is the thoracoacromial artery (a. thoracoacromialis), branching into acromion, deltoid muscle (m. deltoideus), clavicle, and pectoralis major (m. pectoralis major). Another branch is the lateral thoracic artery – a. thoracica lateralis, passing down in linea axillaris mediana up to m. serratus anterior while nourishing it. In women, it branches to the breast gland – rr. mammarii laterales.

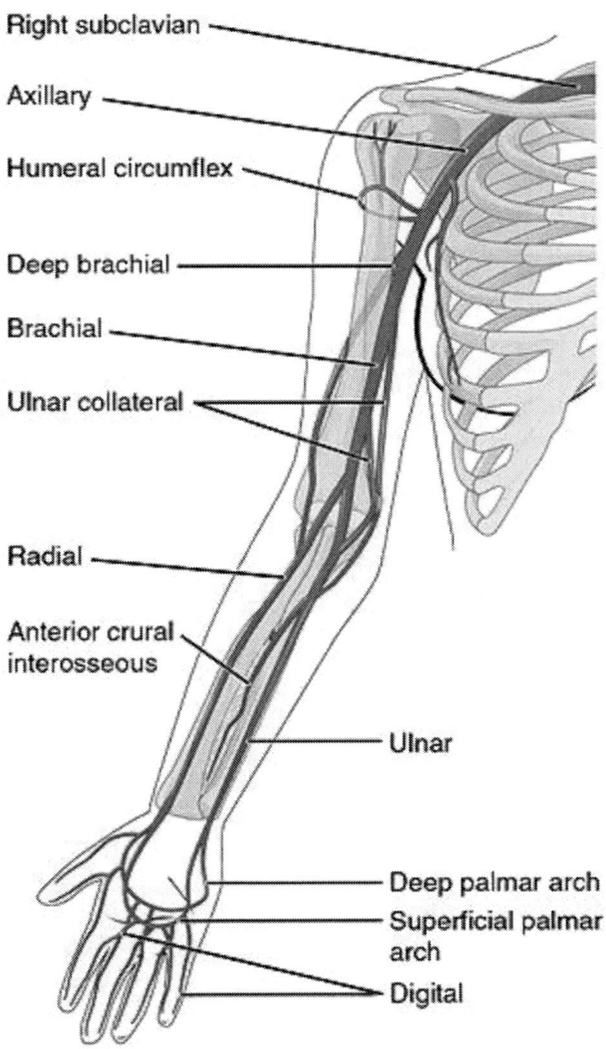

Figure 1. Arteries of the upper limb (source: WikiSkripta).

In the third section, a. axillaris branches into three parts. The most significant branch of a. axillaris is the subscapularis artery – a. subscapularis (divided into a. thoracodorsalis and a. circumflexa scapulae). Other branches are the anterior humeral circumflex artery (a. circumflexa humeri anterior) and the posterior humeral circumflex artery (a. circumflexa humeri posterior).

Direct continuation of the axillary artery – a. axillaris - is the brachial artery – a. brachialis.

It extends in total length in sulcus bicipitalis medialis on the inside part of the arm.

The brachial artery – a. brachialis branches into:

1. Deep artery of the arm – a. profunda brachii – it enters together with the radial nerve (n.radialis) between the lateral and medial head of the triceps muscle (caput laterale et mediale musculi tricipitis brachii) behind the humerus into the sulcus nervi radialis humeri. Deep brachial artery (a. profunda brachii) extends into a. collateralis media and a. collateralis radialis, both to the area of the elbow joint.
2. The superior ulnar collateral artery (arteria collateralis ulnaris superior) arises in the same height as a. profunda brachii. It accompanies the ulnar nerve (nervus ulnaris) first in front of septum intermusculare brachii mediale, further behind the septum into the sulcus nervi ulnaris, behind medial epicondyle (epicondylus medialis) of the humerus. It supplies the muscles on the backside of the forearm and branches in the area of rete articulare cubiti (elbow joint).
3. The inferior ulnar collateral artery (arteria collateralis ulnaris inferior) arises above the medial epicondyle of the shoulder bone and extends along the brachial muscle (m. brachialis) to the forearm. It supplies the muscles of the front side of the forearm and the brachial muscle.
4. Bicipital artery arises in various height and enters the biceps (musculus biceps brachii).

In the area of cubital fossa at the elbow with different variations (proximal/distal), the brachial artery is divided into the lateral branch. radialis and medial branch a. ulnaris. Both arteries give rise to nutrient branches for the elbow area (a. recurrens radialis and a. recurrens ulnaris). A. ulnaris has a short branch of a. interossea communis that branches at the forearm to provide nutrition for the structures in front of and behind the membrana interossea.

Brachial, radial, and ulnar arteries are the most commonly used arteries for AV shunt as of the needs of the dialysis process.

Veins of the Upper Limb

The veins are part of the bloodstream and together with arteries, blood capillaries, and heart they form the closed cardiovascular system.

As a part of the circulatory system, veins also have the role of transporting blood, nutrients, waste, and heat. A unique role of veins compared to the arteries is to carry blood with carbon dioxide from tissues and organs to the heart. In the systemic circulatory system, the veins deliver deoxygenated blood from the capillaries to the right atrium of the heart. In the pulmonary circulatory system, the veins have to take the oxygenated blood from the lungs to the left atrium of the heart.

The walls of veins are thin; their structure is similar to arteries. The veins in the lower part of the body and upper limbs have valves (*valvulae venosae*) that prevent the reflux of the blood caused by gravity.

The veins on the back of the hand form rete venosum dorsale manus and continue as vv. metacarpales dorsales. At the side of the palm, there is a weaker net of veins arcus venosus palmaris superficialis. The vein nets located at the back and at the palm of the hand respectively, are connected by the vv. intercapitulares. Superficial veins at the lateral edge of the hand form v. cephalica antebrachii, the ones at the medial edge form v. basilica antebrachii. Both veins run on the forearm superficially up to the cubital fossa (fossa cubitalis), where they are as v. cephalica and v. basilica mutually connected by the medial cubital vein, v. mediana cubiti.

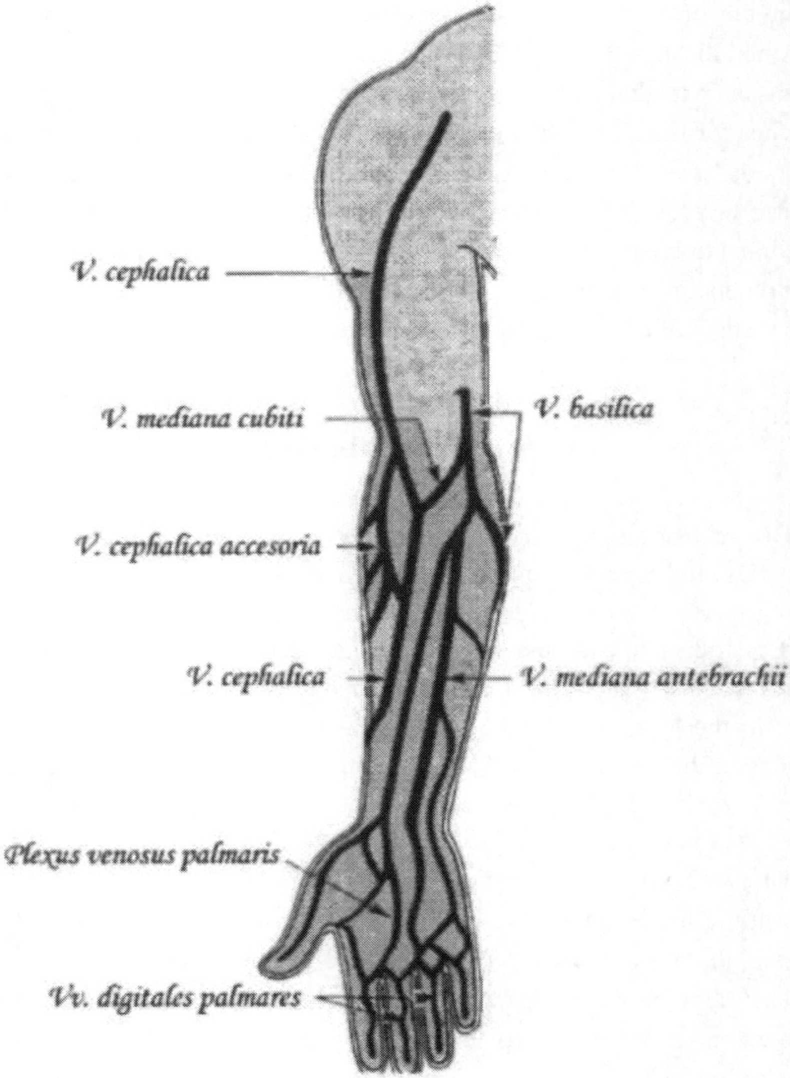

Figure 2. Venous system of the upper limb (source: Morehealthis.com).

The cephalic vein then continues laterally up to the trigonum clavipectorale, where it crosses through the superficial fascia into the depth and joins v. axillaris. V. basilica passes up medially up to the half of the arm, continuing deeper into v. brachialis.

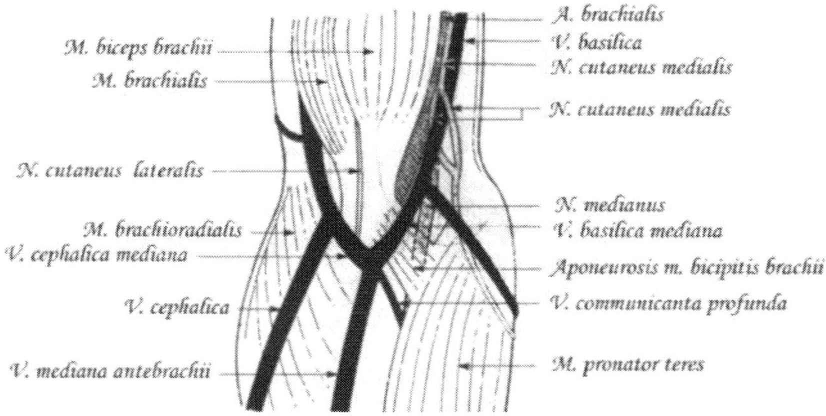

Figure 3. The veins of the forearm and arm used most often to create AV shunt (source: Morehealthis.com).

Deep vein, v. brachialis, is formed by v. radialis and v. ulnaris. At the arm area v. brachialis changes into v. axillaris, subsequently, as v. subclavia that by connection with v. jugularis interna forms v. brachiocephalica on both sides. Vv. brachiocephalicae join as v. cava superior, which enters the right atrium of the heart.

Superficial veins of the upper limb are used not only for venipuncture but also to create AV shunt: at the forearm v. cephalica, v. mediana cubiti in the cubital fossa. In the arm area v. basilica, that is very often the last option to create the vascular access for long term dialysis program, with failure or closure of AV shunts formed in the areas of the forearm and cubital fossa.

References

Borovanský, L. 1978. *Anatomie.* Praha. [*Anatomy*. Prague.]

Čihák, R. 2008. *Anatomie*. Praha: Galén, [*Anatomy*. Prague: Galén].

Kluchová, D. et al. 2018. *Anatómia hlavy a krku*. Košice: UPJŠ. [*Head and neck anatomy*. Košice: Pavol Jozef Šafarik University].

Mráz, P. et al. 2015. *Anatómia ľudského tela.* Bratislava: Slovak Academic Press. [*Anatomy of the Human body*. Bratislava: Slovak Academic Press].

In: Surgeon´s Perspective on Dialysis Patient ISBN: 978-1-53619-262-9
Editor: Maria Frankovicova

Chapter 3

Chronic Kidney Disease from the Surgeon's Perspective

M. Zavacká**, *MD
Department of Vascular Surgery,
East Slovak Institute of Cardiovascular Diseases,
Faculty of Medicine, Pavol Jozef Šafárik University in Košice, Slovakia

Abstract

Chronic kidney disease (formerly also chronic renal insufficiency) is irreversible impairment of renal functions. It is defined as abnormalities of kidney structure and function that are present for more than 3 months. The disease should be classified based on the cause, a category determined by glomerular filtration, and albuminuria. The prevalence of chronic kidney disease has been rising at a rapid pace over the last decades, gaining epidemic proportions and has become one of the major public health problems. The worldwide prevalence varies from country to country, with a prevalence of 10-13%.

---

* Corresponding Author's E-mail: martinazavacka80@gmail.com.

Keywords: chronic kidney disease, proteinuria, blood pressure, acute kidney injury, diabetes mellitus

Abbreviations

CKD	Chronic kidney disease
eGFR	Estimated Glomerular Filtration Rate
ESRD	End-Stage Renal Disease
GFR	Glomerular Filtration Level
KDIGO	Kidney Disease: Improving Global Outcomes
KDQoL	Kidney Disease Quality of Life
MICS	malnutrition–inflammation–cachexia syndrome
NKF	National Kidney Foundation

Chronic Kidney Disease (CKD) is a disease that currently affects a large percentage of the population and represents an enormous social and economic burden. This burden is reflected in many areas of society, starting with the individual quality of life of patients with this disease, the rate of incapacity for work, changing demands on healthcare services, and increasing healthcare costs. The worldwide burden of CKD is manifested in increased mortality, incidence, and prevalence of the end-stage of the disease. Chronic diseases are caused mainly due to unhealthy lifestyles, but factors such as rapid urbanization, lack of exercise and obesity, inadequate eating habits, stress, and risky behaviors such as smoking and alcohol abuse also contribute to their development. Socio-economic factors, which contribute to health inequalities, also influence their development. Diderichsen, Andersen, and Manuel (2012) point to the impact of socio-economic status on health-related behavior and perceive chronic diseases partly as a result of poverty and socio-economic disadvantage. Current trends in dealing with chronic kidney disease include prevention, early detection of the emerging disease, slowing of end-stage progression, reducing the risk of cardiovascular morbidity and mortality, and improving the patient's quality of life. This disease places high demands on the patient's self-management and has a negative impact on both mental and physical health. The ability of patients to overcome this burden and the demands of chronic disease, their level of social support, and other factors on the side of the health system can influence their overall health, wellbeing, and overall quality of life. The treatment of this disease is a significant burden on public finances. Efforts to reduce the enormous costs associated with the treatment of chronic kidney disease lead policymakers as well as health care providers to reconsider using less costly approaches of managing the disease such as patient education, increasing of adherence and the ability of individuals to effectively manage their own disease and participate actively in treatment. The focus is shifting more and more on healthcare providers, to improve the cooperation of the patient and healthcare professionals, and to adjust services to benefit the patient, but also the health system itself, i.e., on the responsiveness of the health system. Since 2006, World Kidney Day is established on the second Thursday of March each year. Through annual worldwide events, it aims to raise awareness of kidney diseases, risk factors, and their prevention and to appeal not only to the general public but also to health care providers and national governments to take steps to prevent and reduce CKD risk and especially in high-risk populations (www.worldkidneyday.org). Jha et al. (2013) recommend that prevention programs become a part of national strategies for non-infectious diseases involving general practitioners, adapting to local needs, as well as the human, material and economic resources available in the region. In 2009, the CKD Prognosis Consortium was set up with the support of KDIGO (Kidney Disease: Improving Global Outcomes) and the NKF (National Kidney Foundation) to monitor more than 50 cohorts (including Slovakia) to improve the definition and classification of CKD in relation to the prognosis of CKD and monitor various indicators such as overall mortality, cardiovascular mortality, end-stage progression and others. However, for the prevention and treatment of chronic diseases, it is important, from a public health perspective, to address other relevant health-related factors and inequalities in access to healthcare and they should be taken into account in policy-making. These include factors such as social group membership, gender, ethnicity and geographical affiliation, and other social determinants. From the perspective of individuals, the important factors are education, employment, and financial income.

Chronic kidney disease (formerly also chronic renal insufficiency) is irreversible impairment of renal functions. It is defined as abnormalities of kidney structure and function that are present for more than 3 months. These include albuminuria, urinary sediment abnormalities, structural abnormalities, histological abnormalities, and decreased glomerular filtration of the kidneys. The disease should be classified based on the cause, a category determined by glomerular filtration, and albuminuria. Estimated Glomerular Filtration Rate (eGFR), i.e., determination of calculated glomerular filtration rate from serum creatinine concentration, is considered to be one of the key indicators of renal function. Based on this indicator, 5 stages of chronic kidney disease were identified, that correspond to eGFR categories (Table 1). However, the estimated glomerular filtration rate is not considered to be a reliable criterion for the evaluation of kidney function and differences in diagnostic tests, or respectively in criteria may lead to a failure to recognize renal impairment or fluctuation in prevalence at different stages of the disease, which may impact clinical practice, policies, and funding. The glomerular filtration rate is influenced by several indicators, such as age, sex, and muscle mass.

Table 1. Categories of calculated glomerular filtration of CKD (KDIGO, 2012)

GFR category	GFR (ml / min) 1.73 m^2	Glomerular Filtration Level (GFR)
Category 1	> 90	Normal or high
Category 2	60-89	Slightly reduced
Category 3a	45-59	Slightly or moderately reduced
Category 3b	30-44	Moderately or seriously reduced
Category 4	15-29	Seriously reduced
Category 5	*<15*	Kidney failure

Later studies on the relation of estimation of glomerular filtration rate and albuminuria with disease progression to end-stage disease and mortality, have provided evidence that both indicators are adequate to define and determine stages and prognosis of renal disease. Albuminuria has, therefore, become a part of the revised classification KDIGO (2012) (Table 2).

Table 2. Categories of albuminuria in chronic kidney disease KDIGO, 2012

Category	A1	A2	A3
Original name	Reference albuminuria	Microalbuminuria	Proteinuria
Degree of albuminuria	Normal or slightly elevated	Moderately increased	Significantly increased
mg of proteins / g of creatinine (range)	<30 mg / g	30-300mg / g	> 300 mg / g

Thanks to a more precise classification of chronic kidney disease, it is possible to distinguish the different stages of CKD more effectively. The disease is asymptomatic or oligosymptomatic in the earlier stages and can only be detected by changes in biochemical parameters. Stage 3 is divided into stages 3a and 3b reflecting the increased cardiovascular risk. This stage includes the largest number of patients overall, approximately 80-90% of cases. Stage 5 of Chronic Kidney Disease (formerly referred to as End-Stage Renal Disease (ESRD) in foreign literature) is a stage of renal insufficiency where renal replacement therapy, such as dialysis or kidney transplantation, is necessary to maintain human life. The most common causes of CKD development are diabetes mellitus and hypertension, especially in developed countries. It can be said that any kidney disease may progress to the end stage of kidney disease and the progression depends on many factors and indicators. The progression of chronic kidney disease is gradual and is affected by several risk factors, some of which are influenceable, such as obesity, hypertension, and proteinuria. Risk factors for chronic kidney disease, according to KDIGO (2012), include acute kidney injury, diabetes mellitus, smoking, arterial hypertension, dyslipidemia, and sedentary lifestyle. Hypertension, diabetes mellitus as well as obesity are among the emerging non-infectious diseases. Diabetes mellitus accounts for up to 50% of cases of CKD in developed countries. The world prevalence of hypertension was up to 26% in 2000, and the prevalence of diabetes in 2030 should be as high as 7.7%. The prevalence of obesity is also increasing rapidly and obesity is considered to be another important target for screening and prevention of CKD. Weight loss can make a significant contribution to reducing proteinuria, blood pressure, and slowing down the degradation of renal function. Other specific factors of progression and complications include inflammation, oxidative stress and malnutrition, anemia, bone diseases, and a decline of cognitive functions.

The prevalence of chronic kidney disease has been rising at a rapid pace over the last decades, gaining epidemic proportions and has become one of the major public health problems. The worldwide prevalence varies from country to country, with a prevalence of 10-13%. Some sources report an 8-16% prevalence in Asia, Australia, Europe, and North America. Hill et al. (2016) conducted a systematic review and meta-analysis of studies to determine the global prevalence of chronic kidney disease and the prevalence of individual stages of CKD. The overall prevalence of all stages was on average 13.4% (11.7 - 15.1%), for stages 3 - 5 the average was 10.6% (9.2 - 12.2%). The prevalence rates for the individual stages of CKD, which were assessed by estimated glomerular filtration and albuminuria, were as follows: Stage 1 (2.8 - 4.2%), Stage 2 (2.7 - 5.3%), Stage 3 (6.4 - 8.9%), Stage 4 (0.3 - 0.5%) and Stage 5 (0.1%). The increase in the prevalence of chronic kidney disease is dramatic. In the US, the prevalence doubled between 1990 and 2000. The increasing prevalence of CKD is partly due to the population aging, but the increased prevalence of obesity, diabetes, and arterial hypertension also contribute to a continuous increase in CKD prevalence. The differences between the countries of the world can be attributed to different lifestyles, different living standards, and behavioral habits of the population. Little information is available on the prevalence of early stages of chronic kidney disease because at these stages the disease is asymptomatic and often underdiagnosed. Therefore, it is difficult to determine the extent of disease burden at these stages compared to the final stage of the disease. Speaking of the prevalence of Stage 5 of chronic kidney disease - it represents 0.2% of the population in the United States. In Slovakia, 147 304 patients over 19 years of age (3,378.4 / 100,000) were monitored in nephrology outpatient departments as of 31.12.2015. 4472 patients underwent dialysis treatment, which is the highest number of patients on dialysis between 2006 and 2015.

MORTALITY

According to the Global Burden of Disease Study (2010), chronic kidney disease was the 27th most common cause of death in 1990, but by 2010 it was on the 18th place on the list of causes of mortality in the world. Overall, chronic kidney disease belongs to a group of non-infectious diseases in which the mortality rate has doubled over the two decades under review (as in diabetes mellitus, for example). In 2015, CKD is the 12th most frequent cause of mortality. Overall mortality in 2005 – 2015 has increased by 31.7%, while in other non-infectious diseases (e.g., cardiovascular diseases) we can see a decline of mortality.

Although the demographic indicators of chronic kidney disease patients are heterogeneous across different countries, it can be said that CKD tends to develop and progress to the end-stage disease at an older age. Age is a key predictor of CKD. For example, in the US, up to 11% of patients over 65 years of age (without diabetes and hypertension) had a CKD stage of 3 or more. Worldwide as well as within Slovakia the population is aging, and it is estimated that by 2050 the population over 65 years will make up 37% of the population of Slovakia. Age is related to structural and functional kidney changes, but also vascular changes. Other associated diseases (diabetes, hypertension, and others) aggravate the status, so it is difficult to differentiate the impact of age-related physiological changes and other diseases on CKD development. People with low socio-economic status are particularly at risk of developing chronic kidney disease. They have a 60% higher risk of developing CKD than people with a higher socioeconomic status. Poverty increases the risk of developing diseases that predispose to CKD or contribute to the deterioration of health in people who have already developed CKD.

Chronic kidney disease alone represents a significant financial burden on health care systems worldwide. The burden is the highest in the early stages of the disease due to increased prevalence, which in the UK, for example, covers around 35% of patients over 70 years of age. 2-3% of healthcare spending in developed countries is used to treat patients in stage 5 of the disease, although they account for only 0.1-0.2% of the total population of patients with CKD (Jha et al., 2013). For the treatment and management of end-stage renal disease, 6.7% of total medical costs are consumed in the United States, with costs having increased by 57% between 1999 and 2004. The estimated cost of CKD treatment in the UK in 2009-2010 was 1, 3% of the total spending of the healthcare system, and more than half of these costs were spent on renal replacement therapy for only 2% of CKD patients. Australia predicts that its health system, with such an increase in the number of patients where CKD progresses to the final stage, will not handle this onslaught.

Chronic kidney disease massively affects the patients' lives and also affects their wider social system. The gradually decreasing functional fitness, the increase of comorbidities, the emotional burden, the necessity to orientate in the health system, and adhere to recommendations of health care workers, but also the demands for social support from relatives, all represent a complex change of a patient's life. The high risk of death and the progressive nature of the disease to the end stage where renal replacement therapy is needed exacerbates this burden. Patients' capacities to overcome this burden, their level of social support, and other factors on the health system side can affect their overall health, wellbeing, and overall quality of life.

Many studies on the impact of chronic kidney disease on the patient's life point to the fact that patients with CKD have reduced functional health and physical fitness due to the disease. The patient's functional health decreases gradually as the disease progresses and depends on many factors such as the occurrence of co-morbidities, whether the patient is physically active or with different socio-demographic indicators. A recent study comparing the health of patients at stage 4 and 5 of CKD with a control group of elderly patients in the community showed that patients with chronic kidney disease show worse results in several areas of functional health, in emotional functioning, in cognitive abilities and have a lower level of social support. These patients also had a higher number of co-morbidities, which again affect the management options of this disease. The authors appeal to consider these findings in the management of the patient's disease. Patients with chronic kidney disease often experience weakness, fragility, which manifests as decreased bodyweight, slow gait, exhaustion, decreased physical activity, and overall weakness. A study by Wilhelm-Leen et al. (2009) found a prevalence of fragility of 2.8 - 21.9% in patients with chronic kidney disease with a higher prevalence in advanced disease stages. Several studies have shown that fragility in CKD patients is related to impaired health outcomes and mortality. Walker et al. (2015) investigated the incidence and progression of fragility in CKD patients in 600 non-dialysis patients at stages 4 and 5 over two years and found impaired physical health and fitness in 56% of them. An older study by Murtagh et al. (2007) looked at the prevalence of symptoms in the elderly, non-dialysis patients who were on conservative treatment. More than half of the patients observed experienced pain, dry mouth, convulsions, swelling in more than 60% and fatigue and drowsiness, and loss of total energy in more than 70% of cases.

Pagels et al. (2012) have also addressed health-related quality of life in patients at different stages of the disease. They found that impaired quality of life affects patients at all stages prior to starting the dialysis treatment, and cardiovascular problems and infections of patients are considered to be significant predictors for the observed population. Patients at different stages of the disease differed mainly in physical health indicators and less in mental health. Patients in stage 5 disease showed the lowest level of health-related quality of life. Also, Cruz et al. (2011) monitored the health-related quality of life using the SF-36 scale in 191 younger CKD patients (average age was 52 years). They found that these patients scored worse in domains, related to physical health and fitness as well as emotional functioning and overall health compared to other domains under review (e.g., pain, mental health, and others). Comparing the quality of life in patients at different stages of CKD (stages 1-5) did not reveal significant differences in these parameters. They also found that patients with higher education and professionally active ones scored better. Older patients with a higher number of comorbidities showed worse results. Several studies point to the link between the poor quality of life and increased mortality and worsened clinical outcomes (e.g., Mapes et al., 2003; Porter et al., 2016; Jesky et al., 2016) and the need to assess patients' quality of life and include this aspect into disease management. In a study on predictors and health-related quality of life outcomes in patients with chronic renal disease, Porter et al. (2016) evaluated the quality of life based on a population-specific questionnaire (KDQoL-36, Kidney Disease Quality of Life) filled in by 3837 patients. This questionnaire provides scores in five subscales - physical health, mental health, kidney disease burden, the impact of kidney disease, and the symptoms and difficulties associated with the disease. This study examined the relationship of poor quality of life related to health and indicators such as disease progression, the incidence of cardiovascular disease, and mortality. They found that poor quality of life was associated with cardiovascular problems and mortality, but not with disease progression. In this study, they also identified a link between the lower quality of life and socio-demographic indicators such as older age, female gender, and lower education. Jesky et al. (2018) investigated the quality of life in non-dialysis patients and found that up to 75.7% of patients experienced difficulties in one or more domains related to the quality of life (for example, the self-care domain). The lower quality of life was significantly related to mortality. However, decreased quality of life has not been shown to be a risk factor for disease progression to end-stage, consistent with the findings of the above study. Nor have they established a link between health-related quality of life and socioeconomic status. However, they point to the need to identify patients with difficulties with self-care and with lower quality of life, aiming to positively influence the quality of life and reduce the risk of mortality.

Patients with chronic kidney disease often suffer from loss of appetite, malnutrition, and are at risk of a protein-energy deficit, also referred to as malnutrition–inflammation–cachexia syndrome (MICS). Malnutrition is considered to be a serious complication, especially in the elderly. The state of the protein-energy deficit is one of the strongest predictors of mortality in this population of patients. Chronic kidney disease places specific demands on food and fluid intake. Reduction of salt and phosphorus and control of protein intake are standard adjustments in the diet of a CKD patient. The degree of restriction of fluid intake depends on the degree of maintenance of renal function. Difficulties to comply with drinking and dietary regimes may sometimes be insurmountable, especially in the summer months (fluid intake), but also due to a lack of social support in this area. Non-adherence to the prescribed measures regarding dietary and drinking regimes is reflected in the overall status of the patient and can worsen the course of the disease as well as boost the progression of the disease.

Life with chronic illness also affects mental health and the mental condition of patients with chronic kidney disease, and mental status is associated with other health indicators. Research has shown that depressive symptoms are common in patients with CKD. In dialysis patients, more than 30% prevalence of clinical depression has been reported. Depression and mental health impairment are considered to be a risk factor for higher morbidity and mortality in the end-stage patient population may be related to omission of dialysis, poor adherence to recommendations, impaired nutritional status and weight gain between dialysis, factors that are potentially modifiable and further research is needed to clarify how these factors affect the relationship of depression and mortality. Further research is also needed to investigate whether preventive interventions and depression treatment could increase the quality of life and reduce the risk of death in CKD patients. Martini et al. (2018) found about 25% prevalence of depressive symptoms in elderly CKD patients and appeals to early diagnosis of depression in these patients as it may affect treatment adherence rates and self-management levels. However, they also point to the differential diagnosis of depression and cognitive deficit, which is common in the elderly and may distort the patient's clinical status and point to different needs in relation to disease management. Kurella et al. (2009) identified a positive correlation between cognitive impairment and the severity of kidney disease with a higher prevalence in the elderly. Fischer, Porter, and Lash (2013) discuss treatment options for depression in dialysis patients. Drug treatment appears to be the most effective in some ways, but the interaction of different drugs may be a problem. The question is also whether frequent dialysis does not contribute to the worsening of depressive symptoms in terms of the perception of their own health, lifestyle changes but also because of the demands placed on the patient and supportive social system. The authors question whether long-term hemodialysis treatment is sustainable and how it affects the overall functioning and life of the patient with the disease.

REFERENCES

Bagolan P, Spagnoli A, Ciprandi G, Picca S, Leozappa G, Nahom A, Trucchi A, Rizzoni G, Fabbrini G. 1998. "A ten-year experience of Brescia-Cimino arteriovenous fistula in children: technical evolution and refinements." *J Vasc Surg* 27:640–644.

Beanes SR, Kling KM, Fonkalsrud EW, Torres M, Salusky IB, Quinones-Baldrich WJ, *et al.* 2000. "Surgical aspects of dialysis in newborns and infants weighing less than ten kilograms." *J Pediatr Surg* 35:1543-48.

Brittinger WD, Walker G. 1997. "Vascular access for hemodialysis in children." *Pediatric nephrology* 1(XI):87–95

Burger H et al. 1995. "Survival of arteriovenous fistulas and shunts for hemodialysis." *Eur J Surg.* 161(5):327-334.

Bouquelot P. 2006. "Vascular Access in Children: The Importance of Microsurgery for Creation of Autologous Arteriovenous Fistulae." *Eur J Vasc Endovasc Surg* 32(6):696-700.

Brescia MJ, Cimino JE, Appel K, Hurwich BJ (1966) "Chronic hemodialysis using venipuncture and a surgically created arteriovenous fistula." *N Engl J Med* 275:1089–1092.

Garcia de Cortazar L, Gutierrez E, Delucchi MA, Cumsille MA. 1999. "Vascular accesses for chronic hemodialysis in children (in Spanish)." *Rev Med Chil* 127:693–697.

Goldstein SL, Macierowski CT, Jabs K. 1997. "Hemodialysis catheter survival and complications in children and adolescents." *Pediatr Nephrol* 11:74–77.

Gradman WS, Lerner G, Mentser M, Rodriguez H, Kamil ES. 2005. "Experience with autogenous arteriovenous access for hemodialysis in children and adolescents." *Ann Vasc Surg* 19:609–612.

Fischer MJ, Porter, AC, Lash JP. 2013. "Treatment of depression and poor mental health among patients receiving maintenance dialysis: are there options other than a pill or a couch?" *American Journal of Kidney Disease*. 61(V):694-7.

Frankovičová M. et al. 2018. *Cievna chirurgia*. Košice: Univerzita Pavla Jozefa Šafárika v Košiciach. [*Vascular Surgery*. Košice: Pavol Jozef Šafárik University in Košice]

Frankovičová, M. 2000. *Chirurgia tepnožilových spojení pre potreby dlhodobej hemodialýzy*. Bratislava: Herba. [*Surgery of arterio-venous junctions for the needs of long-term hemodialysis treatment*]

Hakaimhakaim AG, Scott TE. 1996. "Durability of early prosthetic dialysis graft cannulation: results of a prospective non-randomised clinical trial." *J Vasc Surg* 25:1002-5.

Hill, NR, Fatoba, ST, Oke, JL, Hirst, JA, O'callaghan, CA, Lasserson, DS, Hobbs, FD. 2016. "Global Prevalence of Chronic Kidney Disease - A Systematic Review and Meta-Analysis." *PLOS One* 11(VII). doi: 10.1371/journal.pone.0158765.

Chand DH, Valentini RP, Kamil ES. 2009. "Hemodialysis vascular access options in pediatrics: considerations for patients and practitioners." *Pediatr nephrol* 24(6): 1121-1128. doi: 10.1007/s00467-008-0812-3.

Janoušek L a kol. 2008. *Hemodialyzační arteriovenózní přístupy*. Praha: Grada. [*Hemodialysis arteriovenous approaches*. Prague: Grada.]

Jesky, MD, Dutton, M, Dasgupta, I., Yadav, P., NG, KP, Fenton, A., Kyte, D., Ferro, CJ, Calvert, M., Cockwell, P., Stringer, SJ. 2016. "Health-Related Quality of Life Impacts Mortality but Not Progression to End-

Stage Renal Disease in Pre-Dialysis Chronic Kidney Disease: A Prospective Observational Study." *PLoS One* 11(11). doi: 10.1371/journal.pone.0165675.

Jha, V, Garcia-Garcia, G., Iseki, K, Li, Z, Naicker, S., Plattner, B., Saran, R., Wang, AY, Yang, CW. 2013. "Chronic kidney disease: global dimension and perspectives." *Lancet* 382(9888):260-72.

Kidney Disease Improving Global Outcomes. 2013. "KDIGO 2012 clinical practice guideline for the evaluation and management of chronic kidney disease." *Kidney International* 3(1):1-150. https://kdigo.org/wp-content/uploads/2017/02/KDIGO_2012_CKD_GL.pdf.

Kestlerová M. 1991. "Arteriovenózní píštěle na dolní končetine" In *Cévní chirurgie,* edited by Firt P. et al. 323. Praha: Avicenum. ["Arteriovenous Fistula on the Lower Limb" in *Vascular Surgery*, edited by Firt P. et al. 323. Praha: Avicenum.]

Kurella Tamura, M, Covinsky, KE, Chertow, GM, Yaffe, K, Landfeld, CS, Mcculloch, CE. 2009. "Functional status of elderly adults before and after initiation of dialysis." *The New England Journal of Medicine*. 361(16):1539-47.

Konner K. 2002. The anastomosis of the arteriovenous fistula-common errors and their avoidance. *Nephrol Dial Transplant* 17:376.

Mak RH, Warady BA. 2013. "Dialysis: vascular access in children--arteriovenous fistula or CVC?" *Nat Rev Nephrol* 9:9–11. doi: 10.1038/nrneph.2012.265.

Murtagh, FE, Marsh, JE, Donohoe, P., Ekbal, NJ, Sheerin, NS, Harris, FE. 2007. "Dialysis or not? A comparative survival study of patients over 75 years with chronic kidney disease stage." *Nephrology Dialysis Transplantation* 22(1):1955– 1962.

Martini, A, Ammirati, A, Garcia, C, Andrade, C, Portella, O, Cendoroglo, MS, Sesso, R. 2018. "Evaluation of quality of life, physical, and mental aspects in longevous patients with chronic kidney disease." *International Urology and Nephrology* 50(4):725–731.

Mapes, DL, Lopes, AA, Satayathum, S, Mccullough, KP, Goodkin, DA, Locatelli, F, Fukuhara, S, Young, EW, Kurokawa, K, Saito, A, Bommer, J, Wolfe, RA, Held, PJ, Port, FK. 2003. "Health-related quality of life as a predictor of mortality and hospitalization: the Dialysis Outcomes and Practice Patterns Study (DOPPS)." *Kidney International* 64(1):339-49.

National Kidney Foundation. 2002. "Clinical practice guidelines for chronic kidney disease: evaluation, classification and stratification. K/DOQI clinical practice guidelines." *American Journal of Kidney Disease*. 39(2):1–S266.

National Kidney Foundation. 2006. "NKF KDOQI guidelines. Clinical practice guidelines and clinical practice recommendations. 2006 updates. Haemodialysis adequacy, peritoneal dialysis and vascular access." *Am J Kidney Dis* 48(1):1–S322. http://www2.kidney.org/professionals/KDOQI/guideline_upHD_PD_VA/

National Kidney Foundation-Dialysis Outcomes Quality Initiative. 1997. "NKF-DOQI clinical practice guidelines for vascular access." *Am J Kidney Dis* 30:150–S191

Porter, AC, Lash, JP, Xie, D., Pan, Q., Deluca, J., Kanthety, R., Kusek, JW, Lora, CM, Nessel, L., Ricardo, AC, Wright Nunes, J., Fisher, MJ, CRIC Study Investigators. 2016. "Predictors and Outcomes of Health-Related Quality of Life in Adults with CKD." *Clinical Journal of the American Society for Nephrology* 11(7):1154-62.

Pagels, AA, Sőderkvist, BK, Medin, C., Hylander, B., Heiwe, S. 2012. "Health-related quality of life in different stages of chronic kidney disease and at initiation of dialysis treatment." *Health and Quality of Life Outcomes* 18(10):71.

Shroff R, Long DA, Shanahan C. 2013. "Mechanistic insights into vascular calcification in CKD." *J Am Soc Nephrol* 24:179–189. doi: 10.1681/ASN.2011121191.

Sheth RD, Brandt ML, Brewer ED, Nuchtern JG, Kale AS, Goldstein SL. 2002. "Permanent haemodialysis vascular access survival in children and adolescents with end-stage renal disease." *Kidney Int* 62:1864-69.

Shroff R., Sterenborg RB, Kuchta A., Arnold A., Thomas N., Stronach N., Padayachee S., Calder F., Shroff R. 2016. "A dedicated vascular access clinic for children on haemodialysis: Two years' experience." *Pediatr Nephrol* 31(12): 2337–2344. doi: 10.1007/s00467-016-3428-z

Šašinka, MA, Furková, K. 2014. *Chronická obličková choroba. Aktuálne problémy.* Bratislava: Herba. [*Chronic kidney disease. Current issues.* Bratislava: Herba.]

US Renal Data System (2006) *Annual data report: Atlas of end-stage renal disease in the United States.* National Institute of Health, National Institute of Diabetes and Digestive and Kidney Diseases, Bethesda, MD.

Závacká M. 2014. *Cievne prístupy, komplikácie a možnosti ich riešenia u pacientov v dlhodobom dialyzačnom programe.* Residency training thesis. Vascular surgery clinic in Košice. [*Vascular approaches, complications and possibilities of their solution in patients in a long-term dialysis program.* Residency training thesis. Vascular surgery clinic in Košice.]

Zaritsky JJ, Salusky IB, Gales B, Ramos G, Atkinson J, Allsteadt A, *et al.* 2008. "Vascular access complications in long-term pediatric haemodialysis patients." *Pediatr Nephrol* 23:2061-65.

Slezaková, Z. et al. 2020. *Ošetrovateľstvo a legislatíva v praxi*. Martin: Osveta. [*Nursing and legislation in practice.* Martin: Osveta.]

Slezaková, Z. Solgajova, A Zrubcová D. 2020. *Ošetrovateľstvo a konceptuálne modely pre prax.* Nitra: UKF Nitra. [*Nursing and conceptual models for practicing*. Nitra: UKF Nitra.]

In: Surgeon´s Perspective on Dialysis Patient ISBN: 978-1-53619-262-9
Editor: Maria Frankovicova

Chapter 4

External and Subcutaneous Arteriovenous Connections

M. Zavacká*, MD
Department of Vascular Surgery,
East Slovak Institute of Cardiovascular Diseases,
Faculty of Medicine, Pavol Jozef Šafárik University in Košice, Slovakia

Abstract

In this chapter we present the most frequently created vascular accesses: Subcutaneous arteriovenous fistula, Fistula in fossa Tabatiere, Distal radiocephalic fistula, Radiobasilic AVF with transposition, Radiobasilic AVF with transposition, Distal ulnar-basilic fistula, Proximal radiocephalic fistula, Fistula in fossa cubitalis, brachiobasilic AVF with transposition and other options.

Keywords: subcutaneous arteriovenous fistula, cephalic vein, radial artery, brachiobasilic transposition

---

* Corresponding Author's E-mail: martinazavacka80@gmail.com.

SUBCUTANEOUS ARTERIOVENOUS FISTULA

It is important to live up to the principle that a patient who is being prepared for a long-term hemodialysis program by a nephrologist has an A-V fistula created several months in advance. This step prevents the need to create short-term vascular access and can prepare the patient thoroughly for a long-term hemodialysis process.

FISTULA IN FOSSA TABATIERE

In the literature, this type of connection has been described for the first time by Mehigan in 1982 (Mehigan, J. T. et al., 1982). Cephalic vein (v.cephalica pollicis) is dissected from a short 1-2 cm incision in the area of the anatomical fossa, and the radial artery is dissected between the tendons of m. abductor pollicis brevis (Figure 1). End-to-side anastomosis (by continuous suture) up to 7-8 mm in length does not cause a hemodynamic burden for the patient.

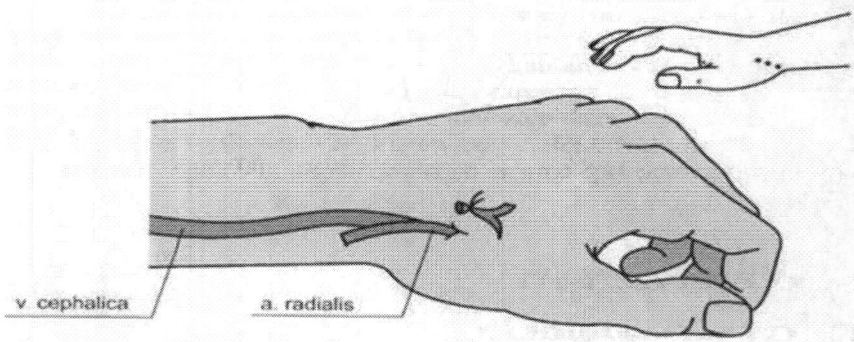

Figure 1. Schematic illustration of AVF in fossa Tabatiere.

DISTAL RADIOCEPHALIC FISTULA

Fistula in this location was mentioned first and described by Cimino and Brescia in 1966 and it is the most suitable way of creating vascular access for the need for long-term hemodialysis (Brescia M. J., Cimino J. E, 1966). Standard arteriovenous fistula expects side-to-side anastomosis between the radial artery and the cephalic vein (Figure 2), however, the modification currently used between these blood vessels is the end-to-side anastomosis (Figure 3), which we perform after distal ligation of v. cephalica. In case of extinction of the distal radiocephalic A - V fistula, there is an option to create a new radiocephalic fistula more proximally on the forearm. The advantages are that this technique is not demanding and it provides good patency results. However, it is necessary to know that one of the main success factors of this type of connection is the diameter of v.cephalica. According to Kherlakian's statistical evaluation, the primary patency is 80% after 6 months, 71% after 12, and 64% after 36 months.

RADIOBASILIC AVF WITH TRANSPOSITION

Another alternative to forming AVF on the radial side of the wrist is to connect the transposed basilic vein to the radial artery. The advantage of this type of connection is to create less of the further proximally mounted connections. The disadvantages are that the basilic vein transposition is a more complicated and time-consuming procedure. We begin by revision and dissection of the basilic vein and subsequently by dissection of a. radialis. We dissect v.basilica on the entire forearm up to the cubital area. We cut it distally and perform gentle hydrodilatation. Through a subcutaneous tunnel, which is created by blunt dissection using a long forceps, we pass the derotated basilic vein to the radial artery (Figure 4). We create a connection in the usual end-to-side way. The patency of this connection is reported at 84% for 12 months and at 69% after 30 months.

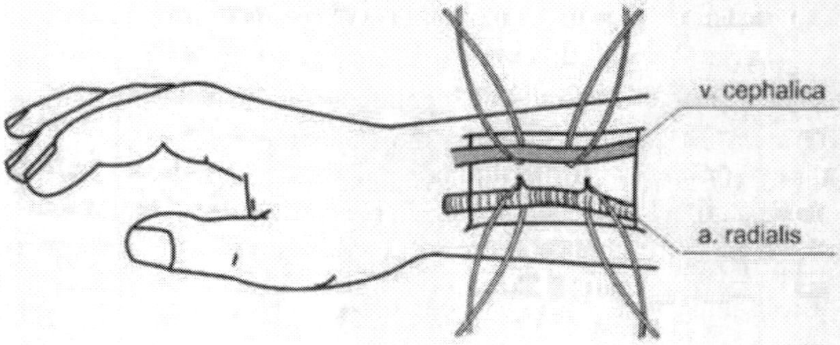

Figure 2. AVF sec. Brescia Cimino by side-to-side anastomosis (before suture).

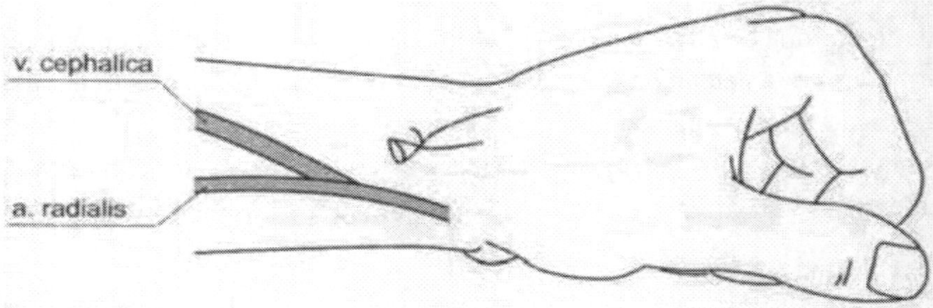

Figure 3. Distal radiocephalic AVF by end-to-side anastomosis.

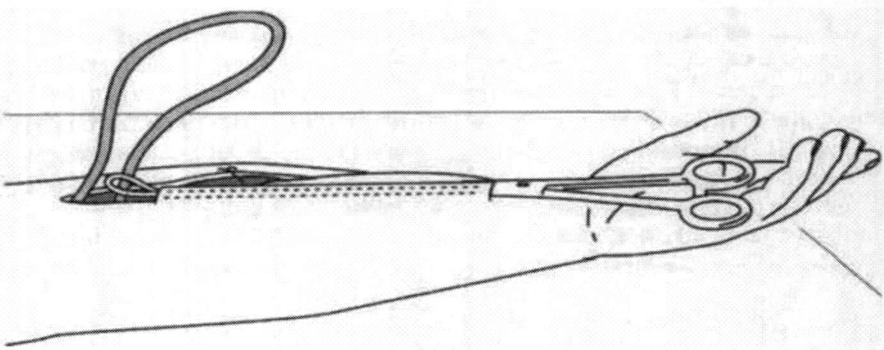

Figure 4. Pulling the basilic vein to the radial artery.

Distal Ulnar-Basilic Fistula

We choose the creation of this fistula in cases of no other possibility of the formation of A - V fistula on the radial side of the forearm and in patients with high quality v. basilica and insufficient blood flow through the radial artery. The prerequisite is a good caliber of v. basilica and a good flow of a.ulnaris while keeping the palmar flow of the arterial arch (negative Allen test). The patency is similar to the radiobasilic AVF with transposition.

Proximal Radiocephalic Fistula

In cases of distal A - V fistula failure, it is possible to attempt to create a proximal radiocephalic fistula, after considering and trying all of the possibilities on the antebrachial region. It is indicated mainly in patients whose A-V fistula failed due to distal insufficiency in the venous system. The disadvantage is the more complicated construction because the radial artery is located deeper. The surgical technique is the same as with the distal radiocephalic fistula.

Fistula in Fossa Cubitalis

It is suitable if the veins in the fossa cubitalis are not damaged by previous punctures. The standard side-to-side brachiocephalic fistula in the fossa cubitalis was described by Cascardo in 1970. This was followed by a modification of this type using vena perforans to end-to-side anastomosis on a.brachialis, published by Gracz in 1977. The advantage of the end-to-side anastomosis is that there is no increase in venous pressure on the forearm and no development of forearm swelling, which is a side effect in the formation of the brachiocephalic fistula by side-to-side anastomosis. The fistula in fossa cubitalis (Figure 5), is sometimes accepted as the first choice in patients with hypoplastic or thrombophlebitically affected venous stream on the forearm. In this type of AVF, however, a higher risk of steal-phenomenon should be considered; therefore, the length of anastomosis should not exceed 4-5mm. The primary patency of the brachiocubital fistula for 36 months is stated at 80%.

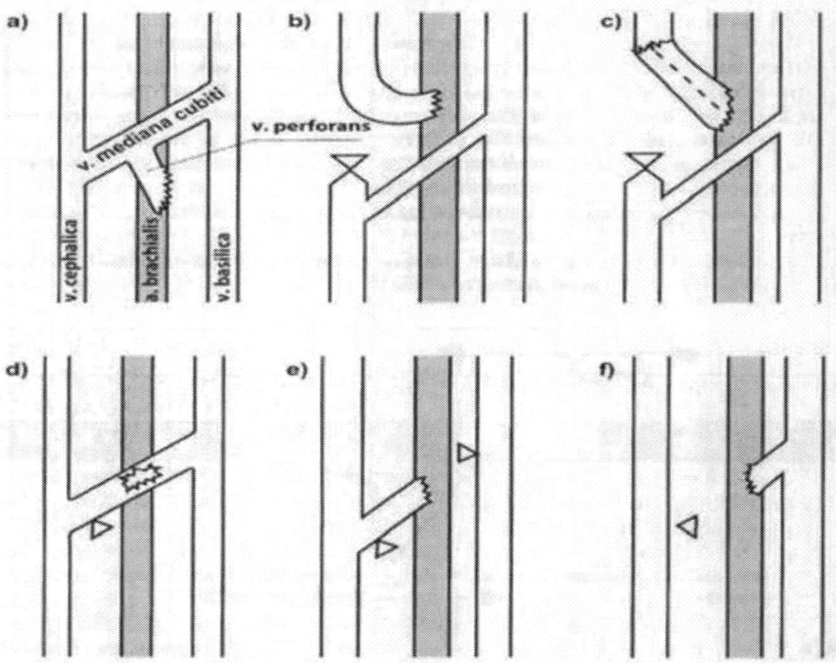

[a] brachiocephalic shunt E-t-S with vena perforans
[b] central brachiocephalic shunt E-t-S
[c] central brachiocephalic shunt E-t-S with interposition
[d] brachiocubital S-t-S
[e] brachiocubital E-t-S ad vena cephalica
[f] brachiocubital E-t-S ad vena basilica

Figure 5. Types of arteriovenous shunt using blood vessels in the fossa cubitalis.

BRACHIOBASILIC AVF WITH TRANSPOSITION

In this type of A - V fistula, the basilic vein is sewn onto the brachial artery in the fossa cubitalis. However, prior to that, for the purpose of hemodialysis, it is necessary to have the vein transposed above the fascia in sufficient length, which requires either general anesthesia or surgery under local anesthesia of the interscalenic nerve plexus. The technique of this operation was described by Dagher in 1976. The basilic vein and the brachial artery are dissected by the curved incision above the medial epicondyle of the humerus. We save n. cutaneus brachii medialis, which lies in the proximity of the basilic vein. After the dissection, we create a subcutaneous tunnel through which the transposed vein after derotation is pulled to the planned site of the anastomosis with the brachial artery (Figure 6) and is sewn by the end to side anastomosis in the length of 4-5mm. There is also a higher risk of local complications due to a long surgical wound.

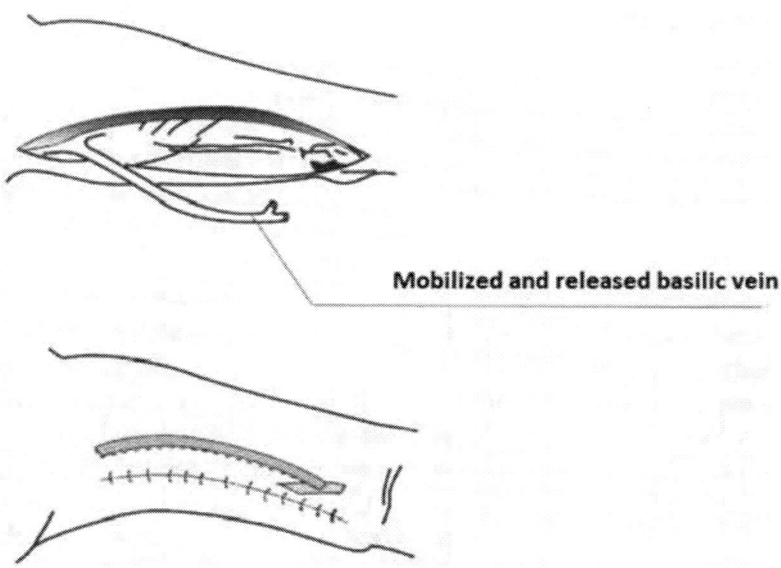

Figure 6. Schematic illustration of transposition of the basilic vein to the formed AVF with brachial artery at the arm.

Using a Venous and Arterial Graft

In the absence of a vein suitable for the creation of the A - V fistula, or in the case of severely damaged veins, the use of an autovenous or arterial graft should be considered. It is possible to use an autologous or heterologous vein. It is also possible to use an autologous, homologous, or heterologous artery.

Using Biografts

One of the options in the absence of a vein is the use of biografts consisting of natural collagen and an outer layer made of a polyester reticulum. Long-term patency results are, however, comparable to artificial materials.

Using Artificial Materials

The PTFE prosthesis is the most commonly used artificial prosthesis. Currently, despite the recommendations, the use of artificial material to create A-V fistula on the upper limb is seen as a last resort, given the higher percentage of complications compared to native veins. If a prosthesis must be used, the most suitable one is the one which is conical at the venous end, which should theoretically reduce the occurrence of the steal phenomenon. The use of a prosthesis is recommended if the outflow vein is at least 4 mm wide.

The indications for the use of prosthetic material to form AVF are as follows:

- insufficiency of the autologous vein stream
- replacement of a damaged section of the native vessel
- solving the stenotic outflow tract
- reducing blood flow through the hyper-functional shunt by adding an interponate or a prosthetic cuff

The upper limbs are the preferred locations for implementing a prosthetic AVF. As with native AVF, the non-dominant upper limb should be chosen first (Figure 7, 8). The shunts on the upper limb can be formed linearly or in the form of a loop. The most common loop-shaped AVF is the brachiobasilic AVF with the insertion of arterial anastomosis on a. brachialis and venous anastomosis implanted on v. basilica.

Alternative Options

If all options to create an A-V fistula on the upper limb fail, it is possible to attempt to construct the A-V fistula on the lower limb, either using the great saphenous vein or using a prosthesis. They are indicated in patients whose vascular access cannot be created on the upper limbs. Their formation is time-limited by hypoplasia and inappropriate branching of the vein. In principle, fistulae can be formed on the lower limb by combining a great saphenous vein with the posterior tibial artery above the inner ankle, with the superficial femoral artery in Hunter's canal region, or with the common femoral artery in inguine. However, it is always necessary to dissect the vein in the length of the skin incision and place it into a subcutaneous tunnel outside the surgical wound. When using a prosthesis, the venous end of the prosthesis is preferably connected to a deep venous system using a short venous conduit (in the case that removal of the fistula is necessary). Another option is to use a prosthesis on the chest.

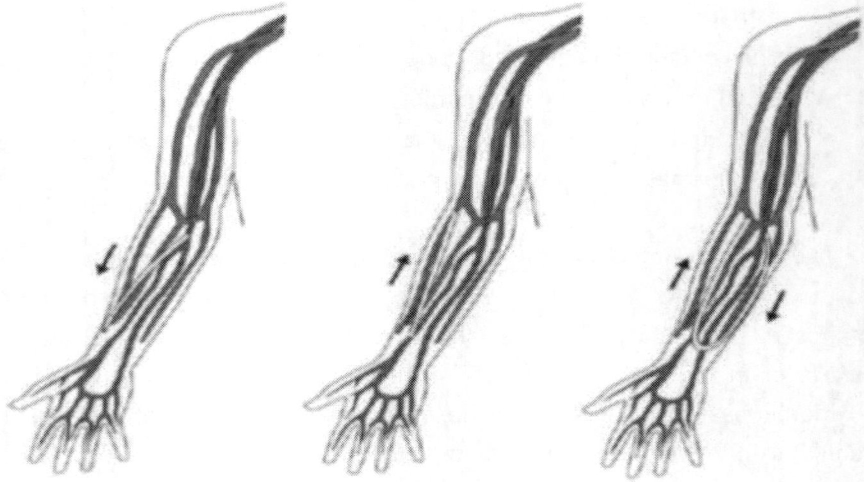

brachiocephalic radiocephalic brachiocephalic
linear graft linear graft “loop“ graft

Figure 7. Types of prosthetic AVF on the forearm.

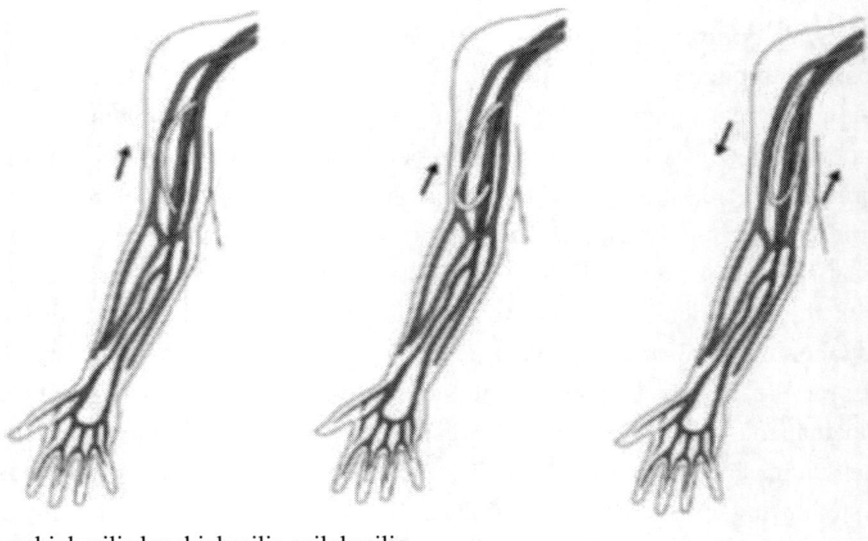

brachiobasilic brachiobasilic axilobasilic
graft “loop“ graft graft

Figure 8. Types of prosthetic AVF on the upper arm.

External Arteriovenous Connection

Regular External Scribner Shunt

The prerequisite is the ligature of the peripheral part of the artery; therefore, it is necessary to examine the arterial system of the upper limb before surgery. The advantages include the possibility of immediate and repeated use. The disadvantages include the limited period of use and the risk of frequent infectious complications. Therefore, it is suitable to convert this shunt into an internal A - V fistula. In the case of acute hemodialysis, it is preferable to introduce a catheter by puncture into the central venous system of the upper or lower limbs.

References

Albers, F. J. 1994. "Causes of hemodialysis Access failure." *Adv. Ren. Replace Ther.* 2:107-118.

Bachleda, P. et al., 2001. *Cévní náhrady v chirurgii arteriovenózních spojek k hemodialýze*. Olomouc: Prodos. [*Vascular prostheses in the surgery of arteriovenous junctions for hemodialysis*. Olomouc: Prodos.].

Ballard, J. L., Bunt, T. J, Malone, J. M. 1992. "Major complications of angioaccess surgery." *Am. J. Surg.* 164(3):229-232.

Bell, D. D, Rosental, J. J. 1998. "Arteriovenous graft life in chronic dialysis." *Arch.Surg.* 123:1169-1172.

Brescia, M. J., Cimino, J. E., Appel, K., Hurwich, B. J. 1966. "Chronic hemodialysis using venipuncture and surgically created arteriovenous fistula." *N. Engl. J. Med.* 275:1089 – 1092.

Brown, P. W. G. 2006. "Preoperative radiological assessment for vascular access." *Eur. J. Vasc. Endovasc. Surg.* 31:64 – 69.

Čertík, B. 2003. *Akútni končetinová ischemie.* Praha: Grada. [*Acute limb ischemia*. Prague: Grada.]

III. NKF-K/DOQI Clinical Practice Guidelines for Vascular Access: Update 2000 *Am. J. Kidney Dis.* 37:137-81.

Ebenová, Š. 2004. *Komplikácie cievneho prístupu a možnosti ich riešenia u pacientov v dlhodobom hemodialyzačnom programe.* Dissertation thesis., Pavol Jozef Šafárik University in Košice. [*Complications of the vascular approach and the possibilities of their solution in patients in a long-term hemodialysis program.* Dissertation thesis, Pavol Jozef Šafárik University in Košice.]

Frankovičová, M. 2000. *Chirurgia tepnožilových spojení pre potreby dlhodobej hemodialýzy*. Bratislava: Herba. [Surgery of *arterio-venous junctions for the needs of long-term hemodialysis*. Bratislava: Herba.]

Frankovičová, M. 1994. "Cievny štep v rekonštrukčnej chirurgii." *Folia Fac. Med. Univ. Šafarikiannae Cassoviensis* 171-177. ["Vascular graft in reconstructive surgery." *Folia Fac. Med. Univ. Šafarikiannae Cassoviensis* 171-177.]

Frankovičová, M. 1996. *Tepenno-žilové spojenia pre potreby dlhodobej hemodialýzy.* Habilitation thesis, Pavol Jozef Šafárik University in Košice. [*Arterio-venous junctions for long-term hemodialysis.* Habilitation thesis, Pavol Jozef Šafárik University in Košice.]

Gade, J., Aabech, J., Hansen, R.I. 1995. "The upper arm arteriovenous fistula- an alternative for vascular Access in haemodialysis." *Scand. J. Urol. Nephrol.* 29(2):121-124.

Janoušek, L., Baláž, P. et al., 2008. *Hemodialyzační arteriovenózní přístupy*. Praha: Grada. [*Hemodialysis arteriovenous approaches*. Prague: Grada.]

Kapoian T., Sherman R. A. 1997. "A brief history of vascular access for haemodialysis: an unfinished story." *Semin. Nephrol.* 3(17):239 – 245.

Kubíková, M., Roland, R. 1995. *Komplikácie pri vyhotovovaní arteriovenóznych fistúl.* Folia fac.med. Univ. šafarikianne Cassoviensis LII. [*Complications in establishing arteriovenous fistulas*. Folia fac.med.Univ. šafarikianne Cassoviensis LII.]

Medricka M., Janecka J., Koranda P., Buriankova E., Bachleda P. 2019. *^{18}F-FDG PET/CT and ^{99m}Tc-HMPAO-WBC SPECT/CT effectively contribute to early diagnosis of infection of arteriovenous graft for* *hemodialysis*. Biomed. Pap. Med. Fac. Univ. Palacky Olomouc. Czech Repub. 163:341-348.

Mehigan, Jr. M. C. McAlexander, R.A. 1982. "Snuffbox arteriovenous fistula for hemodialysis." *Am. J. Surg.* 252-253.

Utíkal, P., Bachleda, P., Sekanina, Z., Král, V. 1996. "Naše skúsenosti se zakladaním arteriovenóznych spojek k dialýze s využitím cévního rečište loketní jamky." *Rozhl. Chir.* 75(2):83-7. ["Our experience with establishing arteriovenous junctions for dialysis using the vascular bed of the elbow socket." Rozhl. Chir. 75 (2): 83-7.]

Zibari, G.B., Rohr, M.S. et al., 1988. "Complications from permanent hemodialysis vascular access." *Surgery* 104(4):681-686.

Slezaková, Z. et al., 2020. *Ošetrovateľstvo a legislatíva v praxi*. Martin: Osveta. [*Nursing and legislation in practice*. Martin: Osveta.]

Slezaková, Z. Solgajova, A Zrubcová D. 2020. *Ošetrovateľstvo a konceptuálne modely pre prax*. Nitra: UKF Nitra. [*Nursing and conceptual models for practicing*. Nitra: UKF Nitra.]

In: Surgeon´s Perspective on Dialysis Patient ISBN: 978-1-53619-262-9
Editor: Maria Frankovicova

Chapter 5

METHODS AND PRINCIPLES OF FORMING ARTERIOVENOUS FISTULAE (PRE-OPERATIVE ASSESSMENT, PATIENT AND OPERATING ROOM PREPARATION, POSTOPERATIVE CARE)

***M. Zavacká**, MD**
Department of Vascular Surgery,
East Slovak Institute of Cardiovascular Diseases,
Faculty of Medicine, Pavol Jozef Šafárik University in Košice, Slovakia

ABSTRACT

The purpose is to create an AV fistula that can be easily cannulated and withstand repeated punctures. The first fistula is introduced in the limb as distally as possible. Doppler ultrasonography **is** a simple examination that will help us map the arteriovenous system on the limbs.

* Corresponding Author's E-mail: martinazavacka80@gmail.com.

AV fistulae are created in super aseptic operating rooms where reconstructive vascular operations are performed.

Keywords: arteriovenous fistula, upper limb, clinical examination, Doppler ultrasonography, phlebography

Abbreviations

AVF	arteriovenous fistula
NKF-DQOI	National Kidney Foundation's Dialysis Outcomes Quality Initiative
UL	upper limb
PTA	percutaneous transluminal angioplasty
PTFE	polytetrafluorethylene
USG	ultrasonography

Surgical creation of arteriovenous connection (arteriovenous fistula, shunt, AVF), which is used for repeated connection of the patient to hemodialysis, is one of the basic vascular surgical procedures. The essence is to create an AV fistula that can be easily cannulated and withstand repeated punctures. It is necessary to ensure sufficient blood flow for the proper functioning of the fistula. Although these operations are considered simpler from a technical point of view, the decision to make the right choice of AVF is sometimes challenging and requires adequate erudition of the vascular surgeon.

According to the rate of progression of renal disease, we classify the need to create dialysis access to acute and elective. Acute access is introduced in the event of sudden renal failure and is expected to be used for less than 3 weeks. The acute dialysis access is currently created by introducing dialysis catheters into the jugular, femoral, or subclavian vein. For the long-term administration of hemodialysis, we establish AVF fistulae in patients electively.

It is necessary to have a strategy of the whole process, including indication, operation, postoperative care, and possibilities of solving complications for the creation of a high-quality AV fistula. Currently, AVF can be formed by joining the patient's own vessels or using prosthetic or allogeneic material. For long-term hemodialysis, subcutaneous arteriovenous fistulae are formed most often as they allow easy cannulation and have the best long-term patency. The second group is the external arteriovenous Scribner arteriovenous fistula, which is currently used less frequently. This fistula was a major advance in the technique of chronic hemodialysis at that time because it allowed long-term treatment, which has been, until then, limited by the reduced possibility of reconnection to the artificial kidney. The outer fistula is a set of Teflon tubes and plastic tubing that permanently connects the peripheral vessels of the limbs above the skin. Immediately after implantation, technically easy, repeatable, and painless connection to the dialysis device is made possible by simply detaching the fistula tubing. Due to frequent complications and limited duration of patency (usually only a few months), the external fistula is no longer used and, if so, only in extreme situations such as temporary vascular access. Scribner's shunt is currently replaced by the introduction of dialysis catheters.

Permanent vascular access can be created in those places where appropriate anatomical conditions are present. The creation of a fistula, the basic surgical strategy for choice of type and location is now more or less clear and follows three basic rules:

1. The first fistula is introduced in the limb as distally as possible, in the case of the upper limb in the area above the wrist. In the case of irreversible failure of the fistula, it is possible to establish another fistula more proximally. To introduce the first AVF, the non-dominant upper limb is selected. In hypoplastic, thrombophlebitis-afflicted veins on the forearm or arteries afflicted by atherosclerosis or mediocalcinosis (often in diabetic and obese patients), we introduce the fistula primarily in the area of the cubital tunnel.
2. The upper limbs (hereinafter referred to as UL) are clearly more suitable for the formation of A-V fistula. Upper limb vessels are

more accessible for puncture and massive atherosclerotic obstruction is less common for upper limbs. The last option for the patient is the formation of the lower limb fistula or the extra-anatomic fistula.

3. A-V fistulae on native vessels have a longer lifetime than synthetic fistulae and are therefore preferred. Only after all the possibilities of autologous connections have been exhausted do we proceed to the creation of the AVF using foreign material and we prefer to use a vascular prosthesis.

Pre-Operative Assessment

All patients indicated for the introduction of AVF require a thorough preoperative examination, which includes a detailed patient history and clinical examination. The examination begins with a detailed medical history of the cardiovascular system, coagulation disorders, the number of AV fistulas established in the past, associated diseases, and the presence of diabetes. We are searching for the history of catheterization of the central venous system, introduction of pacemaker or cardioverter-defibrillator. Subsequently, we can proceed to clinical examination. This examination requires a thorough knowledge of the anatomy of the vascular supply of the upper and lower limbs.

Clinical Examination

This examination is important for choosing the AVF introduction strategy. We begin by examining the arterial system of both upper limbs. We examine the pulse quality of brachial, radial, and ulnar arteries. The examined pulsations will be compared between both limbs and if a suspected lower pulse quality on one limb is identified, the examination of the pressure gradient is indicated. Pressure reduction warns us of atherosclerotic or other arterial diseases. A simple and very important examination is the Allen test. It illustrates the functional state of the collateral circulation of the hand via the arcus arteriosus. After pressing a. radialis, the patient repeatedly clenches the fist and then opens it. A renewed blood flow to the hand within 30 seconds after the fist is open is an indication of sufficient collateral supply from the ulnar artery. In a positive test, the introduction of radiocephalic fistula at the radial artery is contraindicated. Examination of arteries is followed by the examination of the veins (after compression with a tourniquet on the upper arm). After repeated flexion in the elbow, we examine the vein filling on both the palmar and the volar side of the limb. By tapping the filled vein, we follow the pulse wave transmission. The stenosis of the cephalic or basilic vein is indicated by the disappearance of the pulse wave during its course. According to Kalmann, it is necessary to visualize the veins of the limb during the clinical examination before the planned operation. In the authors' opinion, phlebography or ultrasonography mapping is indicated in patients whose veins do not appear even when a tourniquet is applied. In the case of problematic patients, we examine the vascular system on the lower limb, where we focus on the quality of the femoral and popliteal artery respectively, and the condition of the great and small saphenous vein. It is important to warn the patient about a ban on injections and venepuncture into the veins of the operated limb at least 14 days prior to surgery. Some authors describe the protective effect of applying a light bandage to the limbs before the operation is performed.

Imaging Methods

A wide range of imaging methods is currently available, but they cannot be used without a thorough clinical examination. Imaging examinations are available for patients whose basic clinical examination does not provide us with sufficient information about the quality of the vascular system. They will provide the information needed to develop an operational strategy. However, we need to consider the adverse effects of some examinations, especially when the administration of contrast iodine agents is required, the application of which may impair renal function. Therefore, the indication of imaging methods should be well thought over and reserved for cases where the conclusion of the examination is crucial for the patient.

Doppler Ultrasonography

The simple and easy examination will help us map the arteriovenous system on the limbs. Some authors recommend this examination by default in all patients who are indicated for the introduction of AVF. In patients for whom basilic vein transposition is planned, it is generally advisable to supplement the ultrasonographic examination. The acceptable diameter of the cephalic vein on the forearm is 2.5 mm. When planning transposition of the basilic vein in the arm, a diameter of at least 4 mm is acceptable. The table below describes the recommended criteria for introducing fistula with vein transposition (Table 1).

Table 1. Functional state of the vein and artery - suitable for the formation of AVF with transposition

Vein examination	
vein diameter 2.5 mm (v. cephalica)	> 4 mm (basilic vein)
absence of segmental stenosis	continuity with a deep vein system in the upper arm
absence of stenosis or occlusion of the central venous system of the limb	
Artery examination	
artery lumen diameter 2.0 mm	
absence of obliterating calcifications	absence of blood pressure difference between limbs 20 mm Hg
functional palmar arch (negative Allen test)	

Phlebography

Currently, we have the possibility of classical phlebography or computer tomographic phlebography. Both examinations are beneficial in eliminating stenosis of the central venous system in those cases where the ultrasonographic examination was opaque. Both methods require the application of a contrast iodine substance and therefore examination should be reasonably indicated due to the nephrotoxic effect.

Indications for phlebography prior to planned AVF formation

1. limb edema or severe obesity of the patient
2. creation of collateral venous circulation in limbs and suspected stenosis of the central stream
3. different circumference of limbs
4. the intravenous catheter of various types in the central venous system (including in the medical history)
5. prior history of trauma or surgery of the venous system in the upper arm, neck and chest area
6. repeated formation of the AVF in the limb

Native Forearm X-Ray

This examination is indicated in diabetic patients for the exclusion of severe arterial mediocalcinosis. In the picture, we are looking for calcifications in the course of the arteries of the forearm. In the event of a severe finding, we can avoid the affected section of the artery and plan the fistula on the place where the X-ray image is not showing such significant mediocalcinosis.

Surgical Technique

Arterial and vein surgery in vascular surgery requires some special tools, instruments, suture material, and other materials. The operation itself requires a fine scalpel, fine preparation scissors, angled scissors, curved to side scissors, fine short and long Debakey forceps, blunt retractors, large dissector, hooks for tourniquets, vascular clamps: round, slightly curved, strongly curved, angled, wall, aneurysm clamps, straight and curved "bulldog" clips, micro bulldogs, endarterectomy raspatories, flushing cannula, fine needles of varying length, syringes, injection needles, suction tips with flat and round ends, laces for tourniquets, possibly PVC bands, electronic knife (Figure 1).

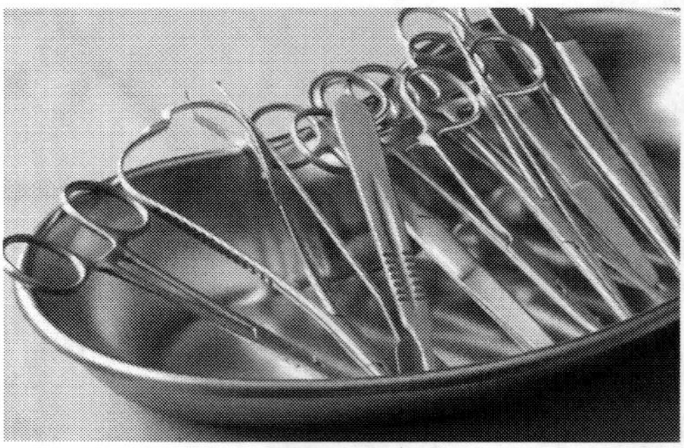

Figure 1. Vascular-surgical instrument set.

Accessories: sewing stitches, Fogarty catheter, Redon drain, intraluminal fistula, aspirator, blood pressure measuring set. Atraumatic vascular sutures from 2/0 to 6/0 with different needle lengths and monofilament fiber (e.g., Prolen) are necessary from the suture material. In principle, we use non-absorbable fibers! Artificial vascular prostheses must be in stock both simple and branched, smooth and corrugated in various sizes and of different designs (woven, knitted, PTFE cast). When sewing fragile vessels, especially with additional stitches because of bleeding from anastomoses, it is advisable to use stitches backed with Teflon felt. Another special feature of vascular surgery is heparinization. Heparin solution for flushing arteries, veins, and prostheses is prepared by adding 2 ml of heparin to 400 ml of Ringer's-lactate solution. For total heparinization we use 2 mg of heparin per 1 kg of the patient's weight, heparin is administered by the anesthetist. Termination of heparinization is achieved by protamine in the ratio of 1.5 mg protamine per 1 mg heparin. For surgery on the blood vessels, it is preferable to apply a self-adhesive film so that the vascular replacement does not touch the patient's skin (Figure 2).

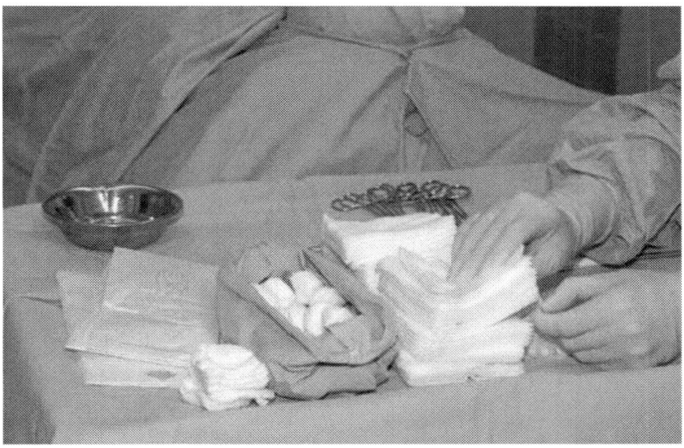

Figure 2. Preparation for surgery.

The surgical plan is prepared during the pre-operative examination of the patient. During the examination, we decide where and how we will carry out the reconstruction. We will instruct the patient and indicate in his documentation where and how we plan to create the fistula and how to protect the blood vessels prior to the surgery. The best way is to protect the limb which is to be operated on with a light bandage. Patients in need of pre-operative preparation are hospitalized and in cases of repeated surgery or predicting a more complicated post-operative period, it is advisable to also hospitalize the patient in the immediate post-operative period. We monitor blood pressure very closely before surgery. In the evening before surgery, the limb should be well washed and bandaged. We will thoroughly shave the location and wide surroundings of the planned operational field. The preparation of the operating room is the same as the preparation before a normal vascular procedure. AV fistulae are created in super aseptic operating rooms where reconstructive vascular operations are performed. After placing the patient on the operating table, the patient's fixation, and attaching the limb to monitor blood pressure and intravenous infusion, we will wash the limb that we plan to operate, from the fingertips to the armpit. We drape the upper arm about 5 cm above the elbow and about 15 cm above the wrist on the other limb. On the wrist, continue with the revision higher, if necessary, in the elbow pit, too. Wrap the hand in a drape and fix it with a bandage or isolate it with a sterile glove. If we are creating the AV fistula in the fossa tabatiere (foveola radialis), leave the thumb free and wrap only the fingers and palm. The whole limb is placed on the table prepared by the instrumental nurse. The limb must lie on the table, free and comfortable. Take care that external pressure does not cause nerve damage during prolonged operations. If we are creating the fistula on the wrist or in the foveola radialis, we sit perpendicularly to the patient. If we plan to make the fistula high on the forearm or in the elbow pit, or if we are considering the transposition of the basilica, we sit on the inner side of the limb in such a way that we have comfortable access to the axilla. Blood pressure and pulse should be monitored during surgery for each patient. The presence of an anesthesiologist depends on mutual agreement with the surgeon. Cover the patient with a sterile sheet. If possible, the patient should lie on a heating cushion. Perchance, you also take care of the patient lying comfortably before the operation, because in the unforeseen situation the duration of the procedure can be prolonged, and uncomfortable placement of the patient tends to result in restlessness, nervousness, which sometimes disproportionately increases the nervousness of the operating team. Therefore, premedication is appropriate for all patients. The operating theatre nurses are responsible for the preparation of the operating theatre. The surgeon should check the instrument set, electrocoagulation function, and aspirator before the operation. Proper seating and adequate height of the desk, auxiliary table, and chair are also an important part of preoperative preparation in the operating room. Local anesthesia follows when the fistula site is selected, the operating field is covered, and the operation preparations are completed.

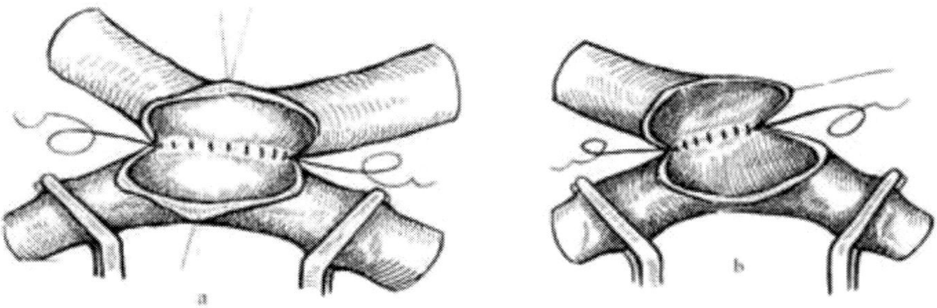

Figure 3. a) anastomosis side to side (wall to wall). b) anastomosis end-to-side (end to wall).

If a fistula is made in foveola radialis, usually a local anesthetic of 5-7 ml of 1% or 2% mesocaine or supracaine, is sufficient. If the fistula is to be placed in a usual place, use 5-10 ml of local anesthetic. Use a fine needle and do not manipulate the needle after injecting it into the subcutaneous tissue to avoid injecting any superficial vein. Instill the anesthetic slowly, with just one puncture. Most often, you should inject the needle distally from the intended incision and direct it proximally with the simultaneous application of the anesthetic (never forget to ask the patient about hypersensitivity to drugs, anesthetics, or complications in the past). When instilling a full dose of anesthetic into the subcutaneous tissue, apply a flat, slight pressure on the site of the instillation with a wet square of gauze, and wait for the anesthetic to slowly absorb. Then it's time to make the incision. If we opt for an elbow fistula, use significantly more anesthetics: 20-30 ml. In the elbow area, after anesthesia of the skin and subcutaneous structures, the second dose of anesthetic is applied preoperatively under visual control so that the artery placed under the fascia is not damaged, and to thoroughly ensure painless preparation of necessary section by anesthesia. If it is necessary to transpose the basilic vein or perform another reconstruction operation on the upper arm, we recommend axillary blockade and also general anesthesia in indicated cases after consultation with a nephrologist.

Surgery is normally performed under local infiltration of anesthesia, although some sites prefer locoregional anesthesia for its vasodilatory effect. The oblique longitudinal or transverse section is made on the palmar side of the wrist between the tendons of m. brachioradialis and m. flexor carpi radialis. The cephalic vein is dissected in the subcutaneous space in sufficient length and the distal end is ligated after cutting. Heparin solution is used to test the venous patency and gentle hydrodilatation. Without this maneuver, there is a higher risk of early AVF thrombosis. After the retinaculum flexorum is cut, the radial artery is dissected, the small branches are ligated. The character of the pulsation on the artery is evaluated (or intraoperatively checked by USG ultrasonography) and the wall quality is evaluated. Significant vascular mediocalcinosis, which is present in diabetics, is not a contraindication to surgery but makes surgery more difficult and the probability of maturation of AVF is lower. After the fine clamps are introduced, an arteriotomy of 8-11 mm is made on the radial side of the artery and is rinsed with a heparin solution. Subsequently, anastomosis with the proximal end of the vein is sewn end-to-side with polypropylene fiber 6/0-7/0 (Figure 3). After releasing the clamps, you can feel the vortex at the site of anastomosis or at the distal part of the cephalic vein. However, its absence may not be indicative of AVF malfunctioning. After checking the functionality of anastomosis and hemostasis, suture the skin with individual stitches or intradermally. The surgical wound is covered with a small sterile cover, never with a circular bandage. If possible, put the limb in an arm sling.

POSTOPERATIVE CARE

The arteriovenous fistula is a predictor of survival in the hemodialyzed population, independently not only of socio-demographic parameters but also of serious and already confirmed comorbidities increasing the risk of death from cardiovascular causes and diabetic complications. Patients dialyzed via the arteriovenous fistula have a 43% higher survival chance compared to respondents with a central venous catheter one year after being enrolled in regular dialysis treatment, regardless of age, gender, nutritional status, time spent on dialysis (months to years), and serious co-morbidities.

This fact, unless there are other significant contraindications regarding the performance of arteriovenous fistula or graft, should be part of the decision to choose long-term vascular access in the hemodialysis population, because in this way we not only increase the chance of the dialyzed population to survive, but at the same time we give them a chance for a higher quality of life and lower morbidity, or complications associated with vascular access (KDIGO, 2013). These aspects are closely linked to a more effective implication of the funds in the health care system and the chance to use them in the prevention or in long-term investments beneficial to the patient not only at a given time but also in the long term.

In addition, arteriovenous fistula not only increases the chance of survival almost by half but also reduces the risk of systemic infections, which are incomparably higher in central catheters. Of course, there are direct and indirect costs of health care, which must cover not only the short-term aspect of the deterioration of health but also the long-term impact, since complex nursing care for a venous catheter is always more costly, including the time without complications (treatment, disinfection, sterile overlapping, regular use of anticoagulant stoppers, etc.).

The unforeseen finding that arterialized vein in the subcutis of the upper limb can withstand often as much as several hundred cannulations without inflammation or thrombosis, greatly improved the prospects of a patient with chronic renal insufficiency and prolonged treatment options by dialysis for several years. The most common cause of vascular access failure is progressive vein stenosis beyond the anastomosis caused by fibromuscular intimal hyperplasia, which leads to graft thrombosis as it progresses. Although methods for diagnosing stenosis are known and allow early detection and correction of an error, stenosis diagnosed only after the previous thrombosis is usually still quite common in our clinical practice.

According to the practical recommendations of the NKF-DQOI /National Kidney Foundation's Dialysis Outcomes Quality Initiative/, the procedure in case of stenosis of A-V fistula is strictly individual and depends on the experience of the workplace. In the case of stenosis of the central venous system, the PTA methodology is preferred, possibly with the introduction of a stent into the affected vascular system. It is the possibility of using early angiography and subsequent PTA that could guarantee better results while maintaining long-term vascular access function. In general, the ideal procedure should be fast, safe, and efficient and should allow the patient to return to the hemodialysis unit as soon as possible with functioning long-term dialysis access. The PTA almost meets these rules almost ideally. It is low morbidity and almost unlimited repeatability of endovascular procedures that in this case favors them in comparison to classical surgical treatment.

It should be also kept in mind that any short-term central venous catheter dialysis access in patients who already require regular hemodialysis carries a risk of stenosis in the central venous system. Thus, if we prefer to correct the malfunctioning AV fistula, either by interventional or surgical method, before creating new access, and if this attempt is successful, we will protect the patient's venous system from two unnecessary procedures

In the case of AV fistula thrombosis, neither percutaneous nor surgical techniques have shown success, and thus the treatment of AV fistula thrombosis has overall unfavorable results. Often, these are elderly patients with cardiac insufficiency, unable to maintain sufficient systolic pressure for A-V fistula functionality. In these patients, the only option is to introduce a tunneled central venous catheter or to perform dialysis through the peritoneal catheter. In the case of infection and removal of the catheter from the central vein, thrombosis usually develops and the vein will be subsequently unusable in the future.

In Europe, unlike the USA, the use of native veins is preferred in the A-V fistula surgery. This also results in a lower number of infectious complications. For fresh AV fistulae using a prosthesis, the method of choice for the treatment of infection is antibiotic therapy in combination with the removal of the prosthesis. In the case of native A-V fistula, 6-week antibiotic therapy is usually sufficient. In cases of A-V fistula infection more than a month after its establishment, we try to preserve the AV fistula as much as possible. Only in extreme cases should the fistula be removed, and the patient receives dialysis via different access.

An important preventive factor in the onset of hemodynamic complications is the correct choice of the type of anastomosis used, where anastomosis end-to-side is preferred. This anastomosis used in the case of the distal radiocephalic fistula on the wrist greatly reduces the risk of developing steal syndrome, on the other hand, consistent skeletonization of the veins while maintaining the exclusively draining branch will prevent venous hypertension when used in the case of A-V fistula in the cubital fossa and brachia. Oftentimes, in order to save the limb, we have no other choice but to remove the A-V fistula and create a new A-V fistula on the other limb, preferably as peripherally as possible.

References

Baláž, P., Rokošný, S., Klein, D., Adamec, M. 2008. "Aneurysmorrhaphy is an easy technique for arteriovenous fistula salvage." *J Vasc Surg* 9:81-84.

Basile, C. et al. 2008. "The relationship between the flow of arteriovenous fistula and cardiac output in hemodialysis patients." *Nephrol Dial Transplant* 23:282-287.

Breza, J., Řezníček, J., Zvara, V. 1985. "Príprava krvného riečišťa pre hemodialýzu vytvorením fistuly medzi a. brachialis a do podkožia ramena transponovanou v. basilica." *Rozhl Chir* 64(11):708-712. ["Preparation of the bloodstream for hemodialysis by creating a fistula between the brachial artery and the subcutaneous are of the shoulder transposed by the basilic vein." *Rozhl Chir* 64 (11): 708-712.]

Brescia, M.J., Cimino, J.E., Appel, K., Hurwich, B.J. 1966. "Chronic hemodialysis using venipuncture and a surgically created arteriovenous fistula." *N Eng J Med* 275:1089-92.

Bourquelot, P., Corbi, P., Cussenot, O. 1989. "Surgical improvement of high-flow arteriovenous fistulas". In *Vascular Access for hemodialysis* edited by Sommer B.G., Henry M.L. 124-130. New York: W.L. Gore & Associates Inc., Pluribus Press Inc.

Bourquelot, P., Rawa, M., Van Laere, O. 2012. "Long- -term results of femoral vein transposition for autogenous arteriovenous hemodialysis access." *J Vasc Surg* 56:440-5.

Cascardo, S., Acchiardo, S., Beven, E.G. 1970. "Proximal arteriovenous fistulae for hemodialysis when radial arteries are unavailable." *Proc Eur Dial Transplant Assoc* 7:42-6.

Dagher, F., Gerber, R., Ramos, E. et al. 1976. "The use of basilic vein and brachial artery as an A-V fistula for long term hemodialysis." *J Surg Res* 20:373-6.

Frankovičová, M. 2000. *Chirurgia tepnožilových spojení pre potreby dlhodobej hemodialýzy*. Bratislava: Herba. [*Surgery of arterio-venous junctions for the needs of long-term hemodialysis treatment*]

Janeckova J., Bachleda P., Utikal P., Jarosciakova J., Orsag J. 2020. "Arteriovenous Grafts' Types of Indications and Their Infection Rate." *Ann Vasc Surg*. 2020 16:S0890-5096(20)30519-7. doi: 10.1016/j.avsg. 2020.06.018.

Jennings, W.C., Miller, G.A., Coburn, M.Z. 2012. "Vascular access flow reduction for arteriovenous fistula salvage in symptomatic patients with central venous occlusion." *J Vasc Access*, 13:157-62.

Malovrh, M. 2003. "The role of sonography in the planning of arteriovenous fistulas for hemodialysis." *Semin Dial* 16:299-303.

Mehigan, J.T., McALexander, R.A. 1982. "Snuffbox arteriovenous fistula for hemodialysis." *Am J Surg* 143(2):252-3.

Robbin, M.L., Gallichio, M.H., Deierhoi, M.H. et al. 2000. "US vascular mapping before hemodialysis access placement." *Radiology* 217:83-88.

Vajó, J. 1996. *Náhle angiochirurgické príhody a akútny ischemicko - reperfúzny syndróm v klinickej praxi Košice.* Košice: TypoPress Košice. [*Sudden angiosurgical events and acute ischemia - reperfusion syndrome in clinical practice*. Košice: TypoPress Košice.]

Wixon, C.L., Hughes, J., Mills, J.L. 2000. "Understanding strategies for treatment of ischemic steal syndrome after hemodialysis access." *J Am Coll Surg* 191:301-310.

Šinák, I., Baláž, P., Zeleňák, K. 2017. "Aneuryzmy arteriovenóznych fistúl pre dialýzu." in *Atlas vaskulárnych aneurzyziem* edited by Mazuch, J. et al, 269-277. Turany: P+M, grafické štúdio. ["Aneurysms of arteriovenous fistulas for dialysis." in *The atlas of vascular aneurysms* edited by Mazuch, J. et al, 269-277. Turany: P + M, graphic studio.]

Frankovičová M. et al. 2018. *Cievna chirurgia*. Košice: Univerzita Pavla Jozefa Šafárika v Košiciach. [*Vascular Surgery*. Košice: Pavol Jozef Šafárik University in Košice]

Slezaková, Z. et al. 2020. *Ošetrovateľstvo a legislatíva v praxi*. Martin: Osveta. [*Nursing and legislation in practice*. Martin: Osveta.]

Slezaková, Z. Solgajova, A. Zrubcová D. 2020. *Ošetrovateľstvo a konceptuálne modely pre prax*. Nitra: UKF Nitra. [*Nursing and conceptual models for practicing*. Nitra: UKF Nitra.]

In: Surgeon´s Perspective on Dialysis Patient ISBN: 978-1-53619-262-9
Editor: Maria Frankovicova

Chapter 6

Monitoring of Vascular Accesses, Causes of Vascular Access Failures, and Prevention and Treatment Options

Norbert Torma*, MD
Angiosurgical Department of the Medical Faculty of
Pavol Jozef Safarik University, Košice, Slovakia

Abstract

Chronic kidney disease is characterized by a gradual loss of kidney function. The most common causes of kidney malfunction are diabetes mellitus, high blood pressure and glomerulonephritis. Chronic renal disease may not be apparent until a kidney function is significantly decreased. Treatment is focused on the treatment of underlying causes to slow progression of kidney dysfunction. Once kidney functions are significantly impaired and progress to end stage kidney failure, patient may need dialysis. There are different types of dialysis, between them hemodialysis with three primary methods to gain access to the blood for

---

* Corresponding Author's E-mail: norko@post.sk.

hemodialysis. This chapter deals with problems with maturation of native arteriovenous access and arteriovenous grafts and possibilities to prevents these complications. In this chapter we also deal with treatments options.

Keywords: AV access, AV fistula, AV graft, central venous catheter, chronic venous insufficiency, maturation of arteriovenous access

ABBREVIATIONS

AV	arteriovenous
AVF	arteriovenous fistula
AVG	arteriovenous graft
CO	cardiac output
CPR	cardiopulmonary recirculation
KDOQI	Kidney Disease Outcomes Quality Initiative
NKF-KDOQI	National Kidney Foundation-Kidney Disease Outcomes Quality
PTFE	polytetrafluoroethylene
USG	ultrasound

INTRODUCTION

By forming an AV fistula or kidney transplantation, it is possible to achieve prolongation of life and many times an increase in workability for a patient with chronic renal insufficiency. However, hemodialysis remains a permanent solution to their disease state for most of them.

If the patient's glomerular filtration rate falls below 25 ml/min., the patient is placed under the care of a team of nephrologists. Regardless of the choice of hemodialysis method, the veins on the upper limbs should be treated for the purpose of making AV fistulae.

The first fistula is placed on the limb as distally as possible, in the case of the upper limb in the area above the wrist. In the case of irreversible fistula failure, it is possible to create another one more proximally. AV fistulae on native vessels have a longer lifetime than synthetic fistulae and are therefore clearly preferred. If urgent dialysis is needed, the subclavian vein cannulation should be avoided as much as possible, as it is ultimately leading to its stenosis, which can seriously limit the possibility of creating functional AV fistulae.

Despite the increasing number of patients with diabetes, peripheral vascular disease, and a large number of elderly patients, a native AV fistula can be introduced in most of them.

However, the lifespan of an AV fistula is limited, and sooner or later, complications develop, such as:

1) stenosis
2) thrombosis
3) infection
4) aneurysm and pseudoaneurysm
5) hemodynamic complications
6) bleeding
7) neuropathy

These are important causes of patients' morbidity in the long-term hemodialysis program and account for a substantial part of their hospitalizations.

Types of AV Fistulae

It is important to adhere to the principle that a patient who is being prepared for a long-term hemodialysis program by a nephrologist should have an AV fistula created several months in advance. This avoids the need to create short-term vascular access and can prepare the patient thoroughly for a long-term hemodialysis process.

Subcutaneous Arteriovenous Fistulae

- Fistula in foveola radialis (fossa Tabatiere)
- Distal radiocephalic fistula
- Distal ulnar-basilic fistula
- Proximal radiocephalic fistula
- Fistula in the cubital pit
- Transposition of the basilic vein
- Use of venous and arterial transplant
- Use of biografts
- Use of artificial materials
- Alternative methods

If all attempts to create an AV fistula on the upper limb fail, it is possible to attempt to construct an AV fistula on the lower limb, either using the great saphenous vein or using an artificial prosthesis. When using an artificial prosthesis, the venous end of the prosthesis is preferably connected to a deep venous system using a short venous conduit (in case of removal). Another option is the use of a prosthesis on the chest, by sewing, using the so-called cross-over technique.

External Arteriovenous Connection

- Classic external Scribner shunt

Central Venous Catheters

- Tunneled
- Non-tunneled

Monitoring of Vascular Accesses, Causes of Vascular Access Failure, and Prevention and Treatment Options

Functional vascular access is necessary for effective dialysis, in the case of AV fistulae, this access should have sufficient patency. In order to ensure this condition, it is necessary to connect the fistula to a suitable artery and vein, preferably both being in close proximity to each other. Unfortunately, such an anatomical configuration is not always present in patients requiring an AV fistula. The most common obstacle and the drawback is the absence of a suitable vein. In these cases, an autologous or synthetic graft with implantation between the artery and the vein can be used to construct the AV fistula. Various materials have been tried in the past to replace native veins. Artificial grafts – prostheses – are now used, with a good use for dialysis, but with a higher complication rate than it is the case in native AV fistulae. Both types of fistulae – native and artificial grafts, have limitations with respect to their maturation. In the case of native fistulae, it is one month on average, in the case of fistulae using artificial material, the period of "incorporation" of the graft is at least a week. During this period, it is not possible to use the AV fistula safely without the risk of complications. If acute dialysis is required, a central venous catheter can be inserted. These catheters can be used when acute dialysis is needed and can be extracted after AV fistula formation and its maturation. They can also be used for chronic dialysis and left in place for several years.

The effectiveness of dialysis is dependent on sufficient blood flow through the AV fistula, or on sufficient blood flow through the catheter during dialysis. Preparation for kidney transplantation or preparation for access to hemodialysis should begin when the glomerular filtration rate drops below 30 ml/1.73 m^2.

The correct technique of creating vascular accesses (fistula, catheter) is a prerequisite in preventing complications, especially thrombosis.

REASONS FOR MONITORING VASCULAR ACCESSES

Vascular access monitoring is performed by clinical examination and non-invasive vascular access monitoring methods. Non-invasive monitoring methods have a high positive predictive value for stenosis greater than 50% for vascular access using grafts. In contrast, for native AV fistulae, these results are unambiguous as the number of thromboses in native AV fistulae is much lower than in fistulae using a graft. Randomized studies have shown that clinical monitoring has a 70% positive predictive value for hemodynamically significant graft stenosis, as opposed to 80% for USG monitoring. Clinical monitoring reveals nearly 70 to 90% of patients with significant hemodynamic stenosis in time. Clinical monitoring is undemanding in terms of time and money and can be performed by a wide range of medical specialists. In contrast, vascular access monitoring involves a number of specialized tracking methods and the need for specialized equipment and specialized personnel.

Unfortunately, studies have shown that despite regular monitoring and early detection of stenosis, preventive angioplasty of stenosis above 50% does not reduce the number of subsequent thromboses and does not prolong the functionality of the vascular access using the graft. The results for native fistulae are ambiguous. Only one study demonstrated the importance of preventive angioplasty in relation to the function of fistulae. Therefore, diagnostic and often also therapeutic angioplasty is indicated only in the following cases:

1) Clinical signs of stenosis in combination with swelling of the limb and/or prolonged bleeding after dialysis needle extraction and/or changes of the murmur and vortex of the fistula
2) “Inexplicable,” prolonged decline in Kt/V
3) Fistula flow drop below 400-500 ml/min
4) A non-invasive finding of an AV fistula abnormality

Angiography reveals changes in the arterial and venous systems as well as on the fistula itself. Almost in 1/3 of the cases, the changes are multifocal lesions. In the same session, PTA can be performed with or without stent implantation.

MONITORING OF VASCULAR ACCESSES

Clinical monitoring includes physical examination and inspection of AV fistulae, monitoring of vascular access problems, and Kt/V monitoring.

1) Physical examination and inspection of the fistulae and the limb itself where the fistula is performed. Palpation of the fistula and the presence of pulsations and vortex on the fistula, auscultation of the fistula and the presence of the murmur, and at each dialysis, recirculation in the fistula can be diagnosed by compression between needles as the first manifestation of low-grade venous stenosis. By inspecting the skin above the fistula and puncture sites, potentially infectious complications can be observed in time.
2) A problem during hemodialysis may be the first sign of a serious complication. Such problems are difficult to cannulate of the fistula, blood aspiration, inability to achieve adequate flow or prolonged bleeding from puncture sites.
3) Decrease of Kt/V by 0.2 units. Kt/V is the preferred method of measuring the adequacy of hemodialysis. This is a dimensionless value, expressing the ratio of the urea-purified volume to the urea distribution volume.

Vascular access monitoring includes monitoring of the flow through the AV fistula or catheter, USG vascular access monitoring, and static venous pressure measurements.

1) AV fistula flow monitoring is most commonly measured by USG dilution, where, after saline application by one of the dialysis needles into the bloodstream, blood flow is measured by sensors. If the flow rate drops (more than 25% below the standard, or below

600 ml/min), it is advisable to perform a fistulogram. Other methods of measuring flow include thermal techniques, glucose infusion test, MRI, or duplex USG.

2) Duplex USG is probably the most valuable and the most accurate method of evaluating the functionality of an AV graft. USG measures the peak systolic velocity (PSV) above and below the putative stenotic lesion. A ratio above 2 is present in patients with severe stenosis in almost 80% of cases.
3) Static venous pressure is measured with a manometer before the start of hemodialysis at the dialysis needle site and after the pump is started. Values below 0.4 are normal, the value above 0.6 is present in cases of severe stenosis in nearly 92%of patients.

Immediate Postoperative Access Monitoring

Rebuilding in the site of the supplying artery, but mainly in the vein site, occurs immediately after the creation of a successful AV fistula due to hemodynamic changes. These changes trigger vascular remodeling, which is referred to as maturation. The flow through the fistula must rise until it is finally sufficient enough for the requirement of hemodialysis. The vein itself must be widened during maturation to allow for its cannulation, and its wall must thicken so that the cannulation can be repeated. The final result of these processes, which include blood flow, vein dilatation, and wall thickening, is the mature AV fistula. Of course, other factors that are specific to each individual patient, the depth of the vein, the course of the vein, affect the success of hemodialysis.

The goal of creating a fistula is the need to gain access for hemodialysis. The whole process can be divided into 3 phases:

1) Creation of AV fistula - preferably between a vein and an artery lying close together, which are approximately of the same diameter and ideally without stenotic lesions in the lumen.

2) Physiological maturation of AV fistula, in which 2 variables play the main role: vein diameter and blood flow through the fistula.

In this second phase, clinical monitoring of the fistula is the most important. According to KDOQI, the "rule of six" applies to newly created AV fistulae. The rule of six says that after **6** weeks of AV fistula formation, it will be suitable for physiological and sufficient hemodialysis if:

a) the outer diameter of the vein is more than 0,**6** cm
b) fistula is more than 0,**6** cm below the skin
c) blood flow through the fistula is greater than **6**00 ml/minute

If the fistula meets these criteria, it is almost always suitable for physiological hemodialysis. According to the American Society of Nephrologists, the Kidney Health Care Initiative - Endpoints for Trials Involving Dialysis Vascular Access - Committee on Fistulas, the vein of a smaller diameter (the inner diameter of the vein from 0.4 cm), can be successfully used for the fistula.

The ideal flow rate for the maturation of the AV fistula is not known, but normally, functional and mature AV fistulae have a flow rate of 352 to 500 ml/min. Flow rates below 400 ml/min lead to a high probability of thrombosis and AV fistula extinction. In the United States Dialysis Outcomes and Practice Patterns Study (DOPPS) Practice Monitor, the average AV fistula flow rate was 417 ml/min (median 400 ml/min). It is assumed that for the maturation of the newly formed fistula, the flow of at least 100 ml/minute more is necessary to avoid recirculation in the AV fistula area. In some studies, blood flow through the newly formed fistula was measured immediately after its creation. The blood flow of the AV fistula as a predictive indicator of its maturation was measured by USG. Subsequently, these values were used to indicate early reintervention to avoid a 6-week waiting period for “non-maturation” of the AV fistula. Individual studies report a flow rate of 120 to 160 ml/min during the first 10 minutes after the formation of the AV fistula as a highly positive predictive factor for its maturation. Normally, blood flow in the fistula is turbulent (turbulent spiral flow). This can also be used as a predictive factor of AV fistula maturation. Using a USG and a transversely placed probe at the fistula site was found to have a sensitivity of almost 91% in the prediction of AVF maturation.

The combination of flow rate (above 500 ml/min) and vein diameter (above 0.4 cm) equals almost 95% success rate of AV fistula maturation and its use for hemodialysis.

It is also possible to measure the wall thickening in the postoperative period, using high-frequency ultrasound (above 30 MHz), since the thickening of the vein wall is one of the maturation factors and is necessary for repeated cannulation without extravasation. A vein wall thickness value above 0.13 mm is present only in AV fistulae suitable for cannulation, without extravasate and prolonged bleeding after a puncture.

3) Clinically functional fistula is a mature AV fistula, ready for puncture. Of course, in order for the fistula to be used for hemodialysis, other factors are also necessary, such as the course of the vein, the depth of deposition, the length of the venous segment, all of which are necessary for the successful course of dialysis. Clinically functional fistula is a fistula that is successfully used for hemodialysis and repeatedly punctured without complications.

Physical monitoring and inspection of AV fistulae can prevent a large number of complications on the patient's side as well as on the AV access side. Physical examination and AV fistula monitoring are very accurate in the early detection of problems. When comparing physical examination, USG, and angiography in the detection of fistula inflow and outflow problems, there was a statistically insignificant difference among these examinations.

As recommended by the National Kidney Foundation, the Kidney Disease Outcomes Quality Initiative (NKF-K/DOQI), a physical AV fistula examination is to be conducted weekly on a regular basis. Since

2008, such monitoring has also been recommended by the Society for Vascular Surgery practice guidelines. In daily practice, the AV access is monitored by dialysis staff at and during each hemodialysis session.

The most common complication associated with AV access is stenosis.

After AV fistula formation, the limb must be elevated during the maturation period to prevent swelling. Symptoms, such as worsening limb edema, or pain, usually require urgent revision. If worsening edema is present in the postoperative period, usually a relevant cause is found in 25% of cases. Most often, it is central venous stenosis or obstruction that has not been diagnosed preoperatively. There are 4 causes of thoracic central stenosis (TCS) in dialysis patients. Most often, it is the damage of the central vein after the previous cannulation. In the second place, it is central vein obstruction due to its thrombosis, its external compression (arterial or musculoskeletal), or due to hemodynamic abnormalities followed by intimal hyperplasia. Sometimes the cause is multifactorial. Regardless of the type of TCS damage, it results in venous hypertension in the limb area and subsequently, in the failure of the AV access. Very often, the cause of TCS is an intravenous foreign body. Either it is the inserted central venous catheter, a peripherally inserted central venous catheter, or an electrode of an established pacemaker. Hemodynamic turbulent flow in the central veins is the cause of intimal hyperplasia. Early stages of this hyperplasia are already present in peripheral veins in the period prior to the formation of AV fistula, to which uremia also contributes. Not only systemic uremia contributes to the worsening of hemodynamic conditions due to endothelial abnormalities, but subsequently, the condition is exacerbated by sewing on the AV fistula and the acceleration of blood flow through the venous system.

The incidence of TCS is unknown, between 3% and 50% of patients are expected, as many of these lesions are overlooked for lack of clinical symptoms in the early stages of the disease. The USG examination of the affected limb itself does not give relevant results due to its inability to thoroughly visualize the central veins. The TCS lesion is definitively diagnosed by a venogram that accurately ascertains its localization in the area of the superior vena cava, brachiocephalic or subclavian vein. Delayed diagnosis of TCS causes deterioration of AV fistula function, eventually its disappearance (thrombosis), and often there is a risk of impossibility to create further access on the affected limb (central pelvic stenosis in the area of the lower limbs). In the early diagnosis of TCS, it is also possible to carry out three-dimensional examination methods (MR and CT), especially when external vein compression is suspected. Treatment of TCS is indicated by clinical or hemodynamic changes in the fistula or in the limb and aims to maintain functional vascular access for dialysis and to prevent limb changes due to central vein occlusion.

Arterial stenosis above the site of the anastomosis is manifested by a non-functioning fistula or by problems with its maturation. It can be caused by stenosis of the supplying artery, or immediately intraoperatively by inappropriate surgical technique directly in the anastomosis, or in the juxta-anastomotic area. Juxta-anastomotic stenosis occurs within 4 cm of anastomosis and is the most common stenosis of AV fistulae in the postoperative period. This stenosis may, in some cases, be combined with anastomotic stenosis, which is clearly the most common arterial stenosis in patients with an AV fistula. Adequate hemodialysis is not possible in the case of insufficient arterial flow with subsequent thrombosis or non-development of fistula. In physical examination, arterial stenosis is manifested by weak or no pulse and/or vortex on the AV fistula, exceptionally by acute ischemia of the affected limb. In the USG examination, the blood flow through the fistula is slowed, in case of thrombosis, the blood flow through the fistula is absent. Inflow stenosis in dysfunctional AV fistulae occurs in 9-26% of patients. Stenosis should be treated at its early stage before any thrombosis occurs in the fistula. In the postoperative period, a surgical revision with correction of the anastomotic and the juxta-anastomotic stenosis is indicated. In cases of inflow stenosis localized above, a DSA angiographic examination with stenosis correction is indicated. In the case of AV fistula thrombosis in the postoperative period, with the disappearance of pulsations and the absence of USG flow through the fistula, acute surgical thrombectomy with correction of the cause of thrombosis (most often stenosis of an anastomosis) is indicated.

Thrombosis of the newly formed AV fistula results in the loss of pulsation and absence of a murmur in the AV fistula area. Complete thrombosis of AV fistula, or only significantly impaired flow are diagnosed by USG examinations. After an urgent thrombectomy, additional intervention is required, depending on the cause. The primary assisted functionality of an AV fistula after 12 months is approximately 60%, and the secondary functionality is up to 90%.

In stenoses of the supplying artery, of the AV fistula itself, or of the drainage vein, endovascular interventions are indicated in cases of hemodynamically significant stenosis above 50% in combination with clinical manifestations of abnormality of the AV fistula. Endovascular treatment is used for fistulas, which are functional and used for hemodialysis, but their functions are deteriorating. The second option is fistulae that have not yet been used for hemodialysis (a maturation problem) or have failed (due to thrombosis).

Causes of Non-Maturation of AV Fistulae

If the AV fistula is formed, it must be developed to the stage that the hemodialysis can be performed. Stenosis, which can be elegantly solved, can be often found in non-maturing fistulae by early diagnosis. If physical examination reveals a problem with the maturation of the fistula, then USG is recommended, followed by an angiographic examination, possibly with its treatment.

The primary failure of the AV fistula is defined as an AV fistula that has never been used for hemodialysis or has ceased to exist within 3 months of its formation. A growing number of dysfunctional and extinct AV fistulas are being described compared to the past. This is mainly due to the increasing age of the patients, the number of associated diseases, as well as faster blood flow through the hemodialysis devices. In the past, a hemodialysis patient was 45 years old with glomerulonephritis, while at present, the average age is higher. Almost 70% of patients have 5 or more associated diseases, nearly 50% are diabetics, and 90% of them suffer from some sort of cardiovascular disease.

Risk factors for non-maturation of AV fistulae are:

- Hemodynamic factors - size and width of blood vessels, blood flow. Echo-mapping is very important for estimating hemodynamic parameters of both the arterial and venous streams. Patients with inadequate width, location, and quality of arteries and veins are not suitable candidates for the creation of a native AV fistula. In these patients, it is possible to use artificial material to create the AV fistula, or to begin to create the AV fistula superiorly – on the brachium. The advantage of using a prosthesis is not only that we obtain a suitable site for the need of hemodialysis, but by increasing blood flow through the venous stream, the veins that were previously unsuitable for AV access are widened. This creates the possibility of creating a secondary, native AV fistula on such a limb, if necessary.
- Demographic factors - age, gender, ethnicity. Most patients with renal impairment are elderly with polymorbidity. The main comorbidities include diabetes mellitus and cardiovascular diseases. Older age is often associated with the non-maturation of AV fistula and early failure of its function. Also, at an older age, renal function failure is significantly faster when compared to younger people, complicating the timing of vascular access for hemodialysis. Based on the 2016 United States Renal Data System (USRDS) study, AV fistula dysfunction in patients over 75 years was 40% versus 32% in patients under 44 years. Also, the secondary assisted functionality of AV fistulae is worse at an older age. According to the USRDS, women have a higher AV fistula maturation rate of nearly 41% compared to men where primary maturation is 31%. Conversely, the time from creating the AV fistula to its first use is shorter in the males (127 versus 143 days). When investigating the functionality of AV fistulae, the primary functionality of AV fistula was slightly lower in females, after a

year of use (55.9% versus 70.6 in men). Females are also indicated for the primary formation of AV fistula a little later than the males and also have a lower overall mortality rate per year per 1,000 patients (104 vs. 123 deaths). The causes are not clear, but for AV fistulae functionality, the difference in artery and vein diameters between men and women is assumed to be a significant factor. Chronic renal insufficiency (hereinafter referred to as CRI) is more common in the black population.

- Clinical factors - the presence of various other diseases. Cardiac and pulmonary diseases, peripheral atherosclerotic disease, diabetes mellitus, and obesity are risk factors for non-maturation and malfunction of the AV fistula. Almost 70% of patients with CRI over 65 years of age suffer from cardiovascular disease. Atrial fibrillation is present in almost 25% of patients, some of the degrees of heart failure in 28% of patients. Mortality in patients with cardiovascular disease and CRI is 10 to 20 times higher than in the general population. According to the Hemodialysis (HEMO) study, 40% of CRI patients have a prior history of signs pointing to cardiac failure, and almost 39% of them suffer from ischemic heart disease. Also, the formation of AV fistula itself may impair cardiac function. The risk of heart failure is directly dependent on the blood flow of the AV fistula and is more common in patients with heart disease before the formation of the AV fistula. Heart failure is also more frequent in patients with AV fistula on the brachium compared to patients with AV fistula on the forearm. There is no difference in the incidence of heart failure in patients with a native AV fistula versus patients with a prosthetic AV fistula. Patients with heart disease and blood flow through AV fistula greater than 2 l/min are at risk. Immediately after AV fistula formation, peripheral vascular resistance decreases, and cardiac output and heart rate increase. Within 2 weeks after AV fistula formation, there is an increase in end-diastolic pressure in the left ventricle and an increase in pressure and flow in the right heart sections. This is one of the factors of increased mortality in dialysis patients within the first 120 days of AV fistula formation. Patients gradually develop pulmonary hypertension, left ventricular hypertrophy, and left atrial dilatation. Clinical symptoms include dyspnea, orthopnea, and fatigue. Physical examination findings include tachycardia, swelling, distension of the jugular veins. According to the 2005 KDOQI recommendation, each patient should be examined for an eventual cardiac disease before establishing the primary AV fistula. We look for signs and symptoms of heart disease, and for risk factors for developing a cardiovascular disease such as diabetes, arterial hypertension, dyslipidemia, smoking, absence of physical activity, anemia, albuminuria. We examine potential atherosclerotic vascular changes by USG, and measure levels of phosphorus, parathyroid hormone levels, signs of inflammation (CRP level).ECG and transthoracic echocardiography should be performed within the first 3 months after the start of hemodialysis. In patients with a left ventricular ejection fraction below 40%, additional examinations should be added, such as non-invasive imaging methods and/or a coronarography examination. In some studies, cardiopulmonary recirculation is monitored, which is given by the ratio of blood flow through the AV fistula to cardiac output. A value above 0.3 indicates a significant risk of heart failure. Another option is to measure cardiac output to the body surface. A cardiac index above 4 L/min/m^2 predicts the development of cardiac failure. Any patient with renal failure should be evaluated by a cardiologist and classified according to the degree of heart failure according to the New York Heart Association functional classification (NYHA I to IV) and the American Heart Association stages of heart failure (ACC/AHA grades A to D). In Grade C and Group I and II patients, radiocephalic AV fistula is indicated. In patients with grade C or D and group III and IV, only catheter access is indicated for hemodialysis.

The peripheral atherosclerotic disease causes changes in the vessel wall, such as calcification and intimal hyperplasia, which reduce vessel elasticity and narrow the vessel lumen. After the AV fistula establishment, the supplying brachial artery must increase blood flow by 10- to 20-times. Alteration of the supplying artery alone leads to a decrease in the artery elasticity, an increase in the resistance index, and may lead to non-maturation of the AV fistula and its disappearance. A correlation is evident between the AV fistula maturation disorder and a degree of intimal hyperplasia. Also, in patients with diabetes mellitus (DM), the finding of mediocalcinosis in an X-ray examination is associated with a lower percentage of primary AV fistula functionality compared to patients without diabetes.

Pulmonary hypertension is often associated with heart disease (various degrees of heart failure), which is associated with an increased risk of cardiovascular events and overall patient mortality. The chronic obstructive bronchopulmonary disease is also a frequent cause of death, with a prevalence of 13.6% in the population of 60-79 years, which is the main group of patients indicated for hemodialysis.

Although diabetes is often described as a risk factor for the non-maturation of the AV fistula, it is more due to comorbidities of this disease. Individuals with DM have a high percentage of cardiovascular disease and peripheral atherosclerotic disease. Most authors agree that diabetes is not significantly associated with non-maturation of the AV fistula when compared to the individuals without DM, and there is no difference in the functionality of the AV fistula on the forearm between these groups of patients.

Obesity affects the functionality and maturation of AV fistulae, both by the course of the vein in the subcutaneous space (depth) and by the frequent occurrence of DM in obese patients. Higher BMI (≥35 kg/m2) is associated with poorer AV fistula maturation, but not with increased AV fistula failure rate. Although the primary functionality of AV fistula is nearly the same in obese and non-obese patients, secondary assisted functionality is worse in obese patients. Technical problems associated with the depth of vein placement can be solved by transposing the vein closer to the skin, possibly by liposuction, or lipectomy.

- Technical factors - surgeon's experience, care for the fistula. Surgical training and experience are crucial in creating an AV fistula and its functionality. The results of a prospective Dialysis Outcomes and Practice Patterns Study (DOPPS) showed that in native AV fistulae, the success of AV fistula functionality was dependent on the surgeon's training intensity and the creation of more than 25 AV fistulae. The experience of selecting AV fistula locations and selecting the type of AV fistula is also increasing. A suitable AV fistula must meet the following criteria:
    - It must be easily accessible in the patient in the sitting position.
    - If located on the forearm, it must be on the volar side.
    - For AV fistulae, which are placed higher, it should be on the front or lateral side of the forearm and brachium.
    - The functional fistula must be suitable for repeated puncturing and use.
    - The AV fistula should ideally be 5-6 mm below the skin and should have a relatively straight section of at least 8-10 cm.
    - The blood flow of the fistula must match the needs of hemodialysis.

According to the recommendations of the National Kidney Foundation Kidney Disease Outcomes Quality Initiative (NKF-KDOQI) Clinical Practice Guidelines and Society for Vascular Surgery of 2008, the order of the AV fistulae should be radio-cephalic, cephalic, brachiocephalic and brachiobasilic (transposition of v. basilica).

Monitoring of Mature Chronic Vascular Accesses

In mature AV fistulae in which thrombosis occurs, the stenotic lesion is almost always found to be the cause. In addition, the causes of thrombosis include damage to the fistula by dialysis, its hematoma, repeated stenosis of the inflow, or of the outflow. Fistulae at risk with a high probability of thrombosis include non-matured AV fistulae, fistulae with pseudoaneurysm, venous stenotic lesions, and secondary AV fistulae. As recommended by the National Kidney Foundation, the Kidney Disease Outcomes Quality Initiative (NKF-K/DOQI, K/DOQI), each hemodialysis workplace should have a program to monitor AV fistulae and monitor the adequacy of hemodialysis. The program should rely mainly on physical examination and monitoring and diagnostic testing of AV fistulae. Venous stenotic lesions in AV fistulae are the result of intimal hyperplasia, which is constantly increasing and, in advanced stages, obliterating the lumen of the vein. During the progression of intimal hyperplasia, vascular resistance increases, and fistula blood flow decreases, leading to, in its final stages, the thrombosis of the AV fistula unless appropriate interventional measures are taken. Stenosis and thrombosis are much more common in AV fistulae using grafts. The most common site of stenosis in AV fistulae with graft is the venous anastomosis. Anatomical lesions are found to be the cause of almost 90% of all thromboses of AV fistulae with graft. Most often (60%), it is a venous anastomosis, followed by changes in the graft itself (38.1%) and in the peripheral drainage vein (37.1%). Only in 3.2% of cases, the cause is found in the central vein, in the inflow artery it is 5%. In almost a third of cases, stenotic changes are present in multiple locations. In native AV fistulae, stenosis manifests itself in the early stages - in the non-maturation of AV fistula, which is seen in almost 20-60% of cases. In native AV fistulae, the most common site of stenosis is the juxta-anastomotic region - 55%, the site of the AV fistula itself - 29%, the peripheral drainage vein - 10% and the supplying artery almost 6%.

Duplex Sonography of AV Fistulae

USG tracking of AV fistulae is a part of the AV fistulae monitoring. It is important mainly for patients with diabetes mellitus (DM), patients suffering from generalized atherosclerosis, and for patients with previous complications of the AV fistula. The aim of the monitoring is to prevent complications of the AV fistula itself as well as to prevent the underdialysis of the patient. Although clinical fistula monitoring is a part of the prevention of complications, compared to USG monitoring, it has very low sensitivity, especially in the diagnosis of early pathological changes in AV fistula itself. USG examination of central veins, mainly in patients after established central venous catheters or pacemaker electrodes, is possible, but it has some limits for which angiographic examination is indicated. The superficial veins suitable for creating an AV fistula must meet the following USG criteria:

1) diameter of v. cephalica at least 2.5 mm
2) localization not more than 6 mm below the skin
3) connection to the deep venous system
4) central venous system without stenosis and occlusion

The artery should be without stenosis with an internal diameter of at least 2 mm. The artery should be without signs of calcification in B-mode with a three-phase Doppler curve. The examination should begin in the subclavian artery up to the anastomosis area of the AV fistula itself. Subsequently, after the AV fistula examination, the examination continues with a venous component to the central vein area. Local stenosis of the venous system, much more frequently in the peripheral venous system (up to 50%), compared to the central venous system (9%), can be detected in USG examinations. Another problem that may stop AV fistula maturation is an accessory vein. Normally, especially in the forearm region, the cephalic vein has a lot of collateral veins. On the brachium, the number of these collaterals is much smaller. Each accessory vein with a diameter of above 70% of the diameter of the cephalic vein, referred to as an accessory vein, is the cause of the non-maturation of AV fistula and should be ligated pre-operatively. In Doppler ultrasonography, the normally matured AV fistulae lose the triphasic curve and change to a monophasic one with continuous flow in both systole and diastole. In the AV fistula itself, blood flow is turbulent with systolic velocities from 100-400 cm/s and end-diastolic velocities of 60-100 cm/s. Subsequently, a pulse flow with a systolic velocity of 30-100 cm/s is present in the drainage vein. Normally, the flow rate through a functional AV fistula is from 350 to 1500 ml/minute. In mature AV fistulae, the blood flow through the brachial artery is 60-150 ml/minute, and the flow through the radial artery is 20-40 ml/minute. In a normal finding in B mode, the vascular wall is smooth, double-lined with a hypoechogenic space between the two lines. In patients with renal impairment and associated diseases, particularly diabetes mellitus, signs of mediocalcinosis, possibly atherosclerotic plaques, prominent into the vascular lumen, can be found in B mode. The calculation of blood flow through the fistula is measured on the brachial artery. For AV fistulae using an artificial prosthesis, the flow through the AV fistula is measured by placing the probe directly on the prosthesis. The flow rate (QVA) is then the result of multiplication of π, multiplied by the squared radius of the vessel (r) multiplied by the timed-average maximum velocity integral (TAMV).

$$QVA = \pi \times r^2 \times TAVM$$

Anatomical abnormalities can also be found when examining the arterial system and measuring the flow, eventually while looking for stenotic sites. These serve as important information for the eventual intervention or for the creation of secondary accesses. In the case of prosthetic AV fistulae we find minor thrombotic changes at the sites of previous punctures, eventually, pseudoaneurysms in the prosthesis itself.

While in native AV fistulas the most common site of stenosis is the anastomosis itself, in prosthetic AV fistulae it is the anastomosis between the vein and the prosthesis. A decrease in blood flow through the AV fistula is a predictor of stenosis and, if not solved, a predictor of the extinction - thrombosis of the AV fistula. Other important predisposing factors for stenosis progression are:

- drop in blood flow below 800 ml/min
- female gender
- condition after previous PTA.

When dealing with complications of AV fistulae (stenosis, not thrombosis), the treatment is considered successful in these cases:

- primary non-assisted 6-month AV fistula functionality of more than 50%
- residual stenosis after PTA less than 30%
- the disappearance of clinical symptoms after the correction of stenosis

ENDOVASCULAR INTERVENTIONS

Endovascular treatment is a method of choice for native AV fistulae, although this treatment is not always indicated and necessary. For treatment, only significant stenoses are indicated in which the lumen is narrowed by more than 50%, and there are clinical signs of its abnormality, or abnormal fistula flows are detected. Fistulas with stenosis but without signs of abnormalities are not indicated for treatment. According to the recommendations of the National Kidney Foundation-Kidney Disease Outcomes Quality Initiative (NKF/DOQI, K/DOQI), the 6-month functionality of the AV fistula after angioplasty should be in at least 50% of the cases. AV fistulae that do not meet these criteria should be indicated for a surgical revision or stent implantation.

In about one-third of patients, despite successful angioplasty, there is no increase in blood flow through the fistula. The causes of these hemodynamic failures are unclear, and likely suspects include stenosis elasticity, residual stenosis, or undiagnosed inflow stenosis. In such cases, the possibility of implantation of stents or stent-grafts is possible after repeated plastics. The results of stent studies vary with the type of the AV fistula, the site of stenosis, and the length of monitoring of patients and the type of stents used. However, the results of the meta-analysis did not show significant differences in the functionality of AV fistulae after angioplasty versus stent/stent graft implantation. The cumulative functionality of AV fistula after interventions is almost 70% after one year, but this is achieved by reintervention. There are very few studies comparing the results after stent implantation against stent graft. The function of the fistula after stent-graft implantation was higher compared to stent implantation, eventually only after angioplasty, in cases of graft - vein stenosis and after stenosis at the site of previous stent implantation. In general, stent-grafts reduce the number of restenosis due to intimal hyperplasia but do not reduce the number of graft thromboses. However, the choice of the type of intervention for stenosis also depends on the resources available and the general condition of the patient. Currently, although stent grafts are used in the treatment of stenosis of the AV fistulae, there are no exact indications for their use yet.

According to the NKF-K/DOQI Guideline Workgroup of 2006, the failure of angioplasty in AV fistulae is defined as any residual stenosis greater than 30% after angioplasty. This stenosis then leads to a rapid relapse and progression of stenosis. Before the eventual application of the stent, the angioplasty should be repeated as long as elastic compliance of the vessel is present. If angioplasty fails, in addition to stent/stent graft implantation, surgical intervention should be considered. In the case of venous stenosis, stents/stent grafts are implanted more often and sooner than peripheral outflows, mainly because of the risk of their rupture. Sometimes a rapid relapse of stenosis is observed after successful angioplasty. According to NKF-K/DOQI, the Guideline workgroup is defined as a relapse of stenosis within 3 months and is believed to be due to residual stenosis after previous angioplasty. Precise technique and use of high-pressure balloons can eliminate these relapses. Successful angioplasty causes damage to the endothelial lining. In rare cases, the intimal flap may interfere with blood flow and be separated. It can be treated by a simple prolonged compression of the balloon or, in case of failure, by stent implantation. A more serious complication in angioplasty is vein rupture with bleeding, with an incidence of 0.9-2% of all interventions. Symptoms and treatment of such rupture depend on the type of vein damage:

1) Subclinical extravasate - a small extravasate near a vein
2) Grade 1 - stable extravasate, without affecting blood flow
3) Grade 2 - stable extravasate, affecting blood flow
4) Grade 3 - unstable extravasate, vascular rupture

Grade 2 and 3 already pose a serious complication of the procedure, and among other complications, there is a risk of extinction of the AV fistula. If necessary, implantation of the stent-graft after transient balloon occlusion of the lesion is possible. The success of angioplasty in central venous stenosis is reported in 70-90% of cases. Its success is 79-99% for peripheral venous system stenosis and 87-98% for AV fistulae. Cephalic stenosis at the inlet to the axillary vein is reported in 15-17% of thrombosed AV fistulae. This is more frequent in patients with a brachiocephalic fistula compared to patients with a radiocephalic fistula. It is believed that the main cause of stenosis is increased blood flow through the cephalic vein of the higher placed fistulae as opposed to the forearm fistula where blood can flow through both the cephalic and basilic streams. Angioplasty in these places is problematic. Angioplasty-resistant stenosis is the most frequent in this site, and when attempting an angioplasty this is a place where the highest number of ruptures happen. The functionality of AV fistula after cephalic vein angioplasty is 41-78% after half a year of observation, and after one year, it drops to 31-45%. The treatment of stenosis in the area of the cephalic vein is accompanied by a higher percentage of failure, a higher number of complications, and a worse long-term functionality of AV fistula compared to angioplasty elsewhere. The solution of venous stenosis in AV fistulae with graft is also problematic. Most often, in this type of fistula, stenosis is localized at the junction of the artificial material and the vein. It is here that the intimate hyperplasia is resistant to angioplasty due to the turbulent flow, which is also complicated by the fact that stenosis involves a non-elastic artificial material. The primary functionality of AV fistula after angioplasty is described between 26-67%.

In the case of angioplasty failure in the treatment of dysfunction of the AV fistula, surgical intervention, or stent/stent-graft implantation is indicated. Meta-analysis comparing stenting/stent graft with angioplasty in treatment did not show significantly different functionality of AV fistulae in the 6-month period of monitoring. The cumulative functionality of the AV fistula within 1 year was nearly 70%, but with the need for aggressive reinterventions (thrombolysis, plastic/atherectomy in-stent stenosis) to manage restenosis. Although the results of AV fistulae after angioplasty and stent-graft implantation are comparable, the stent-grafts are usually implanted after the failure of classical angioplasty. Most studies compare the functionality of AV fistula after angioplasty versus stent or stent-graft implantation. There are only a few studies comparing results after stent implantation when compared to the number of stent-graft implantation studies. When comparing the functionality of AV fistulae after plastic, the best results are seen after balloon cutting angioplasty followed by high-pressure balloon angioplasty and classical, conventional PTA. In the case of AV fistulae with a prosthesis, after comparing the results of the functionality of AV fistulae, the functionality after stent-graft implantation was significantly higher after 2 years compared to the angioplasty itself. Also, the AV fistula functionality after implantation of the stent-graft into the in-stent stenosis, after prior stent implantation, is superior to conventional angioplasty. Generally, there is less restenosis after stent-graft implantation, but the number of thrombotic complications does not decrease. When deciding on the type of procedure (stent – stent-graft - angioplasty), it is necessary to consider the economic aspect and the general condition of the patient (presumed patient survival).

Generally accepted indication criteria for stent/stent graft implantation are:

- early angioplasty failure (residual stenosis of more than 30% after angioplasty - 2006 NKF-K/DOQI Guideline workgroup). In the case of the recoil phenomenon, another angioplasty is indicated prior to stent implantation. Surgical treatment should also be considered before stent implantation. If this is contraindicated, difficult, and uncertain, eventually, the vascular "system" is drained, and stent implantation is indicated. At the same time, the central vein areas are more often stented/stent grafted to peripheral veins. Due to the diameter of the veins in the central area, the possibility of angioplasty is limited, and there is a higher risk of rupture.
- rapid relapse of stenosis (2 x restenosis within 3 months - 2006 NKF-K/DOQI Guideline workgroup)
- rupture, damage to the vein during the angioplasty, unresolvable by conservative measures.

Recirculation of AV Fistulae

Recirculation of the AV fistula means insufficient blood flow to the AV fistula when the cleaned blood from the vein is sucked by the "venous" needle. It is important to diagnose recirculation in a timely manner not only due to the adequacy of hemodialysis but also in order to detect stenoses early where we can prevent thrombosis by treating them early. The repeated flow of dialyzed blood through the device reduces the concentration gradient across the dialysis membrane and thereby reduces the effectiveness of hemodialysis. Significant recirculation thus causes a mismatch between the predicted, required length, and intensity of hemodialysis (Kt/V urea) and its actual application. The degree of AV fistula recirculation can be calculated: Recirculation percentage = ([P-A]: [P-V]) x 100

P, A, V is the amount of solution in the circulation, arterial, and venous one.

In the absence of recirculation, the systemic concentration values of the solution are identical to the arterial, and the result is 0.

The cause of the recirculation is low blood flow through the fistula or lower than the setting of the hemodialysis device (normally 400-500/ml) and the arterial lumen withdrawing blood from the venous lumen. The most common causes of recirculation are venous stenosis, arterial inflow stenosis, or stenosis directly at the AV fistula site. Recirculation of the AV fistula is identified primarily thanks to the inadequacy of hemodialysis. The presence of significant recirculation is an indication for angiographic examination, as recirculation is caused by stenoses. Correction of stenosis will increase the efficacy of hemodialysis and "adjust" the target Kt/V without changing the method and number of hemodialysis. Most AV fistulae work without recirculation, so a value of 5-10% of recirculation is an indication for USG followed by an angiographic examination. Monitoring of recirculation is one method of AV fistulae monitoring, but its importance for monitoring AV fistulae functionality is small. A significant decrease of Kt/V happens only during later stages of stenotic changes, which limits the use of this method for fistulae monitoring.

Methods for measuring recirculation are based either on the urea-based dilution method or the urea-free method. Dilution methods are urea-based, but they provide delayed results. In a two-needle stop-flow technique, the urea level is measured from a blood sample taken after stopping extracorporeal circulation from the arterial lumen (needle). In the double-needle slow flow technique, a blood sample is taken from the arterial lumen after slowing the extracorporeal circulation to 50 ml/minute. Both techniques allow for accurate urea measurement, but the second method is preferred. The three-needle technique is based on blood collection from the peripheral blood, the predialysis arterial lumen, and the post-dialysis venous lumen. However, according to the KDOQI's recommendation, this method should not be used in measuring recirculation, as the measurement results are overestimated when compared to actual results. From dilution methods where urea values are not monitored, USG, thermal, optical, conduction, and potassium dilution are used. The recirculation rate between 5-10% is a threshold value for other investigative methods such as USG and angiography.

Ultrasonographic dilution measurement uses two sensors connected to the arterial and venous lumen. A saline bolus is then applied to the venous lumen. The ratio of dilution in the arterial and venous lumen gives us the percentage of recirculation. The thermal dilution method is based on the principle of measuring temperature difference in arterial and venous lumen after temperature difference is applied. After the blood has been cooled by the device, the drop in the temperature of the dialysis solution is detected not only on the venous lumen but also in the arterial lumen during recirculation. The system is fully automated by hemodialysis devices.

Optical dilution method in which the sensor (crit-line) is located on the arterial inflow port of the hemodialyzer. Upon injection of saline into the venous lumen, the sensor monitors the change in blood density on the arterial port during recirculation.

The conduction dilution is based on the principle of measuring the conductivity of blood on both the arterial and venous lumens by sensors after the application of a saline bolus into the venous lumen.

The dilution method for measuring potassium concentration is based on measuring changes in potassium concentration. The first blood sample is taken from the arterial lumen as soon as the AV fistula is injected. The hemodialysis apparatus is then set at a flow rate of 300 ml/minute, and a bolus of saline is administered, and after 10 seconds, a blood sample is taken from the arterial line. During recirculation, potassium values in the second sample are reduced.

Quantitatively, recirculation is expressed as the ratio of the recirculating fraction (QR) to the total flow through the extracorporeal blood flow (QB).

$$R=QR/QB$$

Malfunction of Chronic Hemodialysis Catheters

Tunneled and non-tunneled catheters may be used for hemodialysis. Tunneled catheters are used for chronic dialysis and are mainly used in patients not suited for AV fistula formation. These are mainly critically ill patients, patients with acute renal failure, or injury. Chronic hemodialysis catheters are associated with a high number of complications, the most common being a dysfunction of the catheter in conjunction with poor blood flow, ending with the thrombosis of the catheter. A higher number of dysfunctions is present when the catheter is inserted into the subclavian vein compared to the insertion into the jugular vein. Catheter dysfunction is defined as the inability to provide sufficient extracorporeal blood flow without significantly prolonging the dialysis time. In practice, this means a flow rate below 300 ml/min, at a negative pressure below 250 mmHg. In the case of catheter flow measurements, they may be inaccurate. The first reason is that during hemodialysis, catheters passing through the hemodialysis device heat up with hysteresis (they do not return to their original width), and thus the flow through the device is reduced. Secondly, as the pressure in front of the pump decreases, so does the QB flow decrease. Typical indicators of dialysis catheter dysfunction are:

1) QB decrease by more than 10%
2) Kt/V below 1.2
3) "Arterial" pressure (in front of the device) below 250 mm/Hg and "venous" pressure above 250 mm/Hg

Catheter dysfunction leads to inadequate hemodialysis and a higher risk of septic complications. If catheter thrombosis occurs, the cost of treatment increases, and the patient's quality of life deteriorates. Permanent catheter dysfunctions are classified as early and late. Early dysfunction is defined as a catheter malfunction right after its introduction. Either there is no blood flow through the catheter, or the flow is only intermittent, or QB is insufficient without significantly prolonging the hemodialysis time. The early failure of a chronic dialysis catheter is related to the technical difficulties associated with the placement and location of the catheter. The catheter tip may be placed in an inappropriate location, and the catheter may be bent, sutured, or scar-compressed after replacement. Late dysfunctions are defined as the inability to achieve adequate hemodialysis without prolonging the dialysis time in a previously functioning catheter. The most common cause is complete or partial thrombosis of the catheter, which is also breeding ground for bacterial settlement. Venous system thrombosis with permanent catheters in place is classified by symptomatology (symptomatic/asymptomatic) and by localization to the catheter (external/internal). The division of thrombosis, according to the catheter itself, is divided into extrinsic and intrinsic thrombosis (Table 1).

Table 1. Types of thromboses with established central venous catheters

Intrinsic thrombosis	**Localization**
Intraluminal thrombus	Thrombus in the catheter lumen
Thrombus of the catheter tip	Thrombus located at the tip of the catheter
Fibrin pericatheter thrombus	Thrombus on the catheter surface
Extrinsic thrombosis	
Central venous thrombus	Thrombosis of the venous system around the catheter
Wall thrombus	At the catheter-venous wall contact site
Thrombus in heart atrium	Thrombosis in the right atrium

Thrombosis, with an established central venous catheter, results in its dysfunction and incomplete hemodialysis. In diagnosis, USG is used as the most sensitive examination method. At the central veins inaccessible for USG examination, the patient is indicated for angiographic examination, or phlebography may be performed. In the USG examination, direct visualization of the thrombus is possible, the indirect sign of thrombosis is the absence of spontaneous flow in the central vein or the lack of biphasic blood flow during respiration or dilatation of the collateral venous system. It's the non-occlusive thromboses in the space not accessible directly for a USG examination (located behind the sternum, clavicle) that can be indirectly diagnosed in this way. The sensitivity and specificity of the USG examination in the diagnosis of thrombosis is 80% and 100%, respectively. In the case of incomplete catheter thromboses, phlebography can be performed via the catheter. In complete thrombosis, the clinical signs of thrombosis are also prominent, limb swelling specifically as the first sign of thrombosis. The first treatment option for thrombosis is the flushing of the catheter with saline. If the treatment isn't successful, we have the option of thrombolytic treatment. The success rate of the primary procedure is 85% and decreases in repeated procedures. If, after lytic therapy, the function of the catheter is still inadequate, or if catheter re-thrombosis occurs within 2 weeks of thrombolysis, catheter replacement is indicated. If this therapy fails, catheter extraction with subsequent anticoagulant therapy is indicated. In the case of mural thrombi, the diagnosis is determined phlebographically through a catheter. Sometimes mural thrombi may be symptomatic due to embolization and complications requiring transoesophageal echocardiography or septic embolization. Atrial thrombus can occur in up to 20% of cases and is not uncommon or asymptomatic. They are diagnosed by USG, possibly by echocardiographic examination. In small thrombi up to 1.5 cm, catheter extraction is sufficient, in some workplaces combined with long-term anticoagulant therapy. In larger thrombi, catheter extraction with anticoagulant therapy is indicated. Thrombolytic therapy is indicated only in cases associated with pulmonary embolism or ineffective anticoagulation therapy. In patients with a central catheter, type B thrombus - fixed to the atrial wall – is usually found during echocardiography. Fortunately, most atrial thrombi are small, with a diameter of up to 1.5 cm. Patients with a larger thrombus require hospitalization, initiation of anticoagulant therapy, and catheter extraction. In the case of massive thrombi (over 6 cm), the patient may also develop syncope with heart failure. Antibiotic therapy is indicated for symptoms of infection. The replacement of the catheter itself is the most appropriate method for intrinsic thromboses. Replacing a permanent catheter by wire is a simple, highly successful method and saves space for the eventual creation of another venous access. The technical success rate of catheter replacement is almost 100%, and the secondary assisted catheter functionality is nearly 80% after 4 months. The number of infections is reported in 1.1 per 1000 permanent catheters exchanged. In some cases, when the catheter is extracted, a fibrin pericatheter thrombus remains in the venous system, which may cause malfunction of a freshly inserted catheter. Therefore, in some workplaces, this is disrupted by balloon angioplasty during catheter replacement. The diameter of the balloon varies from 8-12 mm, and, if necessary, it is possible to simultaneously resolve the stenosis of the central venous system. Intrinsic thrombosis is the most common cause of catheter failure. Other causes include an insufficient amount of heparin applied to the catheter after hemodialysis, failure to close the catheter prior to removal of the syringe after heparin application, and leaving blood in the catheter after hemodialysis.

Conclusion

Operations of the arteriovenous connections for long-term hemodialysis is an integral part of the field of vascular surgery. Classical wrist radiocephalic fistula, according to Cimino and Brescia remains the first-choice method in our country. With its lowest complication rate and best results, this fistula is always the closest idea of an "ideal fistula."

Patients with chronic renal insufficiency have their vascular system affected by atherosclerosis. Many suffer from the hypoplastic vascular system and vessels damaged by repeated punctures. All this affects the final effect of the fistula and its lifespan.

When developing vascular accesses, we must take into account the patient's clinical condition, their prognosis, and assess the possibilities of their vasculature. Both the physical examination of the patient and the results obtained using conventional imaging methods, whether non-invasive or invasive, will provide us with the information needed to make the final decision.

If complications develop, we try to restore the function of the original AV fistula or at least use some of its parts to create a new fistula, if possible.

References

Aftab S. A., Tay K. H., Irani F. G., et al. 2014. "Randomized clinical trial of cutting balloon angioplasty versus high-pressure balloon angioplasty in hemodialysis arteriovenous fistula stenoses resistant to conventional balloon angioplasty." *J Vasc Interv Radiol* 25:190-8.

Agarwal A., Mantell M., Cohen R., et al. 2014. "Outcomes of single-stage compared to two-stage basilic vein transposition fistulae." *Semin Dial* 27:298-302.

Aimaq R., Katz S. G. 2013. "Using distal revascularization with interval ligation as the primary treatment of hand ischemia after dialysis access creation." *J Vasc Surg* 57:1073-8.

Alkhouli M., Sandhu P., Boobes K., et al. 2015. "Cardiac complications of arteriovenous fistulas in patients with end-stage renal disease." *Nefrologia*; 35:234-45.

Andre J., Parsikia A., Minimo C., et al. 2012. "Soft tissue sarcoma at a dialysis access site in a transplant recipient." *Exp Clin Transplant* 10:410-5.

Argyriou C., Schoretsanitis N., Georgakarakos E. I., et al. 2015. "Preemptive open surgical vs. endovascular repair for juxta-anastomotic stenoses of autogenous AV fistulae: a meta-analysis." *J Vasc Access* 16:454-51.

Atkar R. K., MacRae J. M. 2013. "The buttonhole technique for fistula cannulation: pros and cons." *Curr Opin Nephrol Hypertens* 629-636.

Beaulieu M. C., Dumaine C. S., Romann A., Kiaii M. 2017. "Advanced age is not a barrier to creating a functional arteriovenous fistula: a retrospective study." *J Vasc Access* 18:307-12.

Blum C., Baker M. 2008. "Venous congestion of the breast mimicking inflammatory breast cancer: case report and review of literature." *Breast J* 14:97-101.

Cerneviciute R., Sahebally S. M., Ahmed K., et al. 2017. "Regional Versus Local Anaesthesia for Haemodialysis Arteriovenous Fistula Formation: A Systematic Review and Meta-Analysis." *Eur J Vasc Endovasc Surg* 53:734-42.

Chan M. G., Miller F. J., Valji K., et al. 2014. "Evaluating patency rates of an ultralow-porosity expanded polytetrafluoroethylene covered stent in the treatment of venous stenosis in arteriovenous dialysis circuits. *J Vasc Interv Radiol*; 25:183-9.

Chitalia N., Ross L., Krishnamoorthy M., et al. 2015. "Neointimal hyperplasia and calcification in medium sized arteries in adult patients with chronic kidney disease." *Semin Dial* 28:35-40.

Cooper J., Power A. H., DeRose G., et al. 2015. "Similar failure and patency rates when comparing one- and two-stage basilic vein transposition." *J Vasc Surg* 61:809-16.

Cuthbert G. A., Kirmani B. H., Muir A. D. 2014. "Should dialysis-dependent patients with upper limb arterio-venous fistulae undergoing coronary artery bypass grafting avoid having ipsilateral in situ mammary artery grafts?" *Interact Cardiovasc Thorac Surg* 18:655-60.

D'Amato-Palumbo S., Kaplan A. A., Feinn R. S., Lalla R. V. 2013. "Retrospective study of microorganisms associated with vascular access infections in hemodialysis patients." *Oral Surg Oral Med Oral Pathol Oral Radiol* 115:56-61.

D'Ayala M, Smith R. M., Martone C., et al. 2008. "The effect of systemic anticoagulation in patients undergoing angioaccess surgery." *Ann Vasc Surg* 22:11-5.

DeSilva R. N., Patibandla B. K., Vin Y., et al. 2013. "Fistula first is not always the best strategy for the elderly*." J Am Soc Nephrol* 24:1297-304.

Di Nicolò P., Cornacchiari M., Mereghetti M., Mudoni A. 2017. "Buttonhole Cannulation of the AV Fistula: A Critical Analysis of the Technique." *Semin Dial* 30:32-38.

Dixon B. S. 2012. "Fish oil and hemodialysis graft patency: does time matter?" *JAMA* 307:1859-60.

Dolmatch B. L., Duch J. M., Winder R., et al. 2012. "Salvage of angioplasty failures and complications in hemodialysis arteriovenous access using the FLUENCY Plus Stent Graft: technical and 180-day patency results." *J Vasc Interv Radiol* 23:479-87.

Ene-Iordache B., Remuzzi A. 2012. "Disturbed flow in radial-cephalic arteriovenous fistulae for haemodialysis: low and oscillating shear stress locates the sites of stenosis." *Nephrol Dial Transplant* 27:358-68.

Falk A., Maya I. D., Yevzlin A. S. RESCUE Investigators. 2016. "A Prospective, Randomized Study of an Expanded Polytetrafluoroethylene Stent Graft versus Balloon Angioplasty for In-Stent Restenosis in Arteriovenous Grafts and Fistulae: Two-Year Results of the RESCUE Study." *J Vasc Interv Radiol* 27:1465-76.

Feldman L., Tkacheva I., Efrati S., et al. 2014. "Effect of arteriovenous hemodialysis shunt location on cardiac events in patients having coronary artery bypass graft using an internal thoracic artery." *Ther Apher Dial* 18:450-4.

Fu N., Joachim E., Yevzlin A. S., et al. 2015. "A Meta-analysis of Stent Placement vs. Angioplasty for Dialysis Vascular Access Stenosis." *Semin Dial* 28:311-7.

Georgiadis G. S., Georgakarakos E. I., Antoniou G. A., et al. 2014. "Correlation of pre-existing radial artery macrocalcifications with late patency of primary radiocephalic fistulas in diabetic hemodialysis patients." *J Vasc Surg* 60:462-70.

Haskal Z. J., Saad T. F., Hoggard J. G., et al. 2016. "Prospective, Randomized, Concurrently-Controlled Study of a Stent Graft versus Balloon Angioplasty for Treatment of Arteriovenous Access Graft Stenosis: 2-Year Results of the RENOVA Study." *J Vasc Interv Radiol* 27:1105-14.

Hull J. E., Jennings W. C., Cooper R. I., et al. 2018. "The Pivotal Multicenter Trial of Ultrasound-Guided Percutaneous Arteriovenous Fistula Creation for Hemodialysis Access." *J Vasc Interv Radiol* 29:149-50.

Irish A. B., Viecelli A. K., Hawley C. M., et al. 2017. "Effect of Fish Oil Supplementation and Aspirin Use on Arteriovenous Fistula Failure in Patients Requiring Hemodialysis: A Randomized Clinical Trial." *JAMA Intern Med* 177:184-93.

Jennings W. C., Galt S. W., Shenoy S., et al. 2014. "The Venous Window Needle Guide, a hemodialysis cannulation device for salvage of uncannulatable arteriovenous fistulas." *J Vasc Surg* 60:1024-32.

Kakisis J. D., Avgerinos E., Giannakopoulos T., et al. 2012. "Balloon angioplasty vs nitinol stent placement in the treatment of venous anastomotic stenoses of hemodialysis grafts after surgical thrombectomy." *J Vasc Surg* 55:472-8.

Kitrou P. M., Spiliopoulos S., Katsanos K., et al. 2015. "Paclitaxel-coated versus plain balloon angioplasty for dysfunctional arteriovenous fistulae: one-year results of a prospective randomized controlled trial." *J Vasc Interv Radiol* 26:348-54.

Kundu S. 2010. "Review of central venous disease in hemodialysis patients." *J Vasc Interv Radiol* 21:963-8.

Lai C. C., Fang H. C., Tseng C. J., et al. 2014. "Percutaneous angioplasty using a paclitaxel-coated balloon improves target lesion restenosis on inflow lesions of autogenous radiocephalic fistulas: a pilot study." *J Vasc Interv Radiol* 25:535-41.

Lee T., Thamer M., Zhang Y., et al. 2015. "Outcomes of Elderly Patients after Predialysis Vascular Access Creation." *J Am Soc Nephrol* 26:3133-40.

Leontiev O., Shlansky-Goldberg R. D., Stavropoulos S. W., et al. 2014. "Should all inflow stenoses be treated in failing autogenous hemodialysis fistulae?" *J Vasc Interv Radiol* 25:542-7.

Lok C. E., Rajan D. K., Clement J., et al. 2017. "Endovascular Proximal Forearm Arteriovenous Fistula for Hemodialysis Access: Results of the Prospective, Multicenter Novel Endovascular Access Trial (NEAT)." *Am J Kidney Dis*; 70:486-97.

Lok C. E., Sontrop J. M., Tomlinson G., et al. 2013. "Cumulative patency of contemporary fistulas versus grafts (2000-2010)." *Clin J Am Soc Nephrol* 8:810-18.

Long B., Brichart N., Lermusiaux P., et al. 2011. "Management of perianastomotic stenosis of direct wrist autogenous radial-cephalic arteriovenous accesses for dialysis." *J Vasc Surg*; 53:108-14.

Macrae J. M., Ahmed S. B., Hemmelgarn B. R., Alberta Kidney Disease Network. 2014. "Arteriovenous fistula survival and needling technique: long-term results from a randomized buttonhole trial." *Am J Kidney Dis* 63:636-42.

Makhdoomi K., Mivefroshan A., Abbasi F., et al. 2015. "Angiosarcoma at dialysis fistula site in a patient on continuous ambulatory peritoneal dialysis." *Iran J Kidney Dis* 9:154-7.

Mallios A., Jennings W. C., Boura B., et al. 2018. "Early results of percutaneous arteriovenous fistula creation with the Ellipsys Vascular Access System." *J Vasc Surg*; 68:1150-56.

Miller G. A., Goel N., Friedman A., et al. 2010. "The MILLER banding procedure is an effective method for treating dialysis-associated steal syndrome." *Kidney Int* 77:359-66.

Misskey J., Yang C., MacDonald S., et al. 2016. "A comparison of revision using distal inflow and distal revascularization-interval ligation for the management of severe access-related hand ischemia." *J Vasc Surg* 63:1574-81.

Morselli C., Chiari P., Aliberti T., et al. 2015. "Sharp versus blunt dialysis needle use with buttonhole: opn randomized trial." *J Ren Care* 41:213-21.

Napoli M., Prudenzano R., Russo F., et al. 2010. "Juxta-anastomotic stenosis of native arteriovenous fistulas: surgical treatment versus percutaneous transluminal angioplasty." *J Vasc Access* 11:346-51.

Neuen B. L., Gunnarsson R., Baer R. A., et al. 2014. "Factors associated with patency following angioplasty of hemodialysis fistulae." *J Vasc Interv Radiol* 25:1419-26.

Nguyen D. B., Lessa F. C., Belflower R., et al. 2013. "Invasive methicillin-resistant Staphylococcus aureus infections among patients on chronic dialysis in the United States, 2005-2011." *Clin Infect Dis* 57:1393-400.

O'Hare A. M., Allon M., Kaufman J. S. 2010. "Whether and when to refer patients for predialysis AV fistula creation: complex decision making in the face of uncertainty." *Semin Dial* 23:452-5.

O'Hare A. M., Bertenthal D., Walter L. C., et al. 2007. "When to refer patients with chronic kidney disease for vascular access surgery: should age be a consideration?" *Kidney Int* 71:555-61.

Oskrochi Y., Razi K., Stebbing J., Crane J. 2016. "Angiosarcoma and Dialysis-related Arteriovenous Fistulae: A Comprehensive Review." *Eur J Vasc Endovasc Surg*; 51:127-133.

Quaretti P., Galli F., Moramarco L. P., et al. 2016. "Stent Grafts Provided Superior Primary Patency for Central Venous Stenosis Treatment in Comparison with Angioplasty and Bare Metal Stent: A Retrospective Single Center Study on 70 Hemodialysis Patients." *Vasc Endovascular Surg*; 50:221-30.

Radosa C. G., Radosa J. C., Weiss N., et al. 2017. "Endovascular Creation of an Arteriovenous Fistula (endoAVF) for Hemodialysis Access: First Results." *Cardiovasc Intervent Radiol*; 40:1545-51.

Reque J., Garcia-Prieto A., Linares T., et al. 2017. "Pulmonary Hypertension Is Associated with Mortality and Cardiovascular Events in Chronic Kidney Disease Patients." *Am J Nephrol* 45:107-14.

Russell T. E., Kasper G. C., Seiwert A. J., et al. 2017. "Cilostazol May Improve Maturation Rates and Durability of Vascular Access for Hemodialysis." *Vasc Endovascular Surg* 51:120-4.

Scali S. T., Chang C. K., Raghinaru D., et al. 2013. "Prediction of graft patency and mortality after distal revascularization and interval ligation for hemodialysis access-related hand ischemia." *J Vasc Surg* 57:451-8.

Swinnen J., Lean Tan K., Allen R., et al. 2015. "Juxta-anastomotic stenting with aggressive angioplasty will salvage the native radiocephalic fistula for dialysis." *J Vasc Surg* 61:436-42.

Ulloa J. G., Kirkpatrick V. E., Wilson S. E., Williams R. A. 2014. "Stent salvage of arteriovenous fistulas and grafts." *Vasc Endovascular Surg* 48:234-8.

Vascular Access 2006 Work Group. 2006. Clinical practice guidelines for vascular access. *Am J Kidney Dis* 48(1):176-274.

Vaux E., King J., Lloyd S., et al. 2013. "Effect of buttonhole cannulation with a polycarbonate PEG on in-center hemodialysis fistula outcomes: a randomized controlled trial." *Am J Kidney Dis* 62:81-8.

Wheaton A. G., Cunningham T. J., Ford E. S., et al.: Employment and activity limitations among adults with chronic obstructive pulmonary disease - United States, 2013. *MMWR Morb Mortal Wkly Rep* 2015; 64:289-95.

Wong B., Muneer M., Wiebe N., et al. 2014. "Buttonhole versus rope-ladder cannulation of arteriovenous fistulas for hemodialysis: a systematic review." *Am J Kidney Dis* 64:918-36.

Wong B., Muneer M., Wiebe N., et al. 2014. "Buttonhole versus rope-ladder cannulation of arteriovenous fistulas for hemodialysis: a systematic review." *Am J Kidney Dis* 64:918-36.

In: Surgeon´s Perspective on Dialysis Patient ISBN: 978-1-53619-262-9
Editor: Maria Frankovicova

Chapter 7

COMPLICATIONS OF ARTERIOVENOUS CONNECTION (ARTERIOVENOUS FISTULAS)

M. Zavacká**, *MD
Department of Vascular Surgery,
East Slovak Institute of Cardiovascular Diseases,
Faculty of Medicine, Pavol Jozef Šafárik University in Košice, Slovakia

ABSTRACT

Health care of patients with vascular access for hemodialysis requires the collaboration of a nephrologist, a vascular surgeon, an interventional radiologist, and an angiologist. The vascular access is reported to be one of the six factors determining morbidity and, indirectly, the mortality of dialysis patients. Surgery of arteriovenous connections for the needs of long-term hemodialysis is an integral yet at the same time part one of the most problematic parts of vascular surgery. The principle of care for hemodialysis access is to maintain good function as long as possible with a minimum of complications and interventions.

* Corresponding Author's E-mail: martinazavacka80@gmail.com.

Keywords: arteriovenous fistula, PRAL - proximal radial artery ligation, RUDI - revision using distal flow, TRAL - transposition of the radial artery, PAI - proximalization of the arterial inflow, DRIL - distal revascularization interval ligation, DRAL - distal radial artery ligation

Abbreviations

ATB	antibiotics
AVF	arteriovenous fistula
AVG	arteriovenous graft
CPR	cardiopulmonary recirculation
CVC	central venous catheter
DRAL	distal radial artery ligation
DRIL	distal revascularization interval ligation
DSA	digital subtraction angiography
HD	hemodialysis
IJV	internal jugular vein
IMN	ischemic monomelic neuropathy
LMWH	low-molecular-weight-heparin
MRA	magnetic resonance angiography
PAI	proximalization of the arterial inflow
PTA	percutaneous transluminal angioplasty
PRAL	proximal radial artery ligation
PTFE	polytetrafluorethylene
Qa	access flow
RUDI	revision using distal flow
TRAL	transposition of the radial artery

Establishing good vascular access in patients enrolled in a long-term hemodialysis program is often referred to as an "Achilles' heel" in vascular surgery. This statement is concise, and despite the developed and followed procedure scheme in individual cases, some patients undergo repeated surgeries, adjustments, and modifications.

Even the best fistula can cease to exist over time. It is highly important that the surgeon establishes a precise plan and has sufficient experience in the vascular surgery of arteriovenous connections.

In recent years, there has been significant development of hemodialysis treatment. Health care of patients with vascular access for hemodialysis requires the collaboration of a nephrologist, a vascular surgeon, an interventional radiologist, and an angiologist. Certain conditions must be fulfilled for the successful introduction of fistula. Early indication for the formation of AVF and perfect preoperative examination of the entire venous system in the area of application of the planned fistula is a prerequisite for creating a technically correct autologous fistula. The formation of an autologous arteriovenous fistula for hemodialysis is a standard procedure that should be performed by a vascular surgeon.

Long-term dialysis (including hemodialysis) treatment using standard international criteria is currently needed by about 600 patients per million inhabitants within the Slovak Republic. Accurate statistical data on the morbidity, economic costs, and other circumstances of the need for such treatment and its providing are regularly processed. Although there is no such information at hand in Slovakia, there are data available in the foreign literature concerning the importance of establishing arteriovenous connections from a non-professional perspective. The most accessible data are from studies in the USA. The vascular access is reported to be one of the six factors determining morbidity and, indirectly, the mortality of dialysis patients. In Slovakia, surgically established arteriovenous connections clearly dominate, in Europe, this method dominates historically (its authors are Italians Cimino and Brescia). Recent publications point to a change in favor of classical fistulas with an emphasis on economic benefits (as opposed to a high percentage of prosthesis use, particularly in the USA).

Surgical treatment of thromboses is half the cost of using a thrombolytic treatment. As a treatment option for recurrent thromboses, percutaneous transluminal angioplasty is less suitable as a revision but is much more advantageous for resolving fistula stenosis. Liberalization of accepted dialysis criteria in the older generation has an impact on the more frequent occurrence of thromboses following hypotensive events, cardiac rhythm disorders, and the like.

Creating a good fistula requires well-trained staff, sufficient time, and financial costs. Social and psychological aspect concerns the physician, the dialysis nurse and, first of all, the patient.

An inappropriate fistula has a professional (insufficient flow with secondary insufficient dialysability of the patient with all consequences, in some cases including affecting the patient's survival) as well as a social and psychological impact. High-quality fistula allows for shorter dialysis time, is less painful when injected, reduces the number of surgeries and hospitalizations. Consequently, it affects the possibilities of the patient's diet, the possibility of a patient's long-term stay outside the maternal dialysis center, decreased dependence of the patient on dialysis, increased ability to work and devote themselves to individual hobbies, which reduces the number of reactive depressions.

Due to economic reasons in Slovakia, a specific, so far unknown way for creating a quality and adequate fistula, is the possibility of home dialysis, in which the patient himself connects to the dialysis machine. The time of fistula formation is an important factor for the expected outcome and complications increase the maladaptation of patients in the following dialysis period. Increased adaptability, self-control, optimism not only manifests itself in the patient but allows better acceptance of the disease by the environment and communication with their relatives. Obviously, the importance of these factors is increased in childhood as well as in old age. A high-quality fistula clearly improves the quality of life of a patient on dialysis.

During the year, a number of patients are chronically dialyzed at dialysis centers in the Slovak Republic. Each one of them is connected to the artificial kidney 100 to 160 times in the course of a year. For many of these patients, one of the basic prerequisites for successful dialysis is a high-quality and long-term functioning arteriovenous fistula, which is the most precious property of the dialysis patient. The surgeon who establishes the arteriovenous connections must thoroughly examine the patient prior to surgery, correctly assess their vascular system, and choose the most favorable way of creating vascular access for long-term hemodialysis. The determination of the surgical plan and the most optimal vascular access is done on a strictly individual basis and depends not only on the patient's vascular system but also on the patient's overall condition, age, and prognosis. The quality of the connection should also meet the requirements of the simplest and shortest possible operation using local anesthesia. Underestimating any fact may result in the formation of many non-functional A-V fistulas.

Surgery of arteriovenous connections for the needs of long-term hemodialysis is an integral yet at the same time part one of the most problematic parts of vascular surgery. The number of patients enrolled in the long-term hemodialysis program is increasing. The average age of patients increases as well, the age limit shifts upwards. All these circumstances result in the need to create more and more AV fistulas because their applicability has its boundaries and is also limited. The correct surgical tactic, individual approach to the patient, and precise surgical technique contribute to the improvement of the quality of life of sick patients, of which only a small percentage are lucky enough to have their disease cured by successful kidney transplantation.

The principle of care for hemodialysis access is to maintain good function as long as possible with a minimum of complications and interventions. Each surgeon should endeavor to maintain the function of any normofunctional access because access options are often limited. The most common complications encountered in HD accesses are:

7. stenosis
8. thrombosis
9. infection
10. aneurysm and pseudoaneurysm
11. hyperfunction
12. venous hypertension
13. hand ischemia

1. STENOSIS

AVF/AVG stenosis is the most common cause of HD access hypofunction that we encounter every day. Functional HD access causes myointimal hyperplasia in the venous segment. In native AVF, more than 60% of stenoses occur within 5 cm of anastomosis (the so-called juxta-anastomotic stenoses) and in AVF, the predilection site of stenosis is the area of venous anastomosis and drainage vein. Up to 22% of stenosis occurs in the central venous areas, but these are rarely the cause of reduced function of the HD access.

Stenosis is usually manifested by hypofunction of the AVF, i.e., by reduced flow rate and the inability to carry out adequate hemodialysis. Other symptoms are protracted bleeding after cannulation, swelling of the hand, weakening of the vortex above the vein. Duplex ultrasonography is indicated when AVF stenosis is suspected. It allows us to evaluate the type, location, and extent of stenosis. In addition to the morphology of stenosis, sonography also makes it possible to assess the hemodynamic effect of stenosis. In the case of HD access flow (Qa) dropping below 500 ml/min for AVF and below 600 ml/min for AVG, fistulography, and treatment are indicated. Another indication is a decrease in the flow rate of 20% compared to the previous investigation. Sonographically verified stenosis in normofunctional AVF/AVG without complications during HD is not indicated for DSA and PTA.

In the case of severe stenosis causing hypofunction of the HD access, treatment is indicated. The method of choice is percutaneous transluminal angioplasty (PTA) (Figure 1 a, b, c).

The procedure is the same as for other radiological interventions, but due to the nature of the stenosis, it is necessary to use higher insufflation pressures. These higher insufflation pressures lead to significant vein damage, often resulting in restenosis at the PTA site. Therefore, some authors use "cutting" balloons, which allows for the use of lower insufflation pressures.

Surgical treatment of AVF stenoses is, in the era of interventional radiology, indicated for cases of longer filiform stenoses where blood flow couldn't be restored properly. The affected segment can be bypassed by the venovenous bypass, in the case of AVF on the wrist, it is possible to use transposed basilica antebrachia. In the case of early recurrence of juxta-anastomotic stenosis, the formation of new AVF above this stenosis is indicated. Some authors also recommend this method primarily in the treatment of juxta-anastomotic stenoses, as the long-term results are excellent and, unlike radio-intervention, repeated interventions are not required. In the case of stenosis of a venous anastomosis, AVG can be treated with angioplasty or interposite.

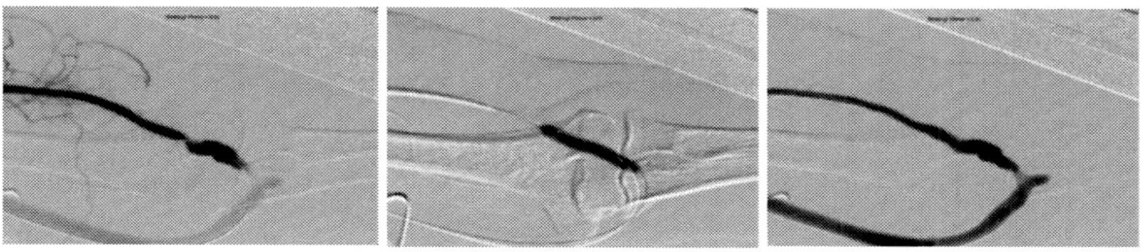

(a) (b) (c)

Figure 1.

2. Thrombosis

Thrombotic occlusion is the most common complication of dialysis access. Large studies suggest that thrombosis occurs 5 times more often in AVG than in native AVF. The most common cause (80%) is stenosis during HD access. Stenosis may be present in the arterial part, in the anastomosis, or anywhere in the venous part of the HD access. In most cases, stenosis is localized in the drainage vein of AVF or the venous anastomosis of AVG, stenosis is less common in the area of an arterial anastomosis. In 20% of cases, thrombosis occurs in the absence of stenosis (external compression, hypotension, dehydration, infection, coagulation disorders, heart failure).

Thrombosis is manifested by the impossibility of HD in the patient. HD access can be restored by radiological intervention or surgery.

Surgical treatment consists of the removal of thrombus by Fogarty catheter no. 2, 3. Thrombectomy of native AVF is difficult because thrombus rarely occurs in a vein without stenosis or another pathological finding. Endothelial damage results in rethrombosis. In the case of native radiocephalic AVF, the best alternative is reanastomosis more proximally because the vein thromboses most often up to the distance of the nearest branch.

AVG thrombectomy has better results because the prosthesis is not prone to rethrombosis, unlike the native vein. Stenosis which caused the thrombosis must also be resolved. Ideally, after AVG thrombectomy, fistulography and PTA of venous anastomosis or drainage vein are performed. If there is no possibility of hybrid performance, it is necessary to treat stenosis by angioplasty or by a short interposite into an intact vein.

3. Aneurysm, Pseudoaneurysm

After the formation of the native AVF, there is a gradual dilatation of the inlet artery and the outlet vein. This dilatation is a normal finding and is not considered an aneurysm. An aneurysm is a localized dilatation of the vessel (Figure 2 a, b) where the wall is made up of all layers of the vessel wall. AVG cannot be dilated, so we only encounter pseudoaneurysms. These arise as a result of the local destruction of the prosthesis followed by the chronic extravasation into the subcutaneous tissue bounded by a fibrous wall. AVF aneurysm is considered to be a localized dilation of the vein (Figure 2 a, b) with a diameter 1.5-2 times larger than the adjacent vein segment.

The incidence of aneurysms/pseudoaneurysms in native AVF is up to 17% and in AVG up to 7%. Native AVFs are almost always associated with stenosis, which can be localized in front of or behind an aneurysm. Other causes are high flow and repeated punctures to the same site. A common cause of pseudoaneurysm is damage to the posterior wall of the vein during cannulation.

Due to the localization of HD accesses, the clinical diagnosis is easy. Duplex ultrasonography distinguishes a hematoma and a perigraft seroma allows for the verification of stenosis in the vein and monitoring the size of the aneurysm.

Aneurysm associated with rapid growth, thin skin, skin erosions, or bleeding is indicated to be treated. Multiple aneurysms that shorten the cannula segment need to be indicated for treatment. A pseudoaneurysm with a diameter greater than twice the diameter of the graft is indicated for surgery.

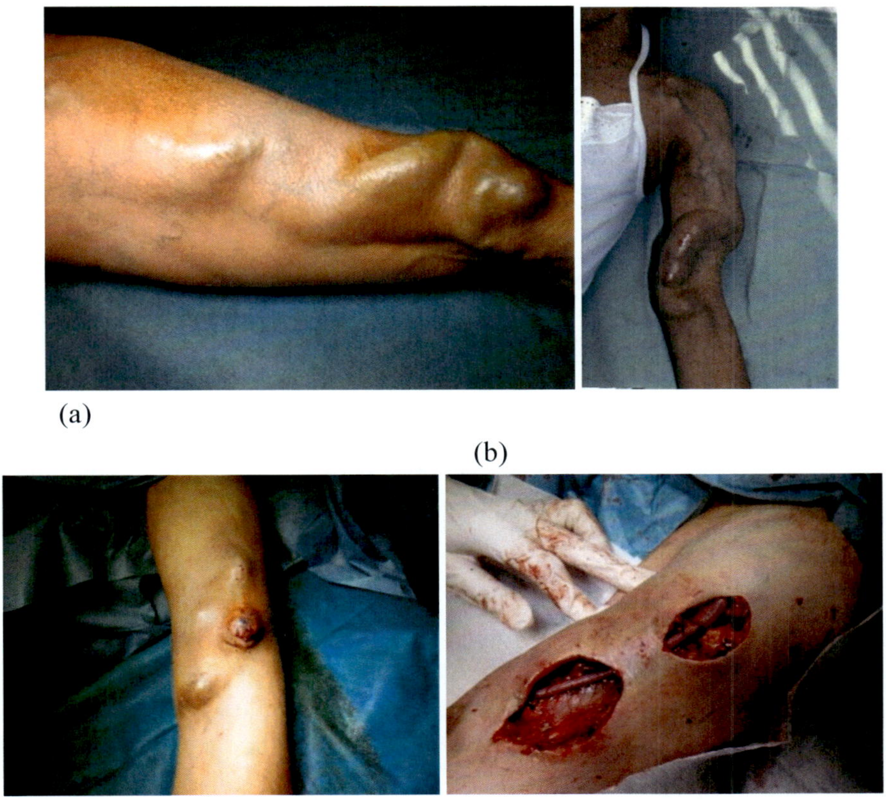

(a) (b) (c) (d)

Figure 2.

Treatment should resolve the aneurysm while preserving the current dialysis access. The aneurysms of AVF on the forearm located just behind the anastomosis are easiest to be treated. In this case, the aneurysm is resected, the artery is reconstructed end-to-end, and the new AVF is sutured proximal to the artery. If the aneurysm is localized on another segment of vein, it can be resected and the vein reconstructed end-to-end. In the case of a major aneurysm, it is possible to make a longitudinal cut of the vein and then reconstruct it with a longitudinal suture (aneurysmorrhaphy). In the case of multiple aneurysms (Figure 2c, d), it is possible to treat them all at once. Bleeding pseudoaneurysm with compartment syndrome is indicated for AVF ligature and fasciotomy.

AVG pseudoaneurysm is resected and the resected part of the prosthesis is replaced by a new interposite, which is inserted into healthy subcutaneous tissue. In the case of an infected pseudoaneurysm, it is best to remove the entire AVG and replace the segment with an autologous or homologous graft.

3. Bleeding

Patients with terminal renal disease are at increased risk of bleeding due to defects in the hemostatic mechanisms of uremia. Another important etiological factor is heparin therapy and the use of low-molecular-weight-heparins (LMWHs), which are often given to these patients. LMWHs are eliminated mainly by the kidneys and their dosage is difficult to estimate in hemodialysis patients.

Bleeding from the HD access cannulation site is a relatively common complication, but in most cases conservatively manageable. The most common cause is platelet dysfunction and the administration of anticoagulants during hemodialysis. Another cause is increased venous pressure due to stenosis in the proximal area of the vein and pseudoaneurysm at the cannula opening site. In the case of bleeding, compressing the injection site for 30 minutes is usually sufficient to stop the bleeding. If bleeding continues despite compression, the cause of the bleeding should always be investigated (pseudoaneurysm, stenosis above the injection site, coagulation disorder, HD access hyperfunction).

Severe bleeding may occur when performing brachial artery cannulation (percutaneous radiological interventions). The most serious complication is the upper limb compartment syndrome, in this case, an urgent surgical treatment should be indicated. The surgical procedure consists of treating the source of bleeding.

4. Venous Hypertension

The most common cause of venous upper limb hypertension in hemodialysis patients is stenosis or occlusion of the central veins of the thorax (subclavian vein, brachiocephalic vein, superior vena cava).

A major etiological factor for stenosis/occlusion is the prior implantation of a central venous catheter (CVC). While the incidence of stenosis is 10% when CVC is implanted in the internal jugular vein (IJV), it is (42-50%) when the CVC is placed in the subclavian vein. The use of CVC use in hemodialysis patients should be as short as possible and it is preferable to implant CVC in the IJV if necessary. Risk factors include prolonged catheter use, repeat cannulation, and catheter infection. Perivenous fibrosis occurs at the site of stenosis and myointimal hyperplasia. The development of stenosis is potentiated by the creation of a functional HD access on the ipsilateral limb since in central vein occlusion, it is almost impossible to create a well-functioning and uncomplicated HD access.

Patients with central thoracic stenosis/occlusion are mostly asymptomatic until the next attempt to create HD access on the ipsilateral side. In mild cases, venous hypertension may be manifested by mild swelling of the limb, development of collateral veins on the anterior, posterior chest and on the shoulder. In more severe cases, massive swelling of the limb develops, with limited movement of the fingers, or even trophic changes and defects. In the case of bilateral brachiocephalic vein occlusion or in the superior vena cava, the patient has swelling of the face, eyelids, neck, both upper limbs, and breasts (Figure 3a).

Venous hypertension may also occur with stenosis of the drainage vein of AVF or AVG, as increased venous pressure results in valvular insufficiency and venous reflux. This is manifested by swelling of the limb distal to the stenosis. In extreme cases, skin changes encountered in chronic venous insufficiency of the lower extremities may occur (Figure 3b).

After AVF/AVG is created in the elbow area, the swelling of the limb is frequent and usually disappears within a few weeks. Treatment consists of elevation and positioning of the limb. If the swelling persists, we look for the cause. In 25% of patients, the cause is a pathological finding in the central veins (stenosis/occlusion of the central veins). If a patient with a prior history of CVC is scheduled to develop HD access, the patient must undergo an ultrasonographic examination of the central veins.

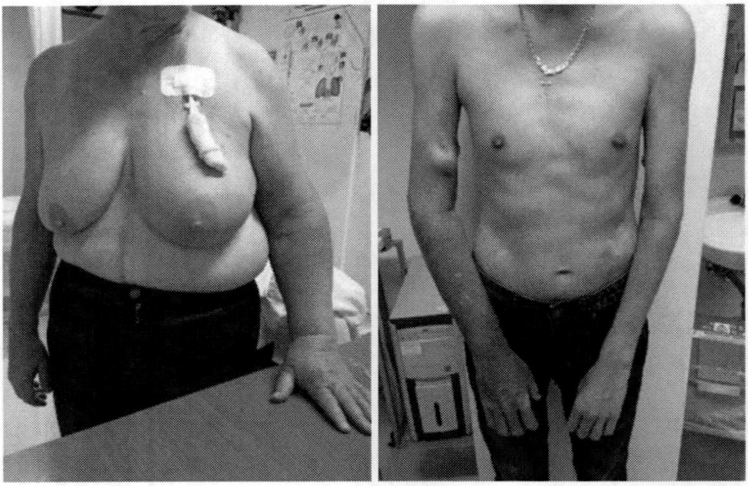

(a) (b)

Figure 3.

Treatment of venous hypertension due to stenosis of the drainage vein is relatively simple and consists of an endovascular or surgical solution. In the case of a centrally located stenosis, the method of choice is endovascular therapy. A stent implantation is indicated in the case of elastic recoil vein after PTA, early restenosis within 3 months or in case of venous rupture during PTA. Although the technical success rate of PTAs in this area is 70-100%, the primary one-year patency is low, and repeated interventions are required. Stent implantation does not improve these results either. Stent graft implantation is a promising option. Given the long-term stenosis/central vein occlusion rate (stent patency of 55% for one year), treatment is indicated only for severe clinical symptoms. The presence of stenosis without clinical symptomatology is not an indication for endovascular or surgical treatment. If a stent is used in a subclavian vein, it should not overlap the IJV in order to be able to implant CVC in the future or to suture distal anastomosis of the axillojugular bypass into the IJV. Similarly, in the case of the implantation of a stent into the brachiocephalic vein, the contralateral vein spacing should remain uncovered.

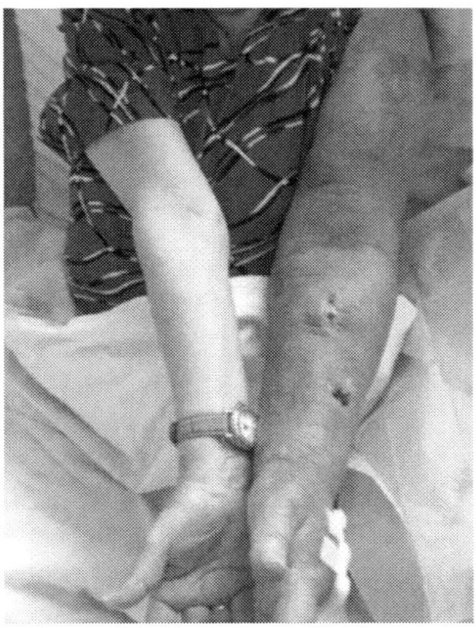

Figure 4.

Surgical treatment is associated with higher morbidity and, therefore, is rarely indicated in the era of endovascular interventions. However, on the other hand, it is the only option of rescuing a well-functioning HD access in a patient with depleted accesses and proximally localized vein occlusion. Extra-thoracic reconstructions are ideal. In the case of occlusion of the subclavian vein, the closure can be bypassed by an axillojugular bypass. In the case of occlusion of the brachiocephalic vein, it is possible to perform an axillojugular cross bypass onto the contralateral IJV. In the case of occlusion of both brachiocephalic veins or of VCS occlusion, the ideal solution is an axilloiliac bypass to the external iliac vein. In all cases, it is necessary to use a reinforced PTFE prosthesis with a diameter of 8-12 mm and to suture sufficiently wide anastomoses (15-20 mm).

Venous hypertension syndrome of the upper limb is often a difficult-to-be-solved complication in hemodialysis patients requiring repeated interventions. This complication should be considered at the start of treatment and implantation should be considered (Figure 4).

5. Infection

Infection is the second most common cause of HD access loss. It is considered early within 30 days of establishing HD access and considered late 30 days post-op. Only 6% of infections are associated with surgery (i.e., early infections), the remaining 94% of infections are a result of HD access use and repeated surgical and radiological interventions. Gram-positive cocci (staph. aureus, staph. epidermidis) are the main etiological agents, Gram-negative bacteria are less common. Some infections are of the polymicrobial nature. AVGs are more likely to be complicated by infection than autologous AVFs (19.7% vs 4.5%). Risk factors include repeated cannulations, poor personal hygiene, frequent hospitalizations, age, diabetes mellitus, location of HD access on a lower limb. Autologous AVF infections are rarely life-threatening. Early deep infection after surgery (formation of AVF) is always an infection at the site of anastomosis. If left untreated, a pseudoaneurysm will develop or rupture and profuse bleeding will occur. Therefore, revision, ligation of AVF, and reconstruction of the artery by venous patch or interposite are indicated. In the case of radiocephalic AVF, the artery can be ligated.

The most common cause of late infection is cannulation and infection of a hematoma. It is manifested by phlegmon, swelling, and pain. The treatment consists of 2-4 weeks of ATB treatment, in case abscess forms it needs to be drained. Stenosis of the vein may develop after the infection has healed. Ultrasound examination is required after the infection has healed. Recurrent infections often require the withdrawal of HD access.

In the case of a dilated vein, a thrombus can be formed in the dilated segment that induces thrombophlebitis, similar to varicophlebitis in the lower extremities. Bacterial inoculation produces septic phlebitis, often complicated by endocarditis and septic pulmonary emboli. The treatment consists of excision of the whole vein segment and long-term ATB treatment.

Prosthetic AVG infection is often associated not only with local signs of inflammation but also with septic symptoms and generally poor condition of the patient. Unlike autologous AVF, the treatment is more complicated. In the case of early infection, anastomoses are always involved, which indicates prosthesis explantation and treatment of arterial anastomosis, similar to in a native AVF. The venous anastomosis is treated after the prosthesis has been explanted with ligature proximal and distal to the anastomosis, with the exception of the axillary vein and larger veins, which are better to be reconstructed. The treatment of late AVG infection depends on the location of the infection and the virulence of the pathogen. In the presence of a staphylococcal aureus infection or gram-negative bacteria, it is better to remove the AV graft because of the higher risk of reinfection, septic complications, and bleeding. The prosthesis is removed completely with a venoplasty of arterial anastomosis (total AVG explantation) or a short cuff from the prosthesis is left in the area of arterial anastomosis (subtotal AVG explantation). The advantage of subtotal AVG explantation is that it is less likely to damage nerve structures and cause bleeding (1.9% vs. 19%). In the case of an infection located outside the anastomoses, it is possible to try to save the HD access. The surgery consists of partial resection of the prosthesis, with a new interposite placed between the proximal and distal ends, which is guided through the healthy subcutaneous tissue. The risk of this procedure is a higher number of relapses (29%), but it avoids CVC in patients with limited HD access options.

6. Hemodynamic Complications, Hyperfunction

The chosen type of hemodialysis approach significantly affects overall morbidity and mortality. Cardiovascular diseases are the leading cause of death in dialysis patients. More than 50% of patients enrolled in a chronic dialysis program are there due to cardiovascular diseases. Normofunctional arteriovenous fistula does not increase cardiac mortality in patients, but patients with an ejection fraction of less than 25% should not have arterial fistula formed because of a high risk of cardiac failure. In this group, the patient is indicated with permanent CVC implantation. An alternative is an artery-artery fistula with a dialysis prosthesis. In the event of an acute inclusion in the HD program, the patient is implanted with a permanent CVC. After recompensating, a portion of the patients will improve their cardiac results and may have an arterial fistula created. The surgeon should endeavor to produce an AVF with a flow rate of up to 800 ml/min, therefore, we prefer an AVF on the forearm. An arteriovenous fistula flow rate of 600-900 ml/min is considered normal and is sufficient for effective hemodialysis. In some patients, the flow rate increases over time. Although this high flow arteriovenous fistula allows easy cannulation and uncomplicated hemodialysis, high flow gradually depletes cardiovascular reserves.

At present, there is a lack of a clear definition of high flow arteriovenous fistula. The Vascular Access Society Guidelines define high flow AVF/AVG when the fistula flow (Qa) is greater than 1.5 l/min and cardiopulmonary recirculation (CPR) is more than 20%. Cardiopulmonary recirculation is defined as the ratio between fistula flow and cardiac output (CPR = Qa/CO). The factors that are responsible and contribute to the development of volumetric cardiac overload into clinically significant cardiac insufficiency are not well known. Cardiac decompensation after the formation of an AVF/AVG is more likely in patients with pre-existing heart disease. There is a higher risk in patients with an arteriovenous fistula on the shoulder. A flow rate above 2.0 l/min has a positive predictive value for the development of congestive cardiac failure. The incidence of high flow arteriovenous fistula is 3.7%. Clinically, a hyperfunctioning arteriovenous fistula may be manifested by aneurysm of the drainage vein, ischemia of the hand, swelling of the upper limb, weakness, dyspnea.

The indication for the solution of hyperfunctioning AVF/AVG is determined not only by Qa and CPR values but also by clinical picture, cardiologic and echocardiographical investigations. In the asymptomatic patient, options of other accesses for HD determine the need for flow reduction too, because any interference with HD access can lead to its failure.

Indications for flow reduction are as follows:

14. Cardiac failure + Qa > 1600 ml/min and/or Qa/CO > 0.3
15. Steal syndrome + Qa for AVF > 800 ml/min, Qa for AVG > 1200 ml/min
16. Prophylaxis of cardiac failure in patients with Qa > 2000 ml/min and/or Qa/CO > 0.3 (2)

Correction operations used in the treatment of AVF/AVG hyperfunction include banding, PRAL (proximal radial artery ligature), revision using distal inflow (RUDI), TRA (transposition of the radial artery). Hyperfunction with aneurysmally dilated drainage vein can be eventually solved by aneurysmorrhaphy with Provena implantation.

7. Banding

Banding is the easiest method. It aims to reduce flow by increasing resistance in the venous part of the arteriovenous fistula. It consists of circular sewing of the drainage vein with a Dacron/PTFE cuff at a distance of 1.5-2 cm above the anastomosis (Figure 5). The goal is to reduce the vein lumen by 60%. The method is blamed for a higher percentage of

AVF/AVG thrombosis. Intraoperative AVF flow monitoring is necessary to properly perform and increase the success of this surgical modality. An alternative is to use a short interposite. In the case of an autologous AVF, a 4 mm PTFE prosthesis is used, in the case of an AVG a conical 4/7 mm prosthesis.

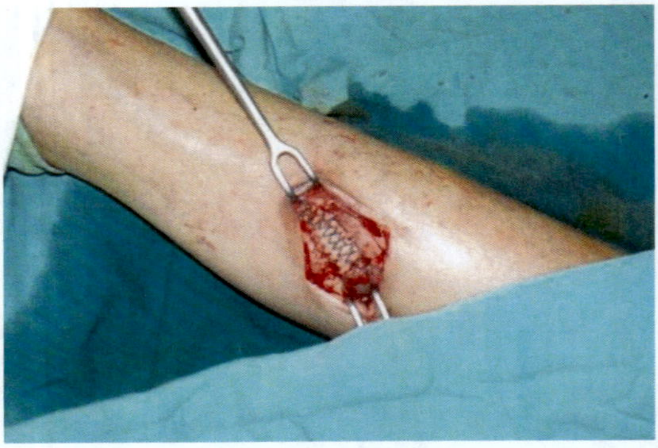

Figure 5.

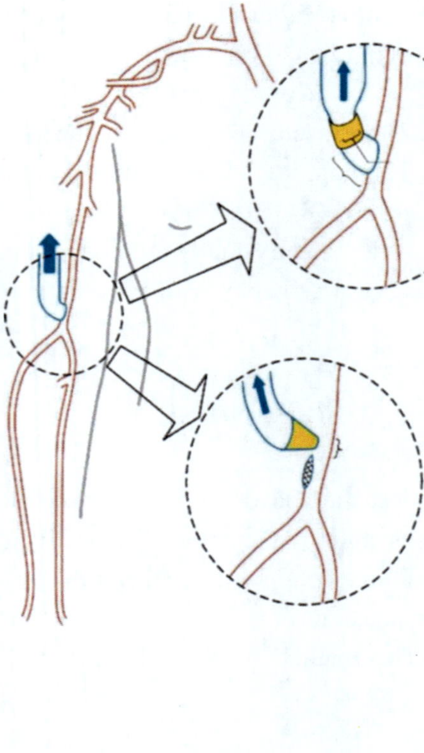

Figure 6.

7.1. PRAL (Proximal Radial Artery Ligation)

The ligature of the proximal radial artery near the anastomosis AVF is an ideal method for distal radiocephalic AVF. The condition is a passable ulnar artery and a palmar arch. This simple operation reduces AVF flow by at least 33%.

7.2. RUDI (Revision Using Distal Inflow)

The principle of this method, which is used in the hyperfunction of cubital AVF, is to move the AVF anastomosis from the brachial artery to the proximal or central portion of the radial artery. The original anastomosis is ligated and a new one is formed between the cephalic vein of the forearm and the radial artery. If the cephalic vein is not suitable, a 6 mm PTFE prosthesis interposite may be used.

By using a thinner inflow artery, the flow through the AVF is reduced, and by using a forearm vein, the cannula segment is extended.

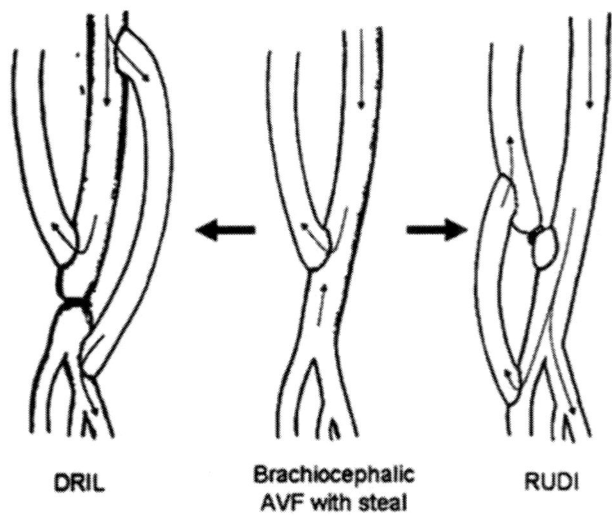

Figure 7.

7.3. TRA (Transposition of the Radial Artery)

Transposition of the radial artery is a relatively demanding surgical method in which the radial artery is mobilized over the entire forearm, is then adjusted, and transposed into the elbow. The original AVF of the brachial artery is abolished and the radial artery is sutured end-to-end or end-to-side onto the vein.

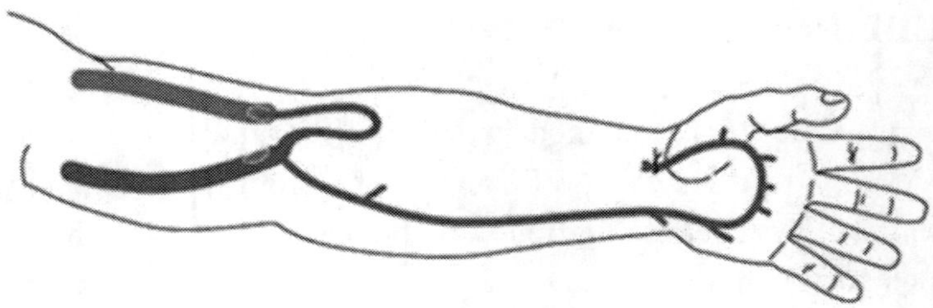

Figure 8.

8. Ischemic Syndrome, Steal Syndrome

Ischemic steal syndrome of the upper limb is a rarer complication of AVF. Patients with proximal localized AVF/AVG (10-25%) have a higher incidence compared to patients with AVF on the forearm (1-2%). Ischemia is most common after arteriovenous fistula formation in the lower limb, with autologous AVF transposed by the superficial femoral vein being more burdened by this complication compared to an AVG on the thigh (20.97% vs 7.18%).

If a steal phenomenon is associated with signs of hand ischemia - ischemic steal syndrome is considered a pathological finding. It may be an indication of insufficient collateral filling through the ulnar artery, peripheral atherosclerotic disease, distal hypoperfusion in high-flow fistulae that eventually cause hand ischemia, even in healthy arteries without atherosclerotic affliction. All these factors interfere with normal compensatory mechanisms, such as peripheral vasodilatation and the increase in flow through the collateral circulation, ensuring adequate perfusion of the distal upper limb. Any disease of the proximal or distal arteries (e.g., atherosclerosis, Buerger's disease, vasculitis) can lead to a reduction in limb blood flow and ultimately to ischemic manifestations of the upper limb in the dialyzed patient.

High flow steal syndrome is the most common form of steal syndrome. From the limb peripherally from the fistula, retrograde blood flow occurs to the extent that ischemia develops. The cause is low venous resistance, which may be technically caused, for example, by a wide anastomosis.

Normal flow steal syndrome should be evaluated as a multifactorial process. In principle, two subgroups of normal flow steal syndrome are distinguished. The two subgroups may overlap one another. In up to 52% it develops due to insufficient collateral circulation, possibly due to numerous stenoses and occlusion of the arterial bed.

Ischemic steal syndrome is primarily a clinical diagnosis. In the case of manifest ischemia, diagnosis can be made on the basis of medical history and physical examination. Clinical manifestations of ischemia include paleness, pain, stiffness, diminished or disappeared pulsation, sensory or motor neuropathy, trophic defects. Other symptoms (paleness, pain, and cold hand) rapidly regress in shunt compression. In fistula compression, pulsation to the radial artery, which was not present before, also occurs. Cold and gentle paresthesia in fingers are described in 10% of newly formed arteriovenous fistulas, but they disappear within a few weeks.

Classification of steal syndrome by Tordoir:

Stage 1: *Pale/blue and/or cold hand without pain, clumsy fingers*
Stage 2: *Pale during activity and/or HD*
Stage 3: *Pain during rest*
Stage 4: *Ulceration, necrosis, gangrene*

After the diagnosis of steal syndrome has been made, the next step is to distinguish what type of syndrome it is depending on the blood flow through the fistula - Qa (either high flow or normal flow steal syndrome). This differentiation is a prerequisite for planning further therapy. There are several non-invasive methods that can be used to measure blood pressure and blood flow at individual levels. These methods determine the risk of developing ischemic syndrome or may provide supportive data for making a diagnosis. Distal limb perfusion is measured by digital plethysmography, finger pressure index (finger to brachial pressure ratio), systolic pressure index (brachial pressure ratio on the AVF side, and on the contralateral side).

Fistula blood flow can be determined by duplex sonography. This examination should be the first examination in any patient with limb ischemia and vascular access established on the affected limb. Another examination is the conventional DSA (under the compression of the AVF) and it is only possible to visualize the arterial limb system under the AVF up to the periphery of the hand. It is also useful to display venous outflow. If contrast administration is not possible, an MRA examination is required.

The aim of steal syndrome treatment is to maintain limb vitality, to reduce the clinical manifestations of ischemia and, if possible, to maintain the patency of the vascular dialysis approach.

Surgical treatment of steal syndrome is a method of choice in patients whose proximal stenosis to the inflow artery has been excluded. Several possibilities of surgical treatment are described. The type of surgical treatment chosen for a particular patient depends on the localization of the arteriovenous fistula and the etiopathogenesis of peripheral hypoperfusion. The principle of surgical treatment is to improve distal flow by redirecting blood flow from the AVF to the hand or by improving the collateral circulation of the hand. In the treatment of high flow steal syndrome, AVF/AVG flow can be reduced by surgical procedures that are also used in hyperfunction (banding, RUDI, TRA). For normal flow steal syndrome, DRIL (distal revascularization interval ligation) or PAI (proximalization of the arterial inflow) is indicated. In steal syndrome based on distal radiocephalic ACF, the method of choice is distal radial artery ligation (DRAL).

8.1. DRIL (Distal Revascularization Interval Ligation, Schanzer's Surgery)

DRIL is the best-known method in the treatment of steal syndrome. The indication is steal syndrome in arteriovenous fistula (AVF or AVG) formed on the brachial artery. The surgical procedure consists of the ligature of the brachial artery under the AVF anastomosis and the revascularization of the limb by a brachio-brachial bypass. A sufficient length of the bypass is required for success, with the proximal anastomosis of the bypass placed at least 7 cm above the anastomosis of the AVF and the brachial artery being ligated just below the AVF.

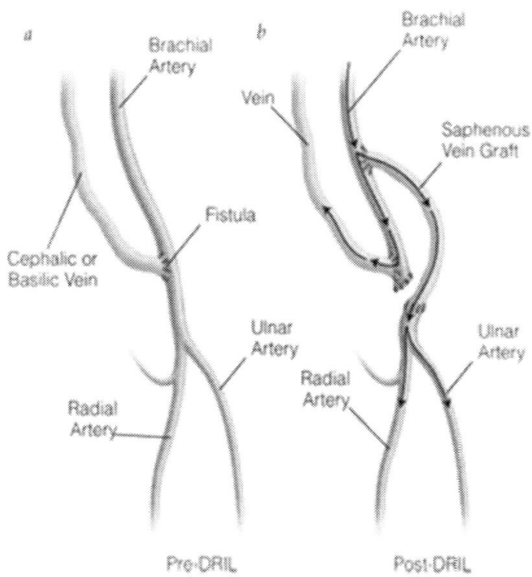

Figure 9.

8.2. PAI (Proximalization of the Arterial Inflow)

Proximalization of the AVF/AVG anastomosis is a suitable alternative to DRIL. The hemodynamic effect is similar. The advantage of this method over DRIL is that it is not necessary to remove a vein, anastomosis is simpler and arterial continuity is maintained. The principle of the method lies in the ligature of the original anastomosis of the arteriovenous fistula and the influx into the original arterialized vein is ensured by the interposite between the vein and the artery located more proximal to the limb. In the case of the cubital fistula, it is the brachial artery in its proximal part, in the case of the brachial artery the axillary artery is used as the inflow. A 4-5 mm PTFE prosthesis is used as an interposite. The hemodynamic effect wlays in connecting to a more centrally located artery with a larger caliber and lower inflow resistance, and hence greater capacity, which means lower arterial pressure under anastomosis. As with DRIL, the original vein can be cannulated on the first postoperative day to avoid CVC. One-year patency is 87%, three-year patency 67%.

8.3. DRAL (Distal Radial Artery Ligation)

Ligature of the radial artery just behind the AVF anastomosis is an ideal solution for ischemic steal syndrome in a distal radiocephalic AVF. The condition is DSA verified patency of the ulnar artery and palmar arch. Under local anesthesia, a longitudinal incision distal to the AVF anastomosis is made. There is no need to prepare anastomosis and the artery is disrupted after the retinaculum flexorum is cut. An alternative is an endovascular therapy in which the radial artery is occluded by embolization.

8.4. AVF Ligature

The abolition of arteriovenous fistula should only be undertaken in indicated cases, as the probability of steal syndrome after fistula formation elsewhere is high. We access it in case of the poor general condition of the patient or after exhaustion of other possibilities.

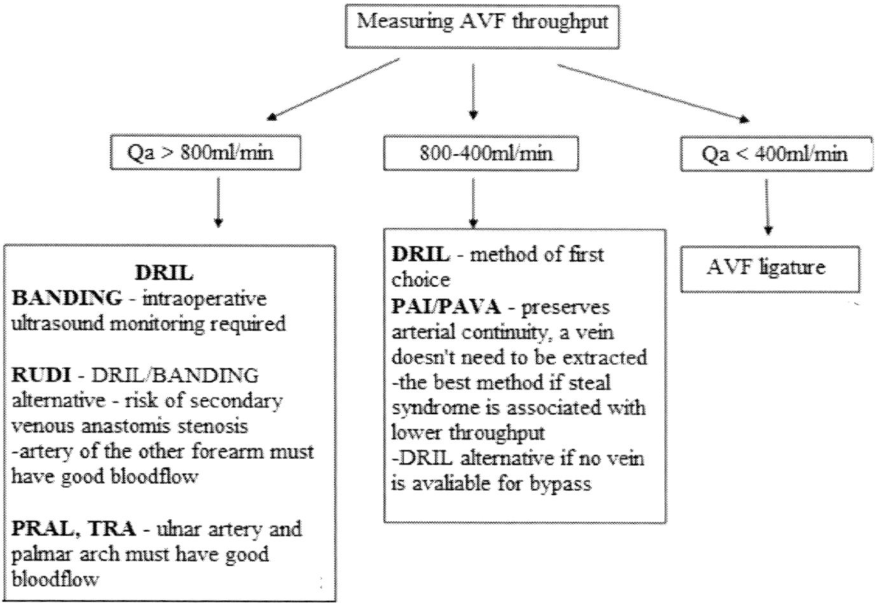

9. Neuropathy

There are several types of neuropathy in dialysis patients. Most commonly, uremic or diabetic polyneuropathy and carpal canal syndrome are present. These neuropathies must be taken into consideration.

Ischemic monomelic neuropathy (IMN) is the most serious complication of the dialysis approach. Incidence is 0.5% of newly created AVFs/AVGs. It is the cause of sensory-motor dysfunction of various degrees on the forearm without tissue ischemia. The clinical manifestations described include sudden and permanent sensory-motor dysfunction involving multiple forearm nerve groups. At the same time, the acral parts of the limb are free of ischemia, the toes are warm and pink. Symptoms appear immediately after suturing the AVF and are believed to be caused by a transient decrease in blood flow that causes vasa nervorum ischemia. Risk factors include diabetes mellitus, atherosclerosis, fistula formation in the cubital pit, and the presence of polyneuropathy. Ischemic monomelic neuropathy should be distinguished from focal nerve injury resulting from an intraoperative or postoperative ultrasound.

As a solution to ischemic monomelic neuropathy, immediate withdrawal of AVF is recommended. If other causes of sensorimotor hand deficiency are ruled out shortly after the fistula has been formed, IMN should be considered and the fistula urgently abolished.

REFERENCES

Bakran, A., Mickley, V., Passlick-Deetjen, J. 2003 *Management of the renal patient: Clinical algorithms on vascular Access for haemodialysis*. Lengerich: Pabst Science Publishers.

Baláž, P., Rokošný, S., Klein, D., Adamec, M. 2008. "Aneurysmorrhaphy is an easy technique for arteriovenous fistula salvage." *J Vasc Surg* 9:81-84.

Basile, C. et al. 2008. "The relationship between the flow of arteriovenous fistula and cardiac output in hemodialysis patients." *Nephrol Dial Transplant* 23:282-287.

Brescia, M.J., Cimino, J.E., Appel, K., Hurwich, B.J. 1966. "Chronic hemodialysis using venipuncture and a surgically created arteriovenous fistula." *N Eng J Med* 275:1089-92.

Bourquelot, P., Corbi, P., Cussenot, O. 1989. "Surgical improvement of high-flow arteriovenous fistulas". In *Vascular Access for hemodialysis* edited by Sommer B.G., Henry M.L. 124-130. New York: W.L. Gore & Associates Inc., Pluribus Press Inc.

Bourquelot, P.: Proximal radial artery ligation (PRAL) for reduction of flow in autogenous radial cephalic accesses for haemodialysis. *Eur J Vasc Endovasc Surg,* 2010, 6, p. 94-99.

Bourquelot, P., Rawa, M., Van Laere, O. 2012. "Long- -term results of femoral vein transposition for autogenous arteriovenous hemodialysis access." *J Vasc Surg* 56:440-5.

Frankovičová, M. 2000. *Chirurgia tepnožilových spojení pre potreby dlhodobej hemodialýzy*. Bratislava: Herba. [Surgery of arterio-venous junctions for the needs of long-term hemodialysis treatment]

Gracz, K.C, Ing, T.S., Song, L. 1977. "Proximal forearm fistula for maintenance hemodialysis." *Kidney Int* 11:71-4.

Chemla, E.S., Morsy, M., Anderson, L. et al. 2007. "Inflow reduction by distalization of anastomosis treats efficiently high-flow high-cardiac output vascular access for hemodialysis." *Semin Dial* 20:68-72.

Janeckova J, Bachleda P, Utikal P, Kocher M, Cerna M, Xinopulos P. 2018. "Surgical Revision vs. Stent-graft to Treat Venous Anastomosis Stenosis Following Surgical Thrombectomy of Hemodialysis Grafts." *Int Angiol* 37(4):315-21.

Kundu, S. 2010 "Central venous disease in hemodialysis patients: prevalence, etiology, and treatment." *The J Vasc Access* 11:1-7.

Mickley, V. 2008. "Steal syndrome. Strategies to preserve vascular access and extremity." *Nephrol Dial Transplant* 23:19-24.

Minion, D.J., Moore, E., Endean, E. 2005. "Revision using distal inflow: a novel approach to dialysis-associated steal syndrome." *Ann Vasc Surg* 19:393-404.

Tordoir, J.H.M., Van der Sande, F.M., Haan, M.W. 2004. "Current topics on vascular access for hemodialysis." *Minerva Urol Nefrol* 56:223-35.

Tordoir, J.H.M., Demmers, R., Van der Sande, F.M. 2004. "Upper extremity ischemia and hemodialysis vascular access." *Eur J Vasc Endovasc Surg* 27:1-5.

Tordoir, J.H.M., Canaud, B., Haage, P., Konner, K. 2007. EBPG on vascular access. *Nephrol Dial Transplant* 22(2):88-117.

Vajó, J. 1996. *Náhle angiochirurgické príhody a akútny ischemicko - reperfúzny syndróm v klinickej praxi Košice.* Košice: TypoPress Košice. [*Sudden angiosurgical events and acute ischemia - reperfusion syndrome in clinical practice.* Košice: TypoPress Košice.]

Zanow, J., Kruger, U., Scholz, M. 2006. "Proximalization of the arterial inflow: a new technique to treat access- related ischemia." *J Vasc Surg* 43:1216-21.

Šinák, I., Baláž, P., Zeleňák, K. 2017. "Aneuryzmy arteriovenóznych fistúl pre dialýzu." in *Atlas vaskulárnych aneurzyziem* edited by Mazuch, J. et al., 269-277. Turany: P+M, grafické štúdio. ["Aneurysms of arteriovenous fistulas for dialysis." in *The atlas of vascular aneurysms* edited by Mazuch, J. et al., 269-277. Turany: P + M, graphic studio.]

Slezaková, Z. et al. 2020. *Ošetrovateľstvo a legislatíva v praxi*. Martin: Osveta. [*Nursing and legislation in practice.* Martin: Osveta.]

Slezaková, Z. Solgajova, A Zrubcová D. 2020. *Ošetrovateľstvo a konceptuálne modely pre prax.* Nitra: UKF Nitra. [*Nursing and conceptual models for practicing*. Nitra: UKF Nitra.]

In: Surgeon´s Perspective on Dialysis Patient ISBN: 978-1-53619-262-9
Editor: Maria Frankovicova

Chapter 8

LONG-TERM CENTRAL VENOUS ACCESS – PERMCATH

J. Pobehová [*]
Department of Vascular Surgery,
East Slovak Institute of Cardiovascular Diseases

ABSTRACT

Long-term central venous access means the introduction of a catheter into the lumen of a vein. Central vein cannulation is also vital in acute life-saving conditions. The permanent catheter is inserted into the superior or inferior vena cava. The most commonly used access paths are subclavian vein, internal jugular vein, external jugular vein. Access path via the femoral vein is associated with a higher incidence of complications.

Keywords: long-term central venous access, subclavian vein, internal jugular vein, deep femoral vein, infection, malfunction

[*] Corresponding Author's E-mail: jana.pastvova@post.cz.

ABBREVIATIONS

ATB	antibiotics
AVF	arteriovenous fistula
CVC	central venous catheter
CT	computed tomography
EJV	external jugular vein
HD	hemodialysis
IJV	internal jugular vein
USG	ultrasound
VS	venous system
VUSCH	East Slovak Institute of Cardiovascular Diseases

Long-term central venous access means the introduction of a catheter into the lumen of a vein. The venous system is divided into the peripheral VS and the central VS. It can be accessed by percutaneous puncture, or surgically, i.e., by vein preparation. Upper and lower limb vein punctures are the simplest and most secure technique for both blood collection and drug delivery as well as infusion therapy. Central vein cannulation is also vital in acute life-saving conditions. In the past, venesection (vein preparation) was performed more frequently than today. However, it was associated with a higher risk of complications. The choice of puncture type is made according to the acute clinical condition of the patient, the therapy currently required, the condition and topographic conditions of the veins as well as the physician's experience.

An adequately functioning vascular access for dialysis should ensure sufficient blood flow - optimally more than 300 ml/min for dialysis to be effective. Nowadays, high-flow central venous catheters (CVCs) are available to ensure higher values without problems. When selecting a catheter, it is necessary to proceed on an individual basis, to assess the constitution of the patient and the duration for which the catheter will be placed in the vein. In the event of acute failure, the introduction of CVC is essential. Acute catheters are also used to measure central pressure, drug delivery, infusion. They are stiffer, with a conical tip, and can be replaced along the conductor.

The permanent catheter is inserted into the superior or inferior vena cava. The most commonly used access paths are subclavian vein, internal jugular vein, external jugular vein. Access path via the femoral vein is associated with a higher incidence of complications (phlebothrombosis, sepsis, pulmonary embolism). Up to 4% of lethality is reported in the literature.

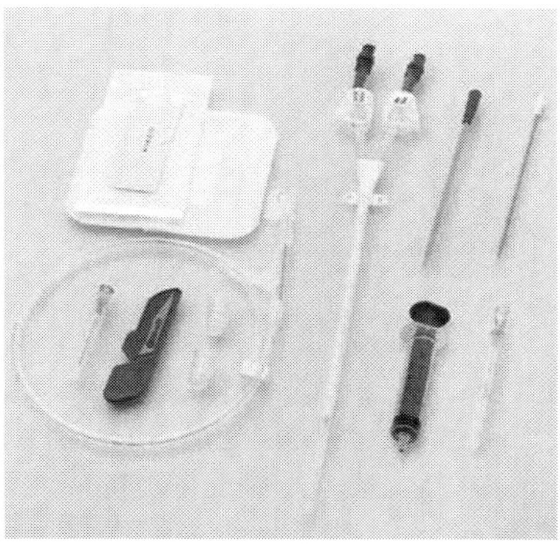

(Source: Department of Vascular Surgery, VÚSCH, a.s.)

Figure 1. Permanent/tunneled catheter set for insertion into the central vein.

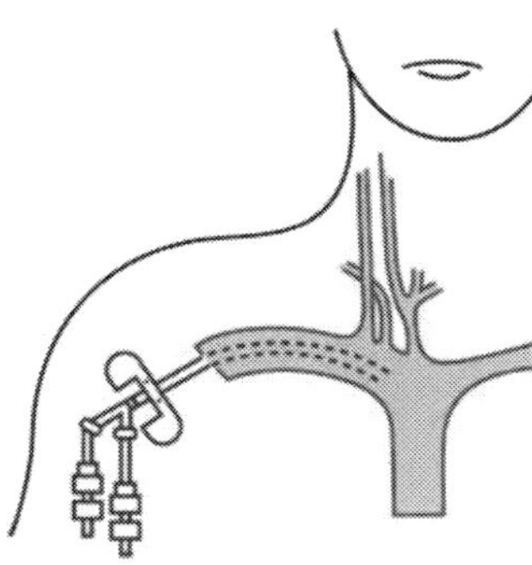

(Source: Department of Vascular Surgery, VÚSCH, a.s.)

Figure 2. Catheter introduced into the right subclavian vein.

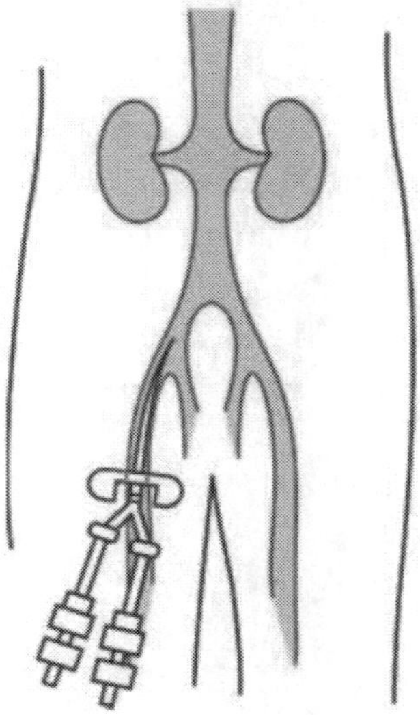

(Source: Department of Vascular Surgery, VÚSCH, a.s.)

Figure 3. Catheter introduced in the right femoral vein.

Central venous catheters (CVCs) are now commonplace for hemodialysis and complement the possibility of peripheral vascular access. Their use began in the 1960s. In 1961, Stanley Shaldon was the first person to have used access via the femoral vessel (Figure 3). In former Czechoslovakia, routine catheters were introduced by prof. Josef Erben into the subclavian vein (Figure 2).

Today these catheters are considered a necessary evil (Figure 1). Their use is when compared to peripheral accesses, associated with higher mortality, higher risk of infection and other complications. In normal practice, however, they cannot be completely avoided. These are, for example, cases of acute or chronic renal failure. In many cases, catheters are used to overcome a period in which peripheral access or another method of renal replacement has failed. The population is aging, patients are polymorbid, often a CVC is the only and definite possibility of long-term vascular access that ensures sufficient blood flow. A frequent reason for the introduction of a catheter is the impossibility of suturing AV fistula due to cardiac insufficiency, poor vascular condition, generally poor condition of the patient, or his poor medical prognosis. Therefore, despite all efforts, the introduction of a catheter is often a life-saving choice.

TYPES OF CATHETERS

CVCs can be classified into two basic types:

1. Acute (non-tunneled) - use for days to weeks
2. Chronic (tunneled with cuff - a barrier to infection) - use for months to years

Catheters are two-way. The arterial line (red) draws blood to the extracorporeal circulation, the venous line (blue) returns the blood back to the bloodstream (Figure 4). They are introduced into the large central veins, optimally into the internal jugular vein. The catheter tip should be located in the right atrium. In the case of an introduction into the femoral vein, the catheter should interfere with the inferior vena cava.

In recent years, there has been a significant shift in the effort to produce an "ideal catheter" that should be: easy to be inserted and removed, cheap, without the risk of infection and fibrin attack, and should not cause venous stenoses and thromboses. It should achieve sufficient blood flow, be acceptable, and pleasant to the patient.

(Source: Department of Vascular Surgery, VÚSCH, a.s.)

Figure 4. Permanent tunneled catheter.

Table 1. Advantages/disadvantages of CVC

Advantages	Disadvantages
Possibility of re-introduction into selected central veins for most patients	High morbidity and mortality of CVC patients
Universal use immediately after the introduction	Common complications - infections and thromboses
Easy replacement	Risk of stenosis or thrombosis of central veins
Usable for several weeks to years	Lower flow rate than AVF
No need for needles and repeated punctures	Limited catheter life
Easy to use, painless connection	Uncomfortable for the patient/aesthetic problem
Low deployment and replacement costs	
Absence of hemodynamic consequences (cardiopulmonary recirculation and hyperkinetic circulation)	
The relatively easy solution of thrombotic complications	
Possible catheter repair without replacement	

There are catheters of various length, luminosity, they differ in construction, design, the material used. They can be two-way, three-way, straight, pre-curved (which reduces the risk of kinking at the site of insertion). The tip of the catheter may be symmetrical with perforations, steppedly terminated. Sometimes the catheter is divided into two separate splits. The development of new catheters is driven by an effort to achieve maximum flow rate with low recirculation and minimization of possible complications. High demands are placed on the material used. It should be biocompatible, flexible, chemically neutral, not influenced by administered drugs, long-term usable, and resistant to chemical disinfectants. The traditional material is a polyurethane, where greater rigidity allows the introduction by the Seldinger technique along the conductor. Silicone is used for the production of tunneled catheters and has a longer lifetime. The material is more flexible and softer. Therefore, it is made with a larger diameter, the walls are thicker to avoid kinking and dysfunction. In order to prevent an increase in the number of infectious complications, catheters are coated with an antimicrobial or antiseptic agent. Heparin-coated catheters are produced to prevent thrombosis. Efficacy has been demonstrated in several studies. Last but not least, the possibilities and habits of the workplace, as well as economic factors all, play a role in the selection of the catheter.

INTRODUCTION OF THE CATHETER

Indication for the introduction is a primarily chronic renal failure if the patient is without a sutured AVF, the so-called "street" suturing, or the native AVF has not yet matured and this period needs to be overcome. Last but not least, the number of patients, in whom fistula formation is primarily excluded due to co-morbidity (cardiac failure, diabetes, arterial sclerosis, venous insufficiency), is still on the rise.

Another indication is the failure of the current vascular access (thrombosis, stenosis, infection) and a catheter is the only solution. Complications can take days, weeks, or even months to resolve. Therefore, the correct catheter type should be selected. We use tunneled cuff if its use is longer than 7-10 days. Indication of catheter insertion is also the need for extracorporeal hemofiltration therapy in intoxication, plasmapheresis, and temporarily after kidney transplantation. It also happens that the patient rejects the fistula and demands the introduction of a catheter, in spite of being informed of the possible risks and complications.

The decision which vein to catheterize is very individual. The most commonly used vein is the internal jugular vein (IJV) on the right side (Figure 5). It is easily accessible and there is a relatively direct entrance to the right atrium when introduced. The introduction in the IJV on the left side is more complicated, where two curves lead to the right atrium. In the case of thrombosis or stenosis of IJV, the external jugular vein (EJV) can also be used. If the catheter is not a definitive solution and maturation of the AV fistula is pending, it is necessary to introduce it to the contralateral side. Deployment onto the femoral vein is particularly at risk for infectious complications in obese patients. The subclavian vein should be catheterized only exceptionally because of stenosis of the central venous bed. When all options are exhausted, it is possible to introduce the catheter into the inferior vena cava via a translumbar access in collaboration with interventional radiology specialists.

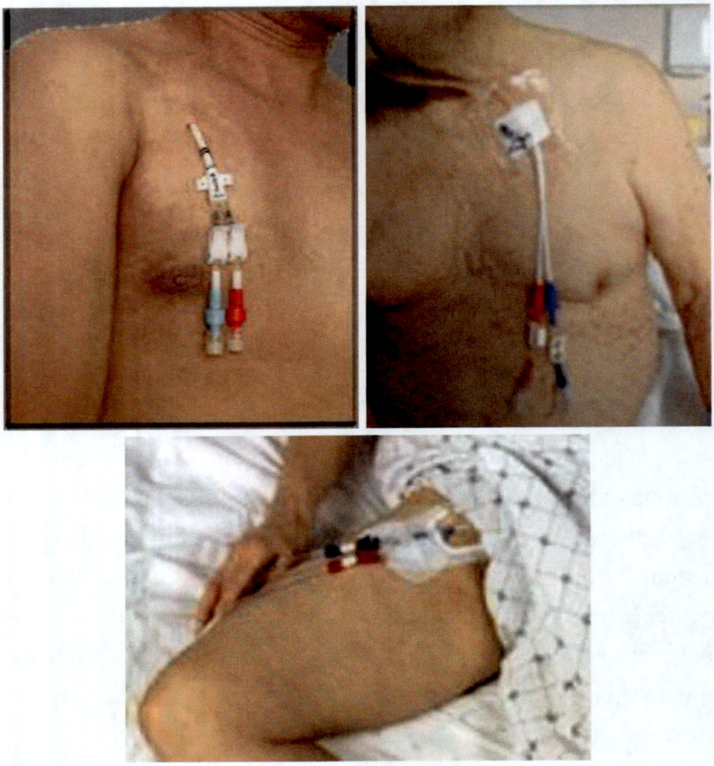

Figure 5. (a) catheter in IJV on the right
(b) catheter in IJV on the left
(c) catheter in the femoral vein on the right (Source: Department of Vascular Surgery, VÚSCH, a.s.).

PREOPERATIVE EXAMINATIONS

The medical history should focus on previous catheterizations, surgeries, and injuries at the site of the planned insertion. Attention should also be paid to allergies and the use of anticoagulants. In patients with a pacemaker, the catheter should be inserted on the contralateral side to avoid damaging the device.

A physical examination can reveal scars, deformities, skin infections. Significant collaterals on the front of the chest or signs of inferior vena cava syndrome may be indicative of poor truncus brachiocephalicus patency.

The most important role is played by imaging methods, especially the USG examination, which will show the patency of the vein, its course, and topographic conditions. In the case of repeated or unsuccessful catheterizations, CT venography or phlebography should be added.

Coagulation parameters should be checked at each examination.

CATHETERIZATION

Catheterization is an invasive procedure with some risks. It begins with the preparation of the surgical field, disinfection, and bandaging. During IJV cannulation the patient is in the Trendelenburg position, the puncture should always be performed under sonographic control (Figure 6). The vein is punctured by the catheter needle during continuous aspiration. Through the lumen of the needle, we insert the conductor, pull the needle out, and the conductor remains in the vein. Along the conductor, introduce a dilatator to relax the subcutaneous tissue (not always necessary). After dilatation, a selected catheter is inserted through the conductor. It is advantageous to use fluoroscopy in which the position of the conductor and the definitive position of the catheter tip are verified.

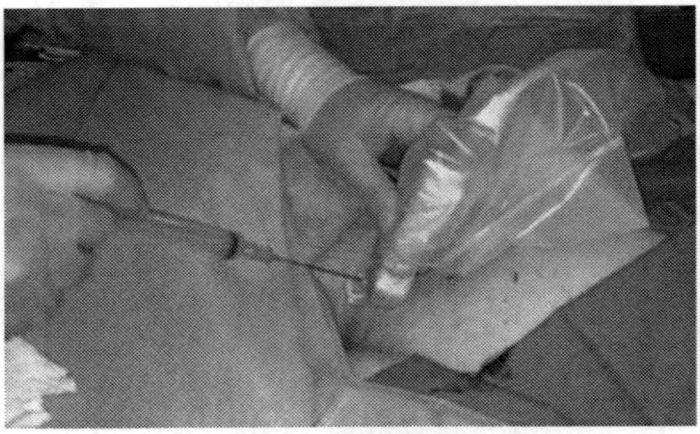

(Source: Department of Vascular Surgery, VÚSCH, a.s.)

Figure 6. Puncture of the vein under sonographic control.

Introduction of a Permanent Catheter According to the Seldinger Technique

The puncture area must be shaved over a large area, the skin must be degreased, disinfected, the puncture area should be wrapped with sterile drapes, sterile gloves, and clothing should be worn during puncture.

In this method, the catheter is inserted through a flexible metallic conductor inserted into the vessel via a puncture needle, percutaneous puncture, or vessel preparation. In this technique, adherence to the principles of asepsis and antisepsis is essential. A metallic conductor or catheter should not come into contact with non-disinfected skin.

The Subclavian Vein and the Innominate Vein

The most commonly used method is an infraclavicular puncture in the subclavian vein, possibly in the innominate vein, that was first carried out in 1952 by Aubaniac.

The subclavian vein is a continuation of the axillary vein, extending in the arch between the first rib and the clavicle through the pleural vault and separates in the area of m. scalenus anterior from the more dorsal and cranial a. subclavia. It connects to the internal jugular vein at about the height of the sternoclavicular articulation with the innominate vein (the brachiocephalic vein). Distance between the left subclavian vein and superior vena cava is 3 times greater than the distance between the right subclavian vein and superior vena cava. At this location, mechanical irritation upon insertion of the catheter, as well as the risk of injury to the ductus thoracicus, is likely to occur, so it is better to puncture the right side. Venous punctures near the heart have the advantage of having a constant wide lumen of 20 mm and a mediastinal fibrous attachment that allows puncture even in the conditions of severe shock. The possibility of damage to adjacent structures is 1-2%, the incidence of erroneous punctures depends on the experience of the doctor, ranging from 5-30%. The risk of thrombophlebitis is 0.4-1.2%.

The Subclavian Vein

Cannulation can be accomplished via several access routes: the supra/ infraclavicular access. The infraclavicular access described by Aubaniac in 1952 and Wilson in 1962 became more prominent. The supraclavicular access according to Yoff (1965) is done in the Trendelenburg position, punctured at an angle between the clavicle and the clavicular attachment of the sternocleidomastoid muscle. The angle of the needle to the skin surface is from 15-20°. The disadvantage of this technique is damage caused to the pleura.

The infraclavicular access is performed in the Trendelenburg position with the head slightly turned to the opposite side. Inferior support of the nape will lower the shoulders dorsally. The puncture region lies in the middle of the clavicle, the puncture is directed towards the upper edge of the sternoclavicular joint and runs tangentially to the pleural vault. Some prefer puncture in the sulcus between the clavicle and the first rib. The angle of the needle to the chest surface is about 30°, although it depends on the body’s constitution. During puncture, the cannula remains in continuous contact with the lower edge of the clavicle. It is necessary to aspire continuously! Maximally after 2-6 cm we reach the subclavian vein and aspirate venous. We insert the catheter in the range of 12-20 cm. The left subclavian vein is 3 times longer than the right one.

When introducing a catheter for long-term use, the procedure is more extensive and invasive. The procedure for puncture and insertion of the conductor is the same, but it is necessary to make an incision on the skin 3-5 cm from the conductor, to dissect the subcutis at the site of the presumed top of the subcutaneous tunnel.

After the measurement, a 1-2 cm incision (cuff width) is made at the site of the presumed ex-site of the catheter at the front of the chest (Figure 7).

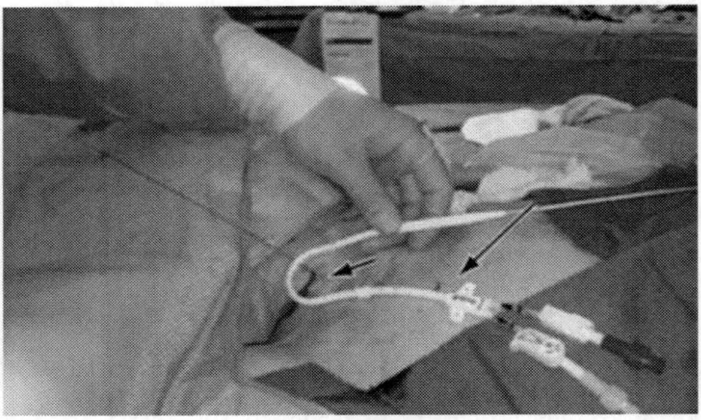

(Source: Department of Vascular Surgery, VÚSCH, a.s.)

Figure 7. Measurement and proper placement of the catheter.

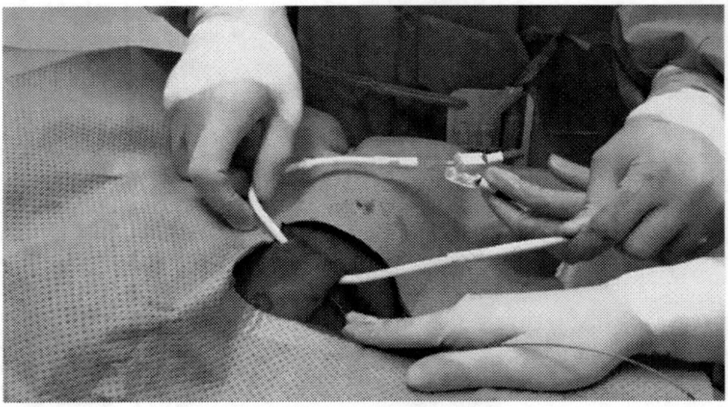

(Source: Department of Vascular Surgery, VÚSCH, a.s.)

Figure 8. Subcutaneous tunneling.

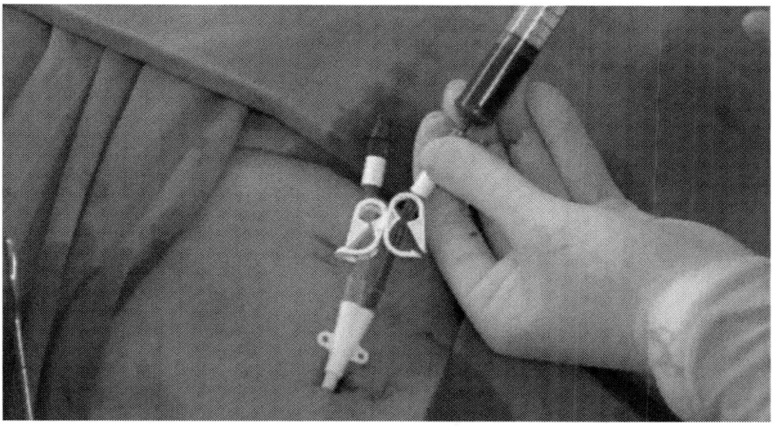

(Source: Department of Vascular Surgery, VÚSCH, a.s.)

Figure 9. Aspiration of both arms of the catheter after its correct insertion.

This place is a catheter with a cuff that has a steel inserter mounted on its tip, extending under the skin and led out at the site of the dissected subcutaneous tissue. The tunnel must be created gently and carefully, as contusions, bleeding and the resulting hematoma are a risk factor for the development of infection (Figure 8).

Along the conductor, a dilator with a breakable sleeve is inserted, and, after its removal, a catheter is inserted into the dilatator. Sleeves with a safety flap reduce the risk of air embolism. After breaking the sleeve, its two upper parts are removed and only the catheter itself remains *in situ*. The course of its storage should be smooth, without breaking. A gentler procedure is without the use of a dilatator when after a slight dilatation of the subcutaneous skin the catheter is inserted directly in the conductor. Check the functionality with a syringe - aspiration and blood return should be without resistance (Figure 9).

If this is not the case, the position of the catheter should be adjusted. Subsequently, both lines are flushed with saline and heparin plugs are applied to the end parts. The skin above the arch is sutured and the catheter is fixed with stitches at the outlet. After the procedure, the patient remains under the supervision of the nursing staff. We monitor pulse and blood pressure. X-ray examination of the chest follows at least 5 hours post-op displays the catheter and reveals a potential complication at injection (pneumothorax, hemothorax) (Figure 10, 11).

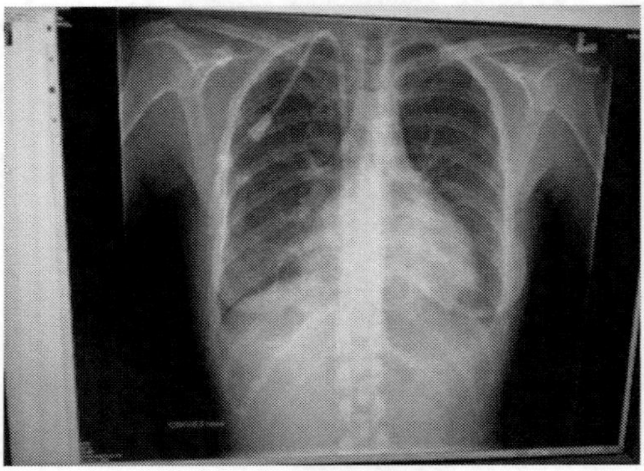

(Source: Department of Vascular Surgery, VÚSCH, a.s.)

Figure 10. Chest X-ray after catheter insertion.

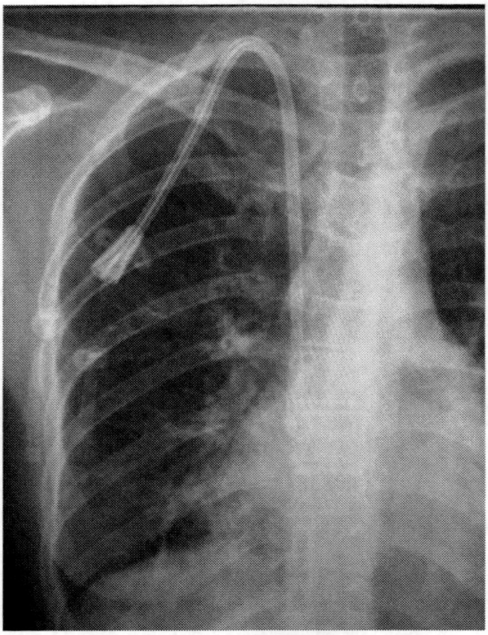

(Source: Department of Vascular Surgery, VÚSCH, a.s.)

Figure 11. Chest X-ray (detail to verify the correct catheter position).

Catheterization of the Femoral Vein

The femoral vein is easily accessible. After you feel the pulse on the femoral artery, puncture the vein that is located medially just below the inguinal ligament (Pouparti). The catheter is inserted along the conductor, deep into the inferior vena cava. This access is more suitable for recumbent patients with limited mobility or when all options are exhausted. During catheterization, the risk of severe soft tissue bleeding without warning symptoms or retroperitoneal bleeding, which may have fatal consequences, should be kept in mind.

The Replacement and Removal of the Tunneled Catheter

Replacements are performed in dysfunction caused by thrombosis, infection. After the catheter is removed, compression is necessary at the catheter entry point into the vein and also in the course of the subcutaneous tunnel. The catheter with the cuff in the subcutaneous tissue is removed surgically, the cuff is removed, the catheter is withdrawn from the vein, which is then compressed. After disinfection, the skin is sutured.

Complications

Acute - arise with interventional power

Chronic - arise when using a catheter

In some cases, complications may occur only after the central catheter is removed.

In recent years, in order to prevent complications, there has been an effort to concentrate patients in specialized centers where a sufficient number of procedures are performed with the necessary equipment (USG, fluoroscopy, vital signs monitoring).

The incidence of complications depends, among other factors, on the choice of the catheterized vein (for example, femoral vein puncture has the lowest number of performance-related complications but has the highest risk of infectious complications). There is also a distinction between temporary and long-term catheters, which have a larger diameter and the complications are related to the long retention time of the catheter. Complications with central venous catheters, especially infections and inadequate flow thromboses, can cause serious complications and death of the patient. In many cases, hospitalization, treatment, and more expensive treatments are required, which increases the cost of treatment.

Acute Complications

These include complications incurred in connection with the procedure, or in the hours following the procedure. Ultrasonographic navigation is used to minimize their incidence, puncture under direct visual control significantly reduces the incidence of periprocedural complications. It is also desirable to perform fluoroscopy during the procedure to check the insertion of the conductor, the catheter, and the direction of the tip.

The most common complication is artery puncture and bleeding, which is solved by a few minutes of compression. Other complications include pneumothorax, hemothorax, hemomediastinum, hemopericardium. Rapid onset of symptoms (tachycardia, dyspnea, hypotension, and others). Further treatment requires cooperation with specialists (vascular surgeon). Others include arrhythmias, up to 42% due to the conductor. They are mostly benign extrasystoles, but they can also be more severe supraventricular tachycardia or persistent ventricular tachycardia. Therefore, the catheter should be pulled out and treatment for arrhythmia should be initiated. Another serious complication is air embolism. This should be considered in dehydrated patients with negative venous pressure. The risk arises when the catheter is inserted, the dilator is pulled out, and when the breakable sleeve is handled. In this case, it is advisable to cover the opening with the fingertip until the catheter is inserted. If air embolism is suspected (tachycardia, tachypnea, hypoxia, hypotension, cyanosis), the patient should be placed on the left side to prevent air bubbles from penetrating the pulmonary artery. Transport the patient to the room with a mechanical respiratory support option.

Other complications associated with catheter insertion include poor placement of the catheter tip (should extend into the right atrium) or malfunction due to kink or subcutaneous tunnel. This complication can be eliminated with the fluoroscopic monitoring during the implantation. Other uncommon complications are also reported in the literature, such as cardiac arrest, perforation of the superior vena cava, perforation of the right atrium of the heart, and nerve damage at the puncture site.

Chronic Complications

They are related to the length and frequency of catheter use. Dysfunction may occur which does not allow sufficient dialysis. This is defined as the inability to achieve an extracorporeal flow rate of more than 300 ml/min. with a vacuum of not more than 250 mm Hg. The dysfunction may be caused mechanically, for example by kinking or bending of the catheter, by incorrect tip position, sometimes by patient position. The most common cause of dysfunction is thrombosis, for which it is necessary to remove up to a third of established catheters. Factors of thrombus formation are decreased flow rate (mechanical failure, hypotension, fibrin coating) and venous wall damage. The thrombus may be intraluminal or extend beyond the tip of the catheter and impair the flow of blood to the arterial line through a flap mechanism. In dysfunction and suspected thrombosis, thrombolysis using rtPa (recombinant tissue plasminogen activator) is recommended. It has a good effect and can be used repeatedly. However, it also has contraindications: thrombocytopenia, coagulation disorders, catheter infection, surgery within the last 48 hours.

Central vein stenosis is related to catheter insertion time and catheterization frequency. The incidence is 20-50%, most commonly in the subclavian vein. Stenosis should be considered when developing collateral circulation or limb swelling. The solution of complications belongs in the hands of vascular surgeons or interventional radiology specialists.

The most serious complication is infection. The risk of bacteremia is 7 times higher and the risk of death associated with infection is twice as high in patients with long-term venous catheters as in patients with an AV fistula. Risk factors for infection include advanced age, comorbidity, skin damage, local trauma, insertion site hematoma. In the context of regular use, the risk factor is the length of use of the catheter, the frequency of manipulation, the number of dialyses, the experience of the staff, the observance of good practice and the care of the catheter. The incidence of infectious complications is from 2.5-5.5 episodes/1000 catheter days, or 0.9-2 episodes/patient/year. With temporary catheters, the risk is 2-3 times higher, so it is better to introduce a tunneled catheter with a cuff as soon as possible. The most common agents are Staphylococcus aureus and Staphylococcus epidermidis, which enter into circulation through the catheter, or by careless handling of catheter tips or entrances into the extracorporeal circulation. The infection may be localized outside the catheter - "ex-site" - or it may spread deeper and affect the tunnel. The most serious complication is sepsis. Bacteremia also causes a high percentage of metastatic involvement: endocarditis, septic arthritis, vertebrate abscess, intervertebral disc inflammation.

Treatment depends on the severity of the disability. Systemic antibiotic administration and follow-up should be considered individually.

In severe infections and their metastatic spread, immediate removal of the catheter is required, and a new catheter is introduced after 48 hours. We treat the patient with antibiotics according to sensitivity for at least 3 weeks. If no other vein is available, make the catheter replacement along the conductor with a newly created tunnel. In individual cases, it is possible to attempt to "rescue" the catheter by targeted antibiotic therapy, including using an antibiotic solution instead of a heparin plug. If the clinical picture does not improve and positive blood cultures persist for another 48-72 hours, the catheter should be removed.

To prevent infection, the catheter must be placed under strictly sterile conditions, and subsequent care and handling must be done using an aseptic technique. Regular monitoring is important, especially the catheter orifice, and treatment must be started at the first signs of redness or secretion. The reduction in the number of infectious complications in the use of antibiotic coated dialysis catheters has not been thus far confirmed. Randomized studies have not shown benefit in prophylactic antibiotics. The best prevention of infection remains to minimize the use of central venous catheters for dialysis.

Mechanical damage to the catheter (rupture, breakage, incision with a sharp object) may cause bleeding, embolism, or require replacement of the catheter. Catheter replacement is not necessary if the end parts are damaged. They can be replaced.

CATHETER CARE

The catheter should be dealt with in compliance with asepsis rules. The place of outlet should be covered in a sterile manner and regularly checked during each dialysis session. It is important to instruct the patient about the need to follow increased hygiene measures, as well as not to touch the bandage. ATB ointment should be applied after catheter insertion, long-term administration may, however, lead to resistance and increase the risk of infectious complications. Each dialysis center should have a precise procedure on how to deal with the catheter. Silicone catheters are damaged by iodine-based disinfectants while well compatible with alcohol and ointments. In contrast, polyurethane may be damaged by ATB ointments.

The catheter plugs on both arms are filled with a solution with anticoagulant and antimicrobial properties. When administering a plug with a high concentration of the antimicrobial agent, the risk of passing part of the agent into the patient's bloodstream should be considered. 15-25% pass into the bloodstream.

In spite of all the recommendations of professional societies and despite the known risks, the number of patients with established catheters does not decrease. An increasing number of patients are starting HD therapy with a catheter and the number of those for whom the catheter is the only access is increasing. The upward trend is thus proof that it is not possible to avoid them, and, thanks to their existence, we are able to provide adequate treatment in acute cases and save lives. The ideal catheter does not exist, but from a wide range, we can individually select one for any given patient. Further developments in the field of catheters can be envisioned. The new materials will be less thrombogenic, more biocompatible, constitutionally superior, but nevertheless, catheters will remain the least suitable long-term access. The situation could be changed by inventing a new type of vascular access, possibly by another technology of renal replacement.

REFERENCES

Chytilová, E. a kol. (2015). *Cévní prístupy pro hemodialýzu.* Praha: Mladá fronta. [*Vascular approaches for hemodialysis.* Prague: Mladá fronta.].

Erben, J., et al. (1969). "Experience with routine use of subclavian vein cannulation in a hemodialysis." *Proc EDTA*, *6*, 59.

Bernadič, M., et al. (2003). "Transformation of the system of education in health care services." *Bratisl Lek Listy*, *104*(11), 367-368.

Trerotola, S. (2000). "Hemodialysis Catheter Placement and Management." *Radiology*, *215*(3), 651-658.

2006. K/DOQI Clinical Practice Guidlines and Clinical Practice Recommendations 2006 Updates Vascular Access. *Am J Kidney Dis*, *48*(Suppl), S176-322.

Bernadič, M., et al. (1985). "The orthogonal electrocardiogram in rabbits after long-term adaptation of the heart to volume overload." *Bratisl Lek Listy*, *84*(6), 683-692.

Rocha, A. (2012). "New tunneled hemodialysis catheter placement preserving the vasculature." *J Vasc Access*, *13*(1), 108-110.

Zavacká, M. & Pobehová, J. (2018). "Aneurysm and pseudoaneurysm arteria carotis interna in our clinical material." *Lekarsky Obzor*, *7*, 32-38.

Vanholder, R., et al. (2010). "Diagnosis, prevention and treatement of haemodialysis catheter-related bloodstream infections: a position statement of European Renal Best Practice." *NDT Plus*, *3*, 234-246.

Niyyar, V. D. (2012). "Catheter dysfunction: the role of lock solutions." *Sem Dial*, *25*, 693-699.

Galloway, S., et al. (2004). "Long-term central venous Access." *BJA*, *92*(5), 722-734.

Zavacká, M. & Dvorožňáková, M. (2018). "Acute limb ischemia: Theory and practice in vascular surgery." *Lekarsky Obzor*, *4*, 22-29.

Gašparec, P., et al. (2009). *Cievne prístupy.* Martin: Osveta. [*Vascular approaches*. Martin: Osveta].

Fissel, R. B., et al. (2006). "Hemodialysis patient prevence for type of vascular Access: variation and predictors across contries in the DOPPS." *J Vasc Access Am J Kidney Dis*, *48*(Suppl.), 264-272.

In: Surgeon´s Perspective on Dialysis Patient ISBN: 978-1-53619-262-9
Editor: Maria Frankovicova

Chapter 9

REPEATED FORMATION OF AN ARTERIOVENOUS CONNECTION

Norbert Torma*, MD
Angiosurgical department of Medical faculty of Safarik University, Košice, Slovakia

ABSTRACT

Patients with chronic kidney disease, where kidney functions are significantly impaired and progress to end stage kidney failure, may require dialysis. There are different types of dialysis, one of which is hemodialysis.

There are three primary methods of establishing vascular access for hemodialysis purposes. Clinical monitoring of AV fistulas, outside and during hemodialysis, can detect AV fistula dysfunction in a timely manner and thus can timely prepare SAVF formation. Any patient with a dysfunctional or non-functional native AV fistula, or with an AV fistula using a prosthesis, is a candidate for SAVF. AV shunt should be monitored at least once a month during hemodialysis and in patients with AV failure SAVF should be considered as the first option for any patient in whom AV fistula has failed.

---

* Corresponding Author's E-mail: norko@post.sk.

Keywords: AV access, AV fistula, AV graft, central venous catheter, secondary AV fistula

ABBREVIATIONS

AV	arteriovenous
AVF	arteriovenous fistula
AVG	arteriovenous graft
SAVF	secondary AV fistula
FFBI	Fistula First Breakthrough Initiative
KDOQI	Kidney Disease Outcomes Quality Initiative
NKF-KDOQI	National Kidney Foundation- Kidney Disease Outcomes Quality
USG	ultrasound

INTRODUCTION

Considering all the options for the dialysis of the patient, the arteriovenous shunt (fistula) is the most suitable. Its advantage over other dialysis options, such as a catheter or peritoneal dialysis, lies in its higher and longer functionality with the need for less intervention and lower mortality and morbidity. The incidence of infectious complications in native AV fistulas is low. Risk factors for infection in native AV fistulas include pseudoaneurysm, hematoma, itching, and scratching of the puncture site, as well as the use of AV fistula in drug addicts.

SECONDARY ACCESS OPTIONS

According to the Fistula First Breakthrough Initiative (FFBI), access via the AV fistula should be the primary choice for a patient in need of dialysis. Despite these recommendations, especially in the United States, nearly 30% of patients have a primary AV fistula using a prosthesis. If an AV fistula with a graft fails, the formation of a native AV fistula should also be considered as the first option in these patients. Currently, secondary AV fistulas are divided into two groups. They are either fistulas using a venous outflow system above the original, non-functional AV fistula (secondary AV fistula - SAVF type I), or another venous outflow system (SAVF type II).

SAVF type I is possible mainly in patients with a primary AV fistula on the forearms. The venous system above the original AV fistula is slightly dilated and partially matured. Most patients are suitable for this type of SAVF. They are either primary patients with a native AV fistula or patients with an artificial prosthesis using the loop technique. In an angiographic examination, the venous brachial system is preserved in almost half of the patients using an artificial prosthesis and is therefore usable for SAVF type I. In cases where it is impossible to create SAVF type I, another option is SAVF type II. Candidates for SAVF type II are also patients with unsuccessful angioplasty, stent implants, stent-grafts in the outflow, the especially central venous system, or with a hypoplastic venous system. SAVF type II is often preferred over repeated interventions in the area of the AV fistula itself or by the inflow and outflow bloodstream. The principles of SAVF formation are the same as for primary AV fistulas. Especially before the planning of the SAVF type II, however, a more precise mapping of the venous system on the other limb is performed to create a new planned AV fistula.

Any patient with a dysfunctional or non-functional native AV fistula, or with an AV fistula using a prosthesis, is a candidate for SAVF. SAVF is the first choice over other methods of hemodialysis. In case of malfunction of AV fistula using a prosthesis, the first choice is a new SAVF without the use of a prosthesis. If the primary AV fistula with the prosthesis is fully functional, without complications, it is never indicated for conversion to a native SAVF.

AV fistula dysfunction often occurs abruptly. In the case of experiments and interventions (angioplasty, stent, stent-graft), which often improve the function of the AV fistula only for a short period, it is always necessary to consider the possibility of later SAVF creation. Therefore, interventions, especially on the outflow tract, should be gentle so as not to "consume" the veins for a later SAVF.

SAVF also takes precedence over reckless and hasty implantation of catheters.

SAVF should be considered by a medical specialist at the first sign of dysfunction of the currently used AV fistula.

Clinical monitoring of AV fistulas, outside and during hemodialysis, can detect AV fistula dysfunction in a timely manner and thus can timely prepare SAVF formation.

Also, early USG examination of the outflow venous tract provides more information about its condition while the flow through the AV fistula and venous system is still dilated.

According to the Fistula First Breakthrough Initiative (FFBI) Change Concept, the outflow tract of the prosthetic AV shunt should be monitored at least once a month during hemodialysis and patients who should have SAVF put in place should be selected timely. According to the 2006 National Kidney Foundation's Kidney Disease Outcomes Quality Initiative (NKF-K/DOQI) Clinical Practice and the 2008 Society for Vascular Surgery Guidelines, SAVF should be considered as the first option for any patient in whom AV fistula has failed. In patients unsuitable for SAVF I, both the arterial and the venous streams should be considered for the suitability of SAVF II by USG examination and, if necessary, by angiography.

EXAMINATION BEFORE SAVF

In SAVF I, the venous system is dilated and better suited to form a SAVF compared to a limb where there was previously no AV fistula. It is possible to use the cephalic or the basilic vein above the site of the original AV fistula to form SAVF type I. If neither of them is adequate to form an AV fistula, other veins meeting the criteria for a new AV fistula may be used. Echo mapping and evaluation of the condition of the arterial and venous streams must be performed. Before developing secondary dialysis access, the overall health condition of the patient must also be considered. Most patients with kidney failure are elderly who are also polymorbid. The main comorbidities are diabetes mellitus and cardiovascular disease.

According to the New York Heart Association functional classification (NYHA I to IV) and the American College of Cardiology Foundation/American Heart Association stages of heart failure (ACC/AHA stages A to D), in patients with heart failure stage C, or D and class III and IV, catheter access only is indicated for hemodialysis. In patients with stage C and classes I and II, radiocephalic AV fistula is indicated. AV fistulas deposited higher with increased flow place high demands on the heart and so their implementation should be carefully considered, as well as the possibility of other accesses. Survival-limiting diseases (e.g., malignancy) also influence the choice of secondary access for dialysis. Furthermore, previous operations on the vascular system also affect the secondary access options for dialysis. Wounds in the neck and chest can damage the vascular system after previous injuries. Likewise, attempts to introduce central catheters at other dialysis sites may limit the choice of secondary access for dialysis. A chest X-ray is also a part of the examination before the SAVF creation. Even in the case of stenosis of the central venous system, swelling of the limb may not be present. Also, stenosis may not be manifested by the presence of a dilated collateral subcutaneous vein system. The thoracic central venous system (TCVS - from (C7 to T1) includes the intrathoracic segment IJV (the internal jugular vein), the subclavian vein (SV), the brachiocephalic veins (BV), superior vena cava (SVC) and the suprahepatic part of the inferior vena cava. TCVS reflects the degree of damage to the venous system (Table 1). At stage 1 and 2, there may be no clinical signs of venous system obstruction, and an attempt to form SAVF results in failure of fistula maturation.

TCVS anomaly may not be detected on the USG examination of both the arterial and venous systems. The central part of SV, BV, and SVC does not have to be shown by the USG at all.

Table 1. Types of obstruction of the central thoracic venous system

Type	Description
I	One of the IJV or SV is obliterated
II	Unilateral obstruction of the BV, or ipsilateral obstruction of the IJV and SV
III	Both BV closed, SVC functional
IV	SVC obstruction, regardless of the status of other TCVS

Possible stenoses and obliterations of these veins can be detected indirectly on the IJV and SV by changing the phases of blood flow during respiration and by changing the heart rate. In these patients, the gold standard is a phlebographic examination - CT phlebography, MR phlebography.

Echomapping is also important in the examination of the arterial and venous systems. Most of the changes and difficulties are caused by the venous system. Examination of the arterial system includes a clinical examination of the pulses, measurement of pressure, and, if necessary, measurement of the pressure difference between the upper limbs, Allen's test, and subsequent USG examination. Examination of the venous system, especially the USG examination, where the course of veins and their diameter and distensibility are determined.

If it is not possible to implement SAVF type I, then SAVF type II is implemented in case of suitable conditions on the limb. (Figure 1) Most patients with SAVF do not require catheter insertion for HD (hemodialysis).

The overall functionality of SAVF is lower than in primary AV fistulas, although the two groups of patients are completely different. In the group of patients with SAVF, each patient had already failed vascular access at least once. Therefore, the primary and secondary functionality is lower in this group. When comparing SAVF type I and SAVF type II, the results are better for SAVF type I. The primary and secondary functionality of SAVF type I and type II, at 6 and at 12 months, is 87% vs. 71%, and 14% vs. 11%.

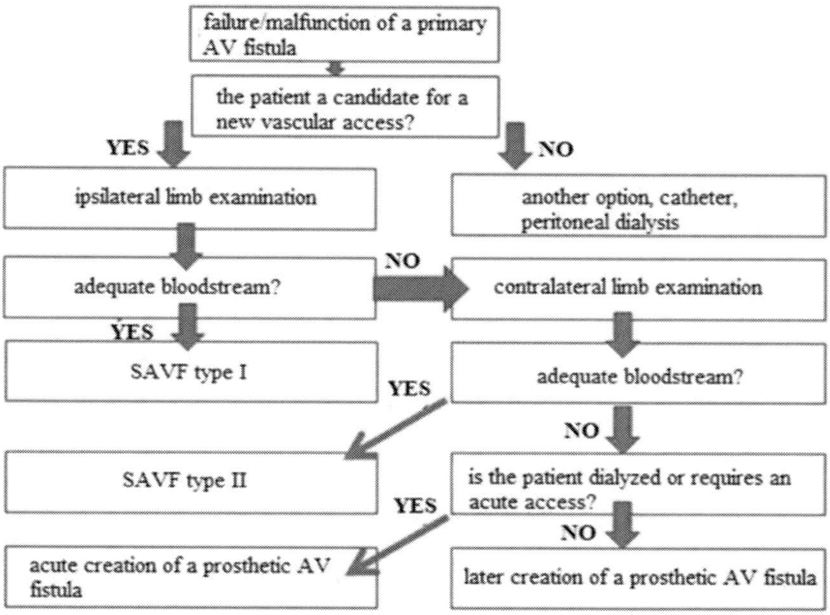

Figure 1. Algorithm for creating secondary access for dialysis.

According to the National Kidney Foundation Kidney Disease Outcomes Quality Initiative (K/DOQI 2006), Canadian Society of Nephrology (2006), European Renal Best Practice (2007) a Kidney Health Australia – Caring for Australasians with Renal Impairment (KHA-CARI 2012), in patients requiring AV access to HD as the first fistula, a radiocephalic fistula should be formed on the forearm. In case of its failure, a radiocephalic and then a radiobasilic native fistula follows. If the venous system is insufficient to form an AV fistula, an AV fistula with a loop-shaped artificial prosthesis on the forearm should be formed. Catheter insertion comes as a last resort.

POSSIBILITIES OF CONSTRUCTION OF AV FISTULAS

There are a large number and variations of fistulas, but the most common are the following: radiocephalic fistula on the forearm, brachiocephalic fistula, and brachiobasilic fistula. The procedure is always to create AV fistulas from the periphery towards the center. The primary fistula is constructed on a non-dominant limb.

A simple, direct AV fistula connects the vein and artery, which remain in their original positions. The distal end of the vein is interrupted and connected to the artery in an end-to-side manner, the end of the cut vein to the incision of the artery wall.

Possible ways of constructing a simple direct AV fistula are:

- hand: AV fistula in fossa tabatiere
- wrist: radiocephalic fistula
- forearm and cubital area: radiocephalic fistula, radiobasilic fistula (often there is a need to transpose the basilic vein), fistula to the median basilic vein, or median antebrachial vein.
- brachium: brachiocephalic
- lower limb: fistula using the great saphenous vein and femoral vein

Transposition leaves the proximal part of the vein in place, but the distal part is moved to the sides or closer under the skin. In this part of the vein, any collateral veins must be tied up and broken. It is also necessary to create a subcutaneous tunnel in which the vein is located. The intervention can be realized in one surgery, or as a two-phase intervention.

The options for vein transposition are:

- Radiocephalic transposition on the wrist in obese patients
- Radiobasilic transposition on the forearm
- Brachiobasilic transposition (transposition of the basilic vein)
- Brachiobrachial transposition
- Brachiocephalic transposition in obese patients
- In the lower limbs – femoro-saphenous and femoro-femoral transposition (in both obese and slim patients)

AV fistula with *translocated vein* - in which the venous section of the vein is transferred to another place and both arteriovenous and venovenous anastomosis are created de novo. The intervention is very similar to the construction of an AV fistula with a prosthesis. Most often, a graft from a great saphenous vein or femoral vein is translocated for the need of the AV fistula.

More about the ways and possibilities of AV fistula formation in Chapter 4 - *External and subcutaneous arteriovenous connections.*

CONCLUSION

When considering all the dialysis options, native AV fistulas have the highest long-term functionality and the least number of complications. These are the method of choice not only as of the primary access to dialysis and HD but also in the case of dysfunction to non-function of the primary AV shunt. Each hemodialysis facility should have a program in place to monitor the functionality of AV fistulas and plan to create a new fistula at the first signs of vascular access dysfunction.

REFERENCES

Huijbregts, H. J., Bots, M. L., Wittens, C. H. et al. 2008. "Hemodialysis arteriovenous fistula patency revisited: Results of a prospective, multicenter initiative". *Clin. J. Am. Soc. Nephrol.,* 3:714 - 9.

Jennings, W. C. 2006. "Creating arteriovenous fistulas in 132 consecutive patients: Exploiting the proximal radial artery arteriovenous fistula: Reliable, safe, and simple forearm and upper arm hemodialysis access". *Arch. Surg.,* 141:27 - 32.

Lynch, J. R., Wasse, H., Armistead, N. C., McClellan, W. M. 2011. "Achieving the goal of the Fistula First breakthrough initiative for

prevalent maintenance hemodialysis patients". *Am. J. Kidney Dis.,* 57:78 - 89.
McClellan, W. M., Wasse, H., McClellan, A. C. et al. 2009. "Treatment center and geographic variability in pre-ESRD care associate with increased mortality". *J. Am. Soc. Nephrol.,* 20:1078 - 86.
Nguyen, V. D., Treat, L., Griffith, C., Robinson, K. 2007. "Creation of secondary AV fistulas from failed hemodialysis grafts: The role of routine vein mapping". *J. Vasc. Access,* 2007; 8:91 - 6.
Oliver, M. J., McCann, R. L., Indridason, O. S. et al. 2001. "Comparison of transposed brachiobasilic fistulas to upper arm grafts and brachiocephalic fistulas". *Kidney Int.,* 60:1532 - 9.
2006. "NKF-K/DOQI Clinical Practice Guidelines for Vascular Access. Clinical Practice Guideline 2: Selection and placement of hemodialysis access, 2.1 the order, 2.1.4. Patients should be considered for the construction of a primary AVF after failure of every dialysis AV access". *Am. J. Kidney Dis.,* 48(Suppl. 1):S248.
Ravani, P., Spergel, L. M., Asif, A. et al. 2007. "Clinical epidemiology of arteriovenous fistula in 2007". *J. Nephrol.,* 20:141 - 9.
Salman, L., Alex, M., Unger, S. W. et al. 2009. "Secondary autogenous arteriovenous fistulas in the "fistula first" era: results of a long-term prospective study". *J. Am. Coll. Surg.,* 209:100 - 9.
Sidawy, A. N., Spergel, L. M., Besarab, A. et al. 2008. "The Society for Vascular Surgery: clinical practice guidelines for the surgical placement and maintenance of arteriovenous hemodialysis access". *J. Vasc. Surg.,* 48:25.

In: Surgeon´s Perspective on Dialysis Patient ISBN: 978-1-53619-262-9
Editor: Maria Frankovicova

Chapter 10

PERITONEAL DIALYSIS

P. Zavacký*, MD
Department of Surgery, Faculty of Medicine, Pavol Jozef Šafárik University in Košice and University Hospital, Košice, Slovakia

ABSTRACT

The essence of PD (peritoneal dialysis) is the exchange of substances between the peritoneal dialysis solution inserted into the peritoneal cavity. The exchange takes place by transport through the peritoneum. PD requires a multidisciplinary approach: a nephrologist, nurses, a surgeon, a dietitian, a social worker, and a pharmacologist, with the patient's connection to the transplant center.

Keywords: peritoneal dialysis, abdominal cavity, peritoneum, peritoneal catheter

* Corresponding Author's E-mail: peterzavacky963@gmail.com.

ABBREVIATIONS

APD	automated peritoneal dialysis
CAPD	continuous ambulatory peritoneal dialysis
CCPD	continuous cyclic peritoneal dialysis
HD	hemodialysis
NIPD	nocturnal intermittent peritoneal dialysis
PD	peritoneal dialysis

HISTORY

The first mention of PD is from 1740 when the English surgeon Christopher Warrich treated a 50-year-old female patient with ascites. He inserted a 1:1 solution of water and red wine into the abdominal cavity through an inserted leather tube. It was used as a rinsing agent with an antibacterial effect. The patient reacted aggressively to the treatment, so the treatment was terminated after 3 procedures.

The first "lege artis" PD was performed in 1923 by the German physician Georg Ganter. He was looking for a substance that removes toxins from the human body and it is not necessary to use an anticoagulant when using it. He prepared a solution of saline, with a normal composition of electrolytes. He added glucose which was supposed to ensure fluid removal. The first patient he treated in this way had suffered from acute renal failure after giving birth. He used 1-3 liters of fluid, which worked for ½-3 hours. Despite the success of the treatment, there was a problem with a safe method of access to the abdominal cavity. Progress did not occur until the year 1952 when A. Grollman developed a new type of catheter that was plastic, flexible, and had small holes at the end that allowed the solution to be filled in and discharged.

ANATOMY

The peritoneum is a thin serous membrane that lines the abdominal cavity and envelopes the organs in it. It is shiny, smooth, its surface is large, it reaches an area of 1.5 - 2.0 m2 (it is as large as the skin). It consists of three layers: on the surface, there is a flat lining of mesothelial cells, located underneath is the interstitium that separates the mesothelial layer from the capillary wall and the third layer is formed by the endothelium of peritoneal capillaries and the membrane of the vascular wall.

The blood supply to the peritoneum is from the mesenteric arteries, the venous blood returns to the portal circulation. The blood flow of the peritoneal stream is 70 - 100 ml/min. The smallest pores in the endothelium of the peritoneum are water-permeable (aquaporins). Larger pores in the interstitium allow small molecules (minerals, urea, creatinine) to pass through. The largest pores, which are of the smallest quantity, are permeable for heavier molecules (beta-2 microglobulins, proteins). Peritoneum permeability increases with peritonitis, resulting in protein loss and lower ultrafiltration ability. The condition resolves after treatment.

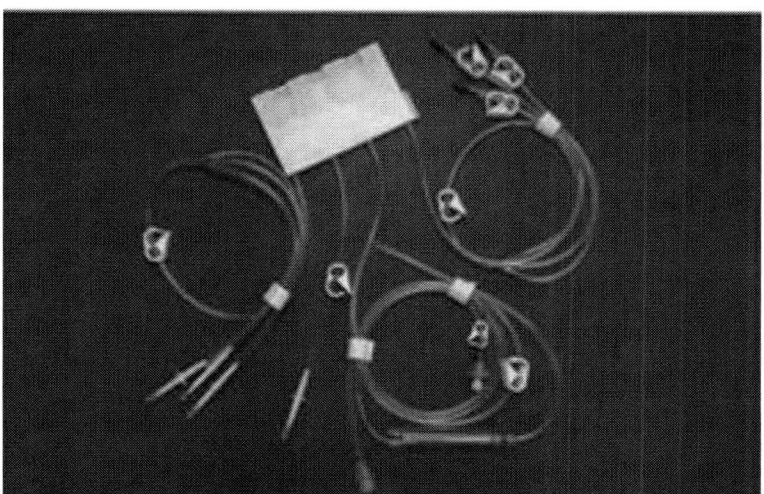

Figure 1. Peritoneal dialysis set (Source: I. Surgical Department UNLP, Košice).

The dialysis solution is injected into the abdominal cavity through a small soft tube, e.g., a Tenckhoff catheter. This solution contains a mixture of minerals and sugars dissolved in water. Sugar - dextrose draws waste products, chemicals, and excess water from the blood vessels of the peritoneal membrane into the dialysis solution. After a few hours, the solution now containing waste products from the blood is drained from the abdomen. The abdomen is then filled with a fresh dialysis solution and the cycle can be repeated. Each change must be done 4-5 times a day. Patients can perform peritoneal dialysis on their own after undergoing training.

TYPES OF PERITONEAL DIALYSIS

There are two main types of peritoneal dialysis: Continuous Ambulatory Peritoneal Dialysis (CAPD) is usually performed during the day and Automated Peritoneal Dialysis (APD), which can be performed at night using a device that fills and empties the abdomen. Both types of peritoneal dialysis can usually be performed by the patients themselves.

Continuous Ambulatory Peritoneal Dialysis (CAPD)

CAPD is the most common type of peritoneal dialysis. It requires no device and can be performed during everyday life. With CAPD, your blood is cleaned continuously. The dialysis solution passes from a plastic bag through a catheter into the abdomen, after sealing the catheter the dialysis solution remains in the abdomen for several hours. You can then drain the dialysis solution back into the bag and discard it. The same catheter can be used to further fill the abdomen with fresh dialysis solution so that the cleansing process can begin again. In CAPD, the dialysis solution remains in the abdomen for 4 to 6 hours (or more). The process of emptying the used dialysis solution and replacing it with a fresh solution takes about 30 to 40 minutes. Replacement should be performed in a clean, well-lit place. Most people change the dialysis solution at least four times a day and sleep with the solution in their abdomen at night. It is not necessary to perform dialysis procedures during the night with CAPD.

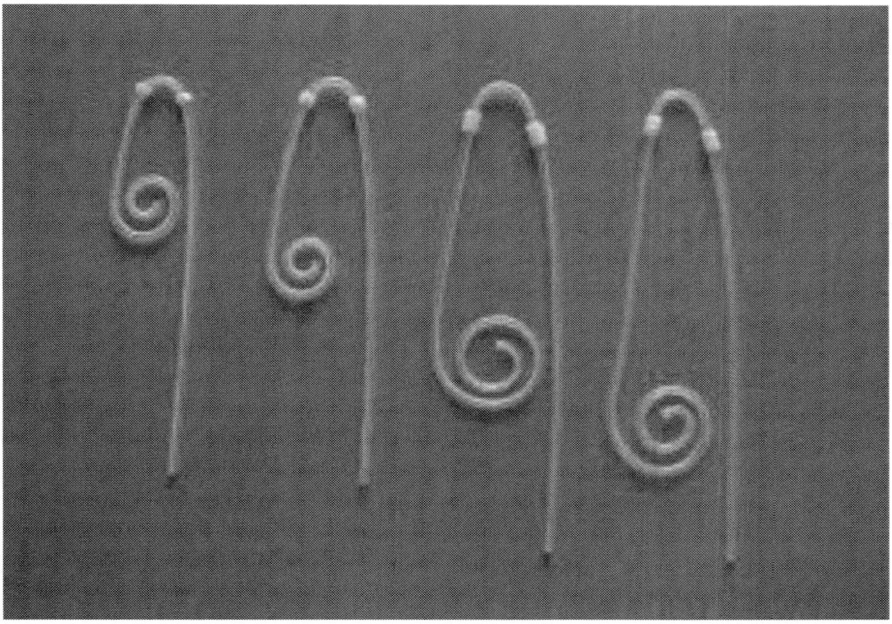

Figure 2. Different types of catheters (Source: I. Surgical Department UNLP, Košice).

Automated Peritoneal Dialysis (APD)

An APD machine called a cycler is used for filling and draining. Filling and emptying of the abdominal cavity occur three to five times during the night. In the morning, the solution is filled in and left inside throughout the day. During this time, patients have the opportunity to perform their daily activities.

A modified form of APD is "PD Plus-therapy," which requires one additional exchange during the day. This type is mainly used in overweight patients or when the peritoneal membrane filters waste products very slowly. If PD Plus therapy is recommended by your doctor, you can use the cycler at night and also make one change during the day. At this time, the cycler can be used as a source of dialysis fluid - if the patient is at home, or you can use the CAPD method. This additional exchange is performed to increase the amount of waste removed and to reduce the amount of fluid remaining in the patient's body.

Peritoneal dialysis is based on the principles of diffusion and osmosis.

Diffusion

Stands for the passage of a substance from a place where its concentration is high (waste substances in the blood) to a place where its concentration is low (peritoneal dialysis solution) through a semipermeable membrane, in our case through the peritoneal membrane to the size of its pores. When the concentration of toxins in the dialysis solution reaches the level of blood toxins, we say that the solution is saturated. This stage is reached after about 4 to 6 hours.

Osmosis

It means the passage of a substance from a place where its concentration is low to a place where its concentration is high across a semipermeable membrane, in our case the peritoneum. This osmotic effect is used in CAPD and is enabled by higher glucose concentrations in the removal of excess water from the blood. The higher the concentration of glucose in the dialysis solution, the more water is excreted from the body. By the action of these two principles, the waste substances up to a certain molecular weight, together with the excess water, pass into the dialysis solution and are then discharged from the abdominal cavity.

The dialysis solution contains osmotically active substances - glucose in various concentrations, when introduced into the peritoneal space, the exchange - diffusion and convection - begins between the plasma and the solution in the abdominal cavity. As soon as the osmotic concentrations equalize (6-8 hours), the ultrafiltration stops, and the effectiveness of PD decreases.

TECHNICAL ASPECTS OF PD

1. Peritoneal dialysis catheter
2. Connector system
3. Bags and sets
4. Peritoneal dialysis solution

The peritoneal catheters provide access to the peritoneal cavity, they are made of 15 cm long silicon rubber, with side holes, they are introduced surgically by mini laparotomy, by puncture.

The catheter has 3 parts: intraperitoneal segment - distal, placed after implantation in the abdominal cavity in the Douglas space, intramural segment - inner, passing through a tunnel in the abdominal wall, the outer segment is connected to the connector system.

The connector system connects the catheter to the dialysis solution. It consists of a titanium adapter and a transfer set. The transfer set has to be changed after peritonitis, every 6 months, the adapter remains permanently. The solution itself is supplied from plastic bags. It consists of two bags, one empty for discharge, and one filled with peritoneal solution, the bags are equipped with a port for drug application and for dialysate collection. The most commonly used solution is glucose in various concentrations (1.3%, 2.27%, 3.86%). The solutions are stable for 3 years, bacteriologically safe, heated to 37 °C before use.

CAPD- continuous ambulatory peritoneal dialysis takes place in such a way that the solution is permanently in the abdominal cavity, 4 exchanges are performed during the day. Discharge and filling happen due to gravity. The solution is left in the abdominal cavity for 4 - 8 hours, the longest interval is overnight, the time for the entire exchange cycle is 45 minutes.

- *CCPD* - continuous cyclic peritoneal dialysis: the solution is changed at night, using a cycler, during the patient's sleep. It usually takes 8 -10 hours, the number of exchanges is 5-7. The procedure ends in the morning, the abdominal cavity remains filled with a solution.

- *NIPD* - nocturnal intermittent peritoneal dialysis: the solution is changed at night using the apparatus, in the morning all the solution is drained, the abdominal cavity remains empty.

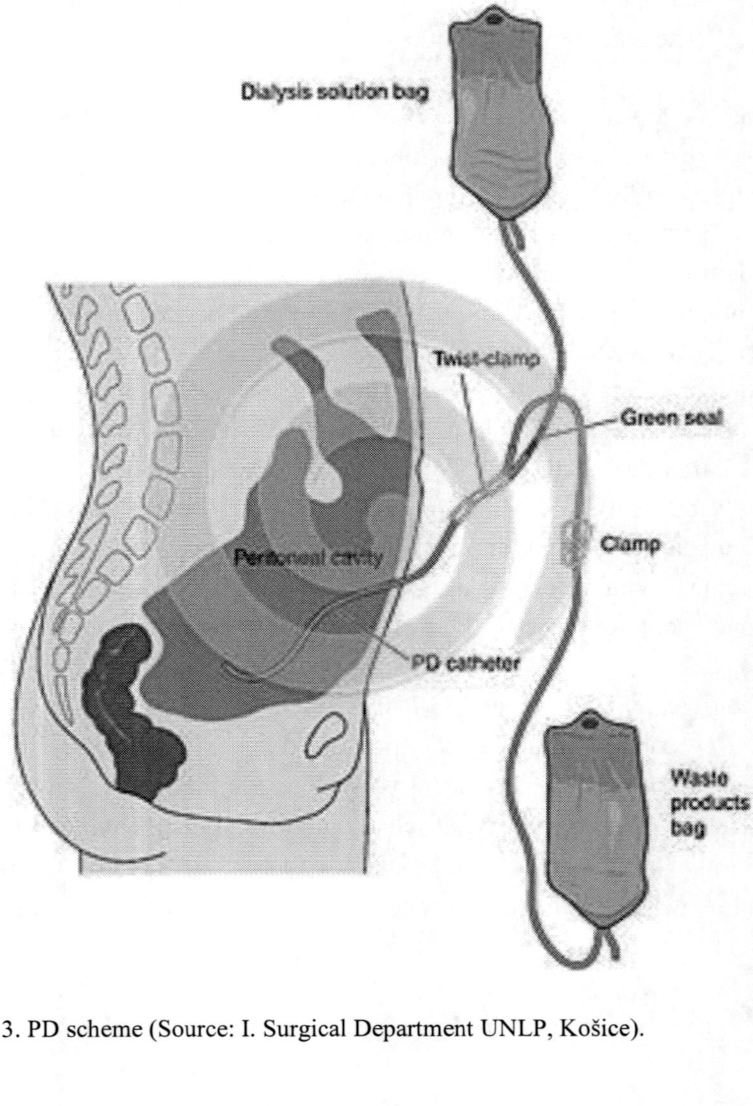

Figure 3. PD scheme (Source: I. Surgical Department UNLP, Košice).

Table 1. Comparison of hemodialysis and peritoneal dialysis

	Hemodialysis	**Peritoneal Dialysis**
localization	Extracorporeal	intracorporeal
access	Synthetic	biological
membrane pore density	High	low
membrane size	influenceable	uninfluenceable
protein loss per week	up to 2 g	up to 60 g
affecting efficiency	flow, area, membrane	amount of solution
the nature of the method	intermittent	continuous
anticoagulation	needed	-
membrane damage	substitutable	irreplaceable
diuresis	minimum	maintained
cardiovascular apparatus	hypertension, anemia, mineral changes	hyperhydration
infection	endocarditis, vascular access, hepatitis B, C	peritonitis
quality of life	device dependence, less freedom, more acute complications	peritonitis, home treatment, freedom - travel, work, diet, the aesthetic aspect

PD INDICATIONS

1. Difficulties with vascular access
2. Decreased function of the left ventricle
3. Poorly tolerated HD
4. Presence of heart valve replacements
5. Age
6. Large distance from the HD center
7. Strong need for autonomy of the patient
8. Cardiovascular diseases
9. Multiple myeloma
10. Labile DM
11. Chronic infection - hepatitis
12. Transplantation results

13. Hyperkalemia
14. Complications in HD (hypotension, arrhythmias)

CONTRAINDICATIONS OF PD TREATMENT

Absolute: loss of peritoneum function, peritoneal fibrosis, carcinomatosis of the peritoneum, acute abdominal inflammation, abnormalities preventing the insertion of a catheter, inability of the patient to perform treatment - mental illness, age, lack of social background.

Relative: pathological obesity, a patient without diuresis, st.p. intra-abdominal surgery, a presumption of adhesions, inflammatory bowel diseases, abdominal cavity infection, stoma, diverticulosis, polycystic kidney disease, malnutrition, immunosuppressive therapy.

Infectious complications: inflammation of the peritoneum, inflammation around the tip of the peritoneal catheter - exit site infection, tunnel infection.

Peritonitis is the most common and the most serious complication. Occurrence: once in 24 months.

Factors determining peritonitis: age, immune status, DM, nutritional status, hygiene requirements, immunosuppression, corticoids, HIV, St.aureus carrier, proton pump blockers, H2 receptor blockers. 2/3 are caused by gram-positive cocci (Staph. Aureus, epidermidis, Enterococcus, Strep. Sp., Klebsiella pneumoniae, Actinobacteria, Pseudomonas aeruginosa, E. coli).

The pathogen enters the peritoneal cavity intraluminally - negligence when handling the catheter, periluminally - along the catheter in the subcutaneous tunnel, during inflammation around the stoma, transmurally from the intestines in diverticulosis or in appendicitis.

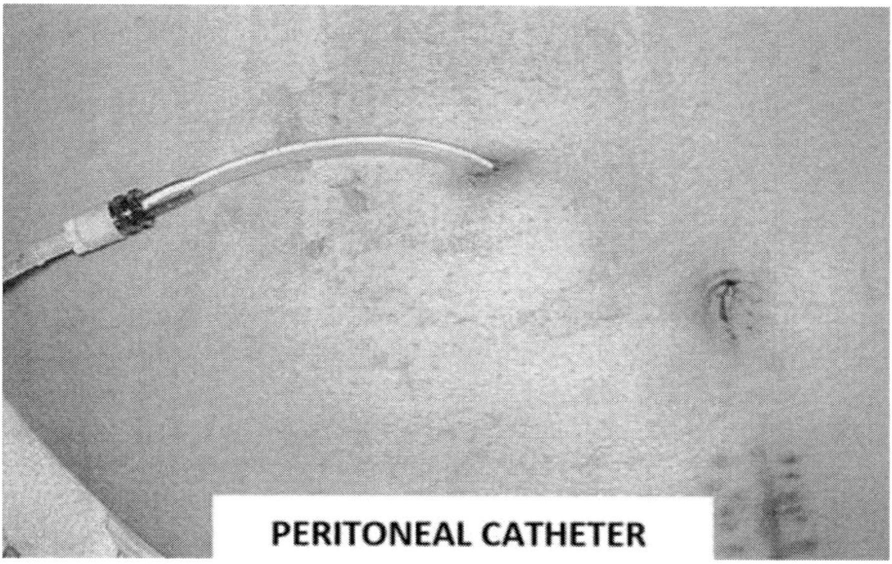

Figure 4. PD Access (Source: I. Surgical Department, UNLP, Košice).

The clinical picture includes cloudy dialysate, abdominal pain, nausea, vomiting, diarrhea, fever, chills, positive culture, increased leukocyte count in the dialysate, increased CRP levels, WBC count in a complete blood count.

Treatment: antibiotics according to the sensitivity, administered intraperitoneally, by addition to a dialysis bag, for 14-21 days, orally after 7-10 days.

Complications of peritonitis include changes of the peritoneum-morphological changes, functional changes of mesothelial cells, increased fibroproduction, metabolic changes - increased peritoneal permeability to glucose, fluid retention, protein loss into the dialysis solution leading to hypoproteinemia, malnutrition, catheter dysfunction, recurring peritonitis.

The prevention is in patient education, analysis of causes, re-education of CAPD procedures, nurse control activities, monthly visits at the patient's home, re-checking of laboratory parameters.

The success of the treatment depends on the patient's abilities, manual skills, strict adherence to treatment procedures, the cooperation of the specialist nurses, their educational skills, theoretical and practical experience, empathy, and communication skills.

REFERENCES

Twardowski Z J, Prowant B F. 1996. "Exit site healing post catheter implantation." *Ferit. Dial. Lntern.*, 16(3):51-70.

Tsimoyanis E C, Siakas F, Glantzounis G, et al., 2000. "Laparoscopic placement of the tenckhoff catheters for peritoneal dialysis." *Surg. Laparosc. Endosc, Percutan. Tech.* 218-221.

Bernardini J, Bender F, Florio T, et al., 2005. "Randomized, double-blind trial of antibiotic exit site cream for prevention of exit-site infection in a peritoneal dialysis patient." *J. Am. Soc. Nephrol.* 16:539—545.

Bachleda P, Janečkova J, Xinopulos P, Smakal O. 2016. "New hybrid procedures in treating occluded arteriovenous hemodialysis grafts." *Biomed. Pap. Med. Fac. Univ. Palacky Olomouc. Czech Repub.* 160(1):149-152.

Özener C, Bihorac A, Akoglu E. 2001. "Technical survival of CAPD catheters comparison between percutaneous and conventional surgical placement techniques." *Nephrol. Dial. Transplant.* 16:1893—1899.

Firano B, Bailie GR, Bernardini J, et al., 2005. "Peritoneal dialysis-related infections recommendations, 2005 update." *Perit. Dial. Lnt.* 25:107—131.

Strippoli G, Tong A, Johnson D, Schena F, Craig J, Cochrane Renal Group. 2004. "Antimicrobial agents for preventing peritonitis in peritoneal dialysis patients." *Cochrane Database Syst. Rey.* CD004679.

Danielson A, Blohme L, Traneus A et al., 2002. "A prospective randomized study of the effect of a subcutaneously "buried" peritoneal dialysis catheter technique versus standard technique on the incidence of peritonitis and exit site infection." *Perit. Dial. Int.* 22:211 —219.

Ash S, Daugirda J T. 2001. "Peritoneal access devices." in*: Handbook of Dialysis, 3rd edn* edited by Daugirdas M. D., John T. Philadelphia: Lippincott Williams and Wilkins.

In: Surgeon´s Perspective on Dialysis Patient ISBN: 978-1-53619-262-9
Editor: Maria Frankovicova

Chapter 11

SKIN COVERING IN DIALYSIS ACCESSES FROM THE POINT OF VIEW OF A PLASTIC SURGEON

M. Vidová Uğurbaş**, *MD
Department of Plastic, Reconstructive and Aesthetic Surgery, Faculty of Medicine, Pavol Jozef Šafárik University in Košice and University Hospital, Košice, Slovakia

ABSTRACT

The number of patients who need a long-term hemodialysis is constantly increasing. The most frequent complications of arteriovenous fistula type subcutaneous vascular accesses include infections, thromboses, and complications due to low blood flow. Complications can include skin necrosis or defects. Skin defects can be most often covered by a flap, a skin transplant or a skin substitute. The flaps are classified according to several criteria as local and distant flaps. The Limberg flap is one of the most commonly used flaps used to cover defects after removal of necrosis in complications of hemodialysis accesses. For

* Corresponding Author's E-mail: vidova.martina@gmail.com.

definitive cover of the skin, we can also use an autograft, for temporary cover using skin substitutes of various origin. Skin substitutes can be divided into biologic, synthetic, biosynthetic, and combined. Reconstruction of tissue defects is needed in case of an extensive defect or a loss of organ function.

Keywords: skin defects, skin flaps, transplantation of skin, skin reconstruction

Abbreviations

AVF	arteriovenous fistula
HD	hemodialysis

Introduction

Multidisciplinary cooperation is essential for the success of the operation and implementation of dialysis access. A plastic surgeon participates in solving various complications, especially complications of hemodialysis approaches.

Hemodialysis (HD) approaches have a high incidence of complications. The most common complications we come across in hemodialysis approaches include stenosis and thrombosis, Steal syndrome, infection, aneurysm, pseudoaneurysm, hyperfunction, venous hypertension, hand ischemia and subsequent skin defects. Repeated invasive techniques to create a suitable HD approaches as well as their complications, such as aneurysms, pseudoaneurysms, lead to skin damage and often to degenerative skin changes (a change of tone, color, nature and characteristics of the skin). Skin necrosis is a severe skin complication caused by the HD approach (Bordils 2010; Frankovičová 2015).

The number of patients who are enrolled in a long-term hemodialysis program is constantly increasing. The average age of patients is increasing as well. These factors have resulted in an increasing number of HD accesses being created. Patients with chronic kidney disease have impaired hemostasis, many of them have diabetes and their vascular system is impaired by atherosclerosis. Many of them suffer from vascular system hypoplasticity and blood vessel damage caused by repeat punctures as well as by thrombosing (Frankovičová 2015). All these factors affect the success rate of the surgery and therefore multidisciplinary cooperation is essential – not only for hemodialysis access but also for resolving the resulting skin defects. The aforementioned infection and thrombosis are the most frequent complications of arteriovenous fistulas (AVF), which are a type of subcutaneous vascular access. The resulting skin defects need to be dealt with by closure, a direct suture is sufficient for uninfected small defects. Extensive skin defects require complex coverage, most often by a flap or a skin substitute.

Reconstruction of tissue defects is needed wherever an extensive defect or loss of function is present. Defect coverage is possible by means of flaps, using skin grafts and tissue expanders.

Defect Covered by Flap

The implementation of flaps into reconstructive surgery marks a significant breakthrough in the development of plastic surgery. Defects that were previously reconstructed only by direct suture or healing by secondary intention could be covered with a fully-fledged tissue. The flap is a composite block of tissue that has its own blood supply. Flaps are used for coverage of defects of various differing etiology and composition. According to the requirements and extent of the defect, we can design the flap and adapt it accurately to fit the recipient site. The flap may comprise of a portion of skin with subcutaneous tissue, or with another tissue (fascia, muscles, bone), which are released from the donor site and transferred to the recipient site (Palenčár 2015).

Classification of Flaps

Classification of flaps is important for understanding the principles of their blood supply, reconstruction options, and composition. The flaps are classified according to several criteria: according to the vascular supply, according to the tissue composition, according to the relationship of the donor and recipient sites, according to the method of transfer and according to the flap time management (Vidová Uğurbaş 2018).

Classification of Flaps According to the Vascular Supply

According to the way of the vascular supply, flaps are divided into random pattern flaps and axial pattern flaps. Random pattern flaps are supplied randomly. Their supply is ensured by subdermal vascular plexus. It is necessary to keep the 1:2 ratio of the flap base to the length. The length of the flap mustn't be more than twice its width. Random flaps contain skin and subcutaneous fat. Their subdermal plexus is supplied by branches of musculocutaneous perforators which pierce the deep muscles and muscle fascia and directly supply the subdermal part of the flap (Figure 1). In comparison with avascular skin grafts, they provide better coverage of defects of different etiology. Their disadvantage is a small range of rotation and insufficient resistance to local infection. An example of a random skin flap is an advancement flap, rotation flap, transposition flap and interpolation flap. Flaps, which have a specific supply are called axial pattern flaps. Axial pattern flaps have a well-defined nutrient artery and committing veins. The axial artery runs below the flap in the intermuscular septum and gives off septo-cutaneous perforators to the skin of the flap (Figure 2). Axial pattern flaps may contain only the skin and subcutaneous fat, or they may include the muscular fascia, which improves the nutritional supply of the flap, and the flap may be greater. Axial flaps do not need to keep the 1:2 ratio, these flaps can be narrow and long (Palenčár 2015; Vidová Uğurbaş 2018).

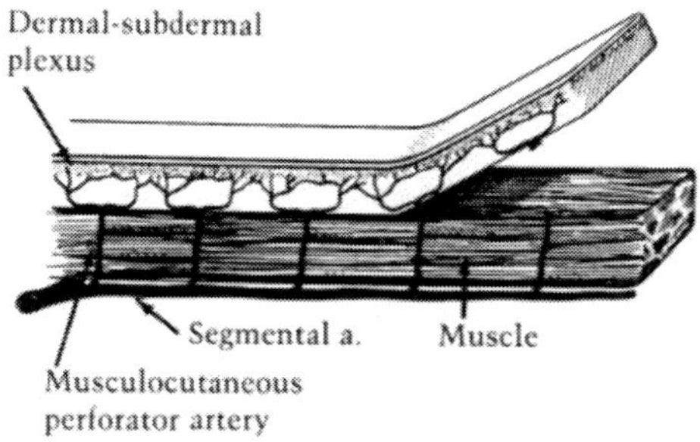

Figure 1. The random pattern flap (Thorne 2007).

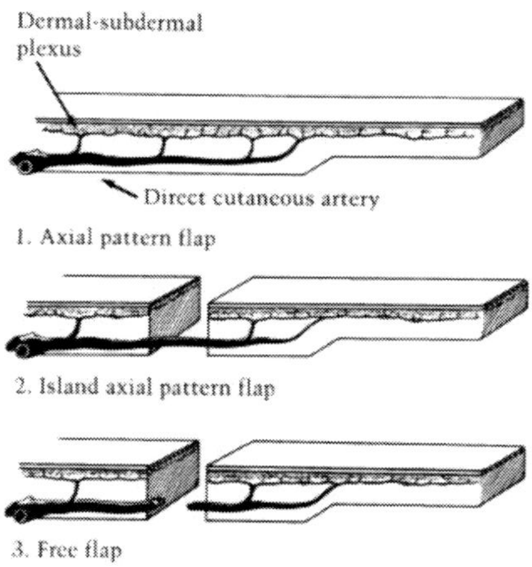

Figure 2. Axial pattern flap (Thorne 2007).

Classification of Flaps According to the Tissue Composition

According to the composition, flaps are divided into simple and compound flaps. Simple flaps contain only one type of tissue: skin, fascial, muscular, osseous, visceral (omentum, colon, small intestine). Compound flaps consist of several types of tissues: fasciocutaneous flaps (comprising skin and fascia), musculocutaneous (muscle and skin), osseous-cutaneous (bone and skin), chondrocutaneous (skin and cartilage), tendocutaneous (skin and tendon), sensory/innervated flaps.

Classification of Flaps According to the Relationship of the Donor and Recipient Sites

According *to donor and recipient sites,* we define local and distant flaps. Local flaps originate from the site which is relatively close to the site of the defect. These include advancement, rotation, transposition, and interpolation flaps. Distant flaps come from a place that is not close to the defect. Their role is to cover distant defects. They can cover the defect directly (without a carrier) - direct flap or indirectly (with a carrier) - indirect flap or they are freely transferred to the defect site- free (microvascular) flap.

Classification of Flaps According to the Time of Reconstruction

Classification according to Listeroly and Asko-Seljavara divides flaps according to the scheduled time as follows: emergency flaps – flaps that are implemented within 24 hours. Acute flaps – flaps implemented within the first seven days after the defect formation. Delayed flaps – which are implemented from day 7 up to the completion of skin healing. A secondary flap can be implemented only after the skin has finished healing after various periods of time have passed (Palenčár 2015; Thorne 2007).

Usage of Flaps

Skin flaps can be used to cover wounds with a compromised vascular bed, to cover wounds located over the exposed bones, tendons, nerves, cartilage, or to cover open cavities. Coverage by flap can be used when there is a later need for surgery of deeper structures. A free skin graft is not suitable as a temporary cover for other operations of tendons, nerves, blood vessels, bones, and cartilages. Such wounds must be covered by a flap. When planning skin flaps the requirements of the recipient tissue must be taken into account and the exact extent of the defect must be determined. It is advisable to plan a flap slightly larger than the size of the defect itself.

Overflapping is a reconstructive method where a new flap is inserted over the original flap, after previous removal of the surface epithelium (e.g., by dermabrasion). This method is used if the original flap gets smaller and its size is inadequate to the place where it is, or if it is below the skin level. Another reconstructive technique is *over grafting*, this method is used when, after some time, the color of the skin flap is different than that of the surrounding skin. It is then possible to perform dermabrasion on the skin of the transferred flap or to remove the entire epidermis and cover the resulting defect by a free skin graft (split-thickness or in full-thickness). The delay phenomenon - the influence of blood flow in the flap (vascular enhancement). Its principle is the partial and gradual separation of the vasculature, which is accompanied by the closure of arteriovenous shunts with an improvement of blood circulation in the capillary bed. The delay phenomenon means that there is an initial delay in the creation of the flap and its conversion into a monopedicle flap by cutting one of the flap pedicles. Maximum blood flow is on the 8th to 10th day, after which a decline in the blood flow level occurs again. The decision to perform a flap delay depends on where the flap is planned, on the patient's age and overall health status.

Factors, which allow for the use of longer flaps include the presence of direct cutaneous arteries and veins directed along the longitudinal axis of the flap - axial pattern flap. Such arterial flaps survive even if they are 50% longer than the flaps which are supplied by musculocutaneous arteries (perforators), located on dermal and subdermal vascular plexuses. Another factor is localization, flaps on the head and neck have good vascularization. Delayed skin flaps survive even if they are 60 to 100% longer than the length of the not-delayed flaps, and whose nutrition depends on the perforating artery of the dermal/subdermal plexus (delay flap). The survival rate of bipedicle flaps is higher than that of monopedicle flaps. Important factors are the age and general health of the patient. A longer flap is more likely to survive in younger patients without diabetes mellitus, atherosclerosis, and other associated serious diseases (Thorne 2007; Vidová Uğurbaş 2018).

Complications

Complications after flap surgery include bleeding, inflammation, wound dehiscence and swelling. Necrosis of a part or of the entire flap occurs as a result of bad flap planning. Flap necrosis is often caused by a local infection in the recipient site, strangulation of flap pedicle, a twisting of the pedicle or excessive pulling of the pedicle. Necrosis may also be caused by overly sharp angles or by a flap that is too small. The flap must be inserted into the defect without tension, breaking, bending or rotating. Similarly, pressure on the flap which prevents venous drainage causes surface necrosis, bullae, or epithelial desquamation. It is also a mistake to insert the flap into suppurative areas because this changes an open wound to a closed one and thus prevents its drainage. The cause of complications may also be incorrect postoperative care. The flap is separated from its innervation, so it loses sensitivity, glandular activity is also limited, and therefore it is necessary to protect the flap from excessive cold or heat (Thorne 2007, Vidová Uğurbaş 2018).

Local Flaps

Local flaps rotate around a pivot point (rotate around the pivot). Two basic principles are applied in the construction of local flaps: mobilize the skin near the defect to the edges of the wound without pulling and perform the suture so that it corresponds with skin lines when the edges of the wound are closer. According to their nutrition, these flaps can be random pattern flaps and axial pattern flaps.

Local flaps include rotational, transposition, interpolation flaps, and the so-called advancement flaps, which are flaps moved into the defect without rotation and lateral movement.

- *Rotation flap* is rotated to the defect from close proximity. The flap has a semicircular shape, healthy tissue is rotated around the pivot into the defect after undermining the surrounding skin. The resulting secondary defect can be closed by direct suture or free skin grafts (Figure 3) (Palenčár 2015; Thorne 2007).

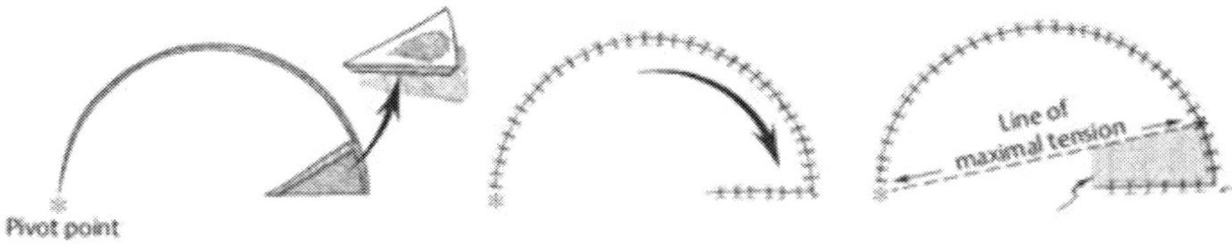

Source: Marre, PlasticSurgeryKey.

Figure 3. Rotation flap (the first scheme shows the defect after the excision of the skin, the arrow in the second scheme indicates the future direction of the rotation of the flap, the third scheme shows a closed rotation flap).

- *Transposition flap* is right-angled, located in close proximity to the defect. The flap should be wider than the defect, the donor site can be directly sutured or covered by another flap (bilobed flap), or it can be covered by a skin graft. The basic shape of the transposition flap is usually a square, rectangle or rhombus. The pivot point is located on the opposite side of the flap base compared to the defect (Figure 4). Examples of the transposition flaps are the "Z"-plasty, "W"- plasty, the Limberg flap, and the Dufourmentel flap.

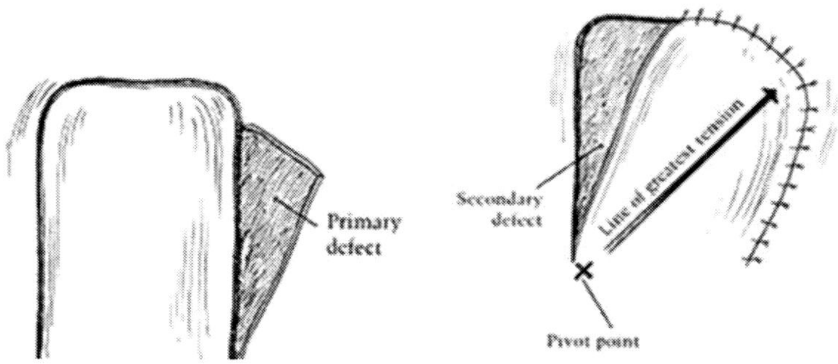

Figure 4. a, b - A transposition flap (Thorne 2007).

The "Z" plasty is a transposition flap surgery in which two adjacent triangular flaps exchange their places. The lateral limbs of Z-plasty must always be the same length as the central limb (median incision above the original scar). Changing the length of the limbs causes wrinkling at the corners and further adjustments are needed to achieve proper closure. The lateral limbs have to form an angle of 30 ° to 90 ° depending on the required lengthening. The limbs of the classic-Z-plasty form a 60° angle and are formed by two equilateral triangles. The central limb should be oriented in the direction of contraction. By the Z-plasty with angles of 60°, we can lengthen the scar by 75%. Angles smaller than 60° are easier to transpose but they lead to a smaller lengthening when using angles larger than 60°, the force required to transpose the flap is increased significantly, making the closure of the defect more difficult (Figure 5) (Salam 2003; Thorne 2007).

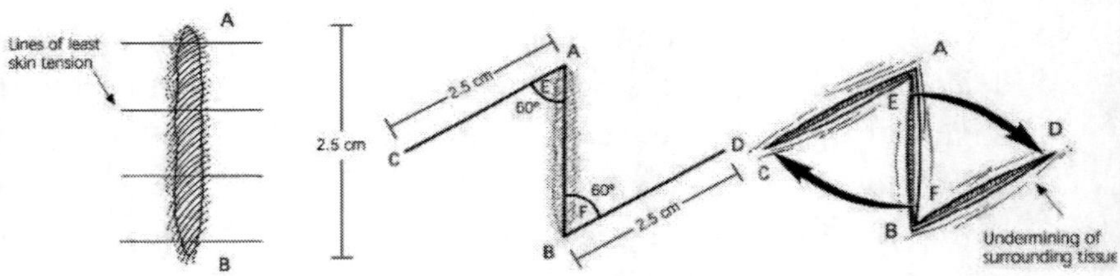

Figure 5. a, b, c - Z- plasty, the scheme indicates that the length of the lateral limbs must be the same as the median incision above the defect. Subsequent transposition of adjacent triangles is shown by arrows (Salam 2003).

The "W" plasty is an excisional technique for the revision of the scar using multiple small triangles. It is used to change the course and shape of a straight linear scar. As Z- plasty, W-plasty is used to change a linear scar into a scar of irregular "accordion" shape. Both techniques significantly lengthen the original scar.

The Limberg Flap

The Limberg flap surgery was first described by prof. A.A Limberg from Leningrad in 1946. It is used to cover rhomboid defects with angles of 60 and 120 degrees. The flap has sides of equal length as the short axis of the rhomboid defect. Flap movement is determined by the line of the maximal extension of skin that is typically perpendicular to the skin tension lines. This flap can be used in all parts of the body. The Limberg flap is one of the most commonly used flaps to cover defects after removal of necrosis in complications of HD accesses. After excision of the necrosis, a rhombus with angles of 60° and 120° is drawn on the skin, in the flap planning process a short diagonal is elongated in one direction by its own length and another incision is performed in parallel with a side of the rhombus. The flap is implemented under local anesthesia, and antibiotic treatment is necessary. The excision of necrotic tissue is performed carefully in order to prevent damaging the vessel (Figure 6, 7) (Chasmar 2007).

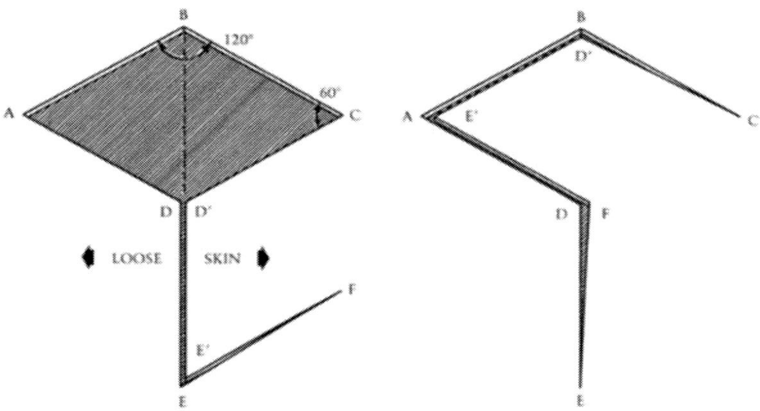

Figure 6. The Limberg flap, a scheme of Limberg flap planning and the subsequent closure of the defect (Thorne 2007).

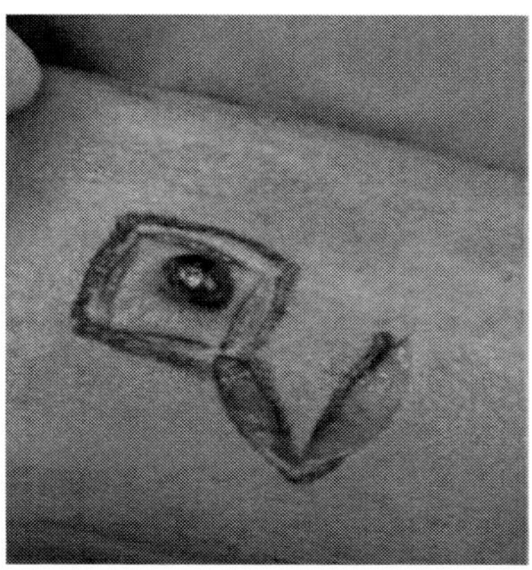

Figure 7. Skin necrosis above the pseudoaneurysm of AVF, a drawing of necrotic tissue excision, and Limberg flap intended to close the defect on the forearm (Pirozzia 2013).

The Defourmental flap is a modification of the Limberg flap. The flap was first described by Defourmental in 1962. It is a variation to the previous flap using larger angles and thus getting a wider pedicle (Figure 8).

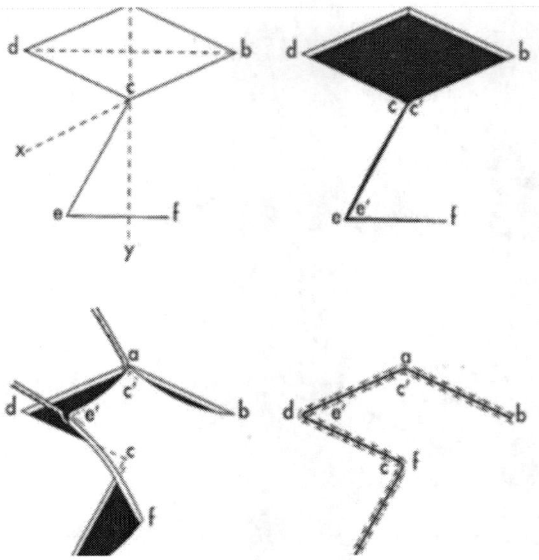

Figure 8. Defourmental flap, diagram of the incision, and the subsequent transposition of the flap to the defect (Osman 2005).

- *The interpolation flap* consists of the skin and subcutaneous tissue. It is rotated around the pivot into the defect from the surrounding area of the defect, but not in its immediate proximity. Interpolation flap is moved in two dimensions, the pedicle goes either above or below the tissue which is located between the flap and the defect. The flap is then interpolated into the defect over or under the bridge of healthy skin. If the flap is sewn into the defect and transposed over a healthy skin, a resection of the flap pedicle is necessary after 21 days. The donor site is sutured or covered by transplanted skin grafts and only the part of the flap necessary to cover the defect remains. The flap which has connected to the defect is fully vascularized from the base and the edges of the defect after disconnecting from the donor site. If the interpolation flap is moved into the defect below the bridge of healthy skin, a part of the flap should be de-epithelized. This procedure is dangerous and may result in a full or partial loss of the flap.

The Peninsular flap has a direct cutaneous artery and vein, and a bridge of the skin and subcutaneous tissue. The exposed area of the pedicle can be covered by a free skin transplant, but it is not usually necessary.

The Island flap is an island of the skin and subcutaneous tissue with its neurovascular pedicle (for hands) or arteriovenous pedicle, it is moved through a tunnel under the skin.

- *The advancement flaps.* The flaps of this type are transposed directly into the defect without rotation or lateral movement (Figure 9). Advancement flaps can be monopedicle or bipedicle. The monopedicle flap is rectangular or right-angled and requires a good skin elasticity for movement. The advancement flaps include V-Y and Y-V advancements.

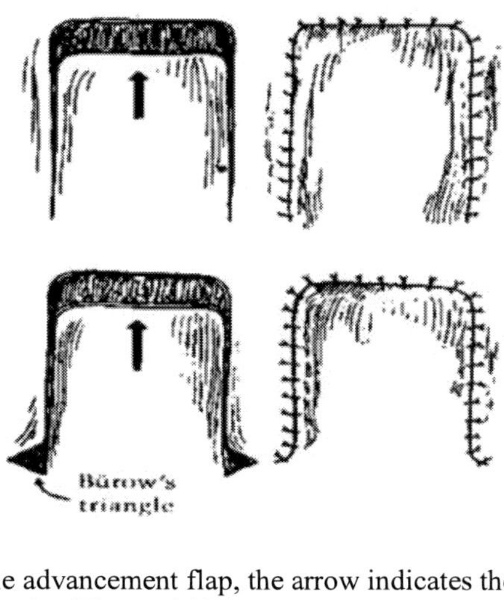

Figure 9. Monopedicle advancement flap, the arrow indicates the next movement of the flap into the defect site (Thorne 2007).

Bipedicle advancement flap is formed by an incision that is parallel to the long axis of the defect. The skin between the incision and the defect is undermined and moved into the defect. The donor site is covered by a free skin graft. The use of advancement flaps is limited by their short length and by the fact that the pulling of the flap reduces its blood supply.

V-Y and Y-V Advancement Flap

The principle of the V-Y advancement flap is that a "V" shape incision is made in the skin, which is then sutured from each of the sides so that the final shape resembles the letter "Y." The Y-V advancement flap is similar, but vice-versa ("Y" shape incision in the skin and subsequent suture in the form of "V") (Figure10) (Thorne 2007, Vidová Uğurbaş 2018).

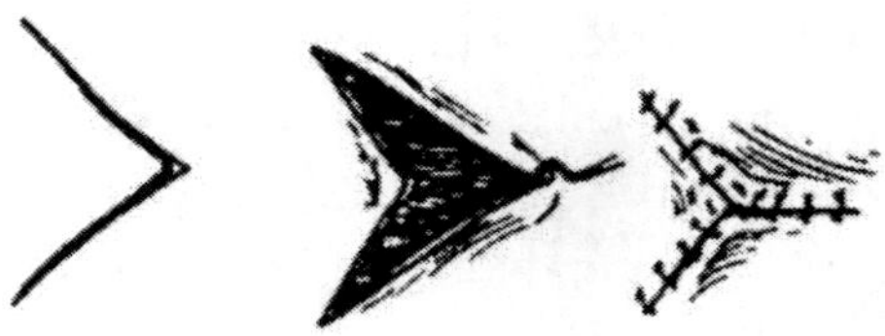

Figure 10. V-Y advancement flap, a scheme of the V-shaped incision and subsequent Y-shaped suture (Thorne 2007).

Distant Flaps

When transferring a distant flap to the recipient site, the donor site, which was created after moving the flap, must be closed. This can be achieved by the following: by putting recipient and donor site closer, by covering the donor site with a thin skin graft, by undermining the edges of the donor site, followed by direct suture, by covering with a rotation flap of healthy tissue.

Distant flaps are divided into direct – e.g., coverage of the defect on the dorsum of the hand by a flap from the torso (Figure 11), indirect - using a carrier - e.g., wrist and free flaps (by microsurgical anastomosis). *Direct distant flaps* are extracted from the chest. In order to cover the defects of the upper limb the flap comes from the other forearm (the cross arm flap).

In order to cover the defects of the lower limb, a flap from the other leg may be used (the cross-leg flap).

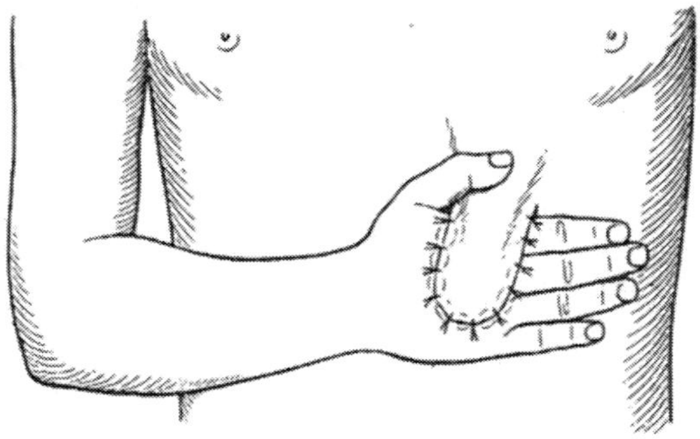

Figure 11. Distant flap surgery from the chest, skin defect on the dorsal side of the hand is covered by direct skin flap from the chest wall.

Indirect distant flap surgery typically tubularize and the flaps are transferred into the defect by the carrier (wrist). These flaps originate from the torso, chest, neck and lower limbs. A tubularized flap is a pedicle flap, whose edges are rolled, which creates a cylinder. Tubularized flaps are used in places where it is necessary to use a greater amount of high-quality skin to cover the defect and where it is not possible to use a direct flap. During the planning process, we must evaluate the defect and the amount of skin necessary to cover the defect, respecting the length: width ratio of 2.5 to 1. We must keep in mind that the skin will retract, so the planned flap should be larger by about 10% (Thorne 2007; Vidová Uğurbaş 2018).

Arterial Flaps

These flaps are supplied by a specific artery (axial pattern flaps). Venous drainage of axial flaps is ensured through the accompanying veins or via the superficial venous drainage system. Arterial flaps are divided into cutaneous (skin), muscular, musculocutaneous, fascio-cutaneous, and free flaps.

- *Skin arterial flaps* are skin flaps whose nutrition is provided by terminal arteries of the skin, which passes in parallel to the skin above the deep fascia. The course of the terminal artery is constant, and the artery is usually accompanied by two veins (venae comitantes). Perfect knowledge of anatomy is necessary in order to use these flaps.

The advantage of skin arterial flaps is the independence of flap's length from its width, as it is in the case of skin flaps supplied by perforators. Their use is wide, they can be used as local flaps (peninsular, island) when they rotate or move around the pedicle. They can also be used as distant flaps, or as free flaps where the pedicle is cut and then joined via anastomosis to another recipient artery and vein by means of microsurgery. Blood supply is determined by the anatomy of the flap, location and size of the blood vessel providing nutrition. Blood flow of the flap can be objectively measured and determined by an ultrasonic flow meter, dilution methods, plethysmography, or photometric methods. Insufficient blood flow leads to ischemia and necrosis of the flap. Ischemia of the flap can be prevented by careful planning of the reconstruction. Blood flow is changing when pulling the pedicle, after twisting the pedicle, with edema, or inflammation, when there is a change of venous blood flow.

- *Muscular and musculocutaneous flaps.* The main component is muscular tissue. Muscle tissue has excellent vascularization. Muscle tissue is resistant to infection and represents a suitable bed for a free skin graft. The basic prerequisite for the use of these flaps is perfect knowledge of the vascular anatomy and the determination of a rotation (pivot) point and arc. The disadvantages of muscular flaps include donor site deformity (which may be closed by direct suture or free skin transplant), loss of sensation, lower mechanical resistance, especially in muscle flaps, and excessive volume in shallower defects. The choice of method depends primarily on the functional and aesthetic needs of the defect itself, on its size, location, and nature. The used muscle flaps are pedicled or free. Muscle flaps are generally indicated to cover chronic, poorly healing infected deep wounds, to cover post-radiation defects, when dealing with open fractures and extensive loss of tissue. The planning process is influenced not only by the local finding of the patient, but also by their overall status, presence of vascular and systemic diseases (diabetes mellitus, lupus, and scleroderma), as well as states of immunodeficiency. There is a number of musculocutaneous perforators in the superficial layer of muscles, which have started to be used as musculocutaneous flaps.

According to the number and size of vascular plexuses (vascular pedicles), Mathes and Nahai classified skeletal muscles into five types (Figure 12):

- Type I. contains a single dominant vascular plexus (pedicle) (medial gastrocnemius muscle, lateral gastrocnemius muscle, tensor fasciae latae muscle).
- Type II. contains a dominant plexus (pedicle) and minor vascular pedicles. This type of muscular flap is used most often (sternocleidomastoid muscle, platysma muscle).
- Type III. contains two dominant pedicles. Ligation of one of them can result in the loss of a part of the muscle, on the other hand, it allows the transfer of half of the muscle (temporal muscle, serratus anterior muscle, rectus abdominis muscle).
- Type IV. contains multiple segmental pedicles, each segmental blood vessel supplies a given part of the muscle. Cutting more than 2-3 pedicles during the flap elevation results in avascular necrosis of the distal part of the muscle (sartorius muscle, tibialis anterior muscle).
- Type V. contains a dominant vascular pedicle and secondary segmental pedicles on the opposite side of the muscle. It is typical for the muscles of the torso. Segmental pedicles enter these

muscles regularly from the midline of the torso (pectoralis major, latissimus dorsi muscle) (Mathes 2007).

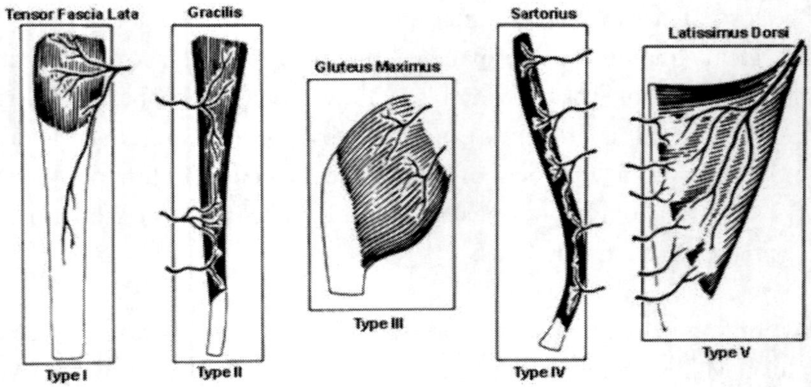

Figure 12. Types of muscular flaps (Classification by Matheas and Nahai).

- *Fascial and fasciocutaneous flaps* contain skin, subcutaneous tissue, and deep fascia. The advantage of these flaps is in maintaining the muscle layer and reinforcement of the skin flap supply by including fascia into the flap. Fasciocutaneous flaps are indicated mainly on the limbs, the use of fascial and fasciocutaneous flaps at other sites of the body is debatable. They can be used as pedicle flaps, but also as free flaps. Fascial and fasciocutaneous flaps are classified according to Mathes and Nahai into three types:
    - Type A Flap supplied by the direct cutaneous vascular pedicle.
    - Type B Septocutaneous perforator
    - Type C Musculocutaneous perforator (Lamberty 1990).
- *Free flaps* are composed of muscle with a dominant artery. The muscle containing the artery is elevated from a distant site and transplanted into the recipient site by vascular microanastomosis of flap artery and recipient site arteries and veins. Free flaps are mainly used in areas where there is a lack of appropriate muscle flaps for a local flap (head, neck, and the distal third of the lower limbs).

Defect Covered by Skin Graft

Skin transplantation is the transfer of skin tissue within one organism or between organisms. The most important role of the skin transplant is to cover skin defects of varying size and extent. The skin can be transplanted as a whole (full thickness) or in individual layers (split-thickness). We distinguish definitive coverage by skin autografts, combined substitutes with autologous keratinocytes, and temporary coverage by skin substitutes of various origin. Skin substitutes can be divided into biologic, synthetic, biosynthetic, and combined.

According to their origin, skin grafts are divided into autologous, homologous (allogeneic) and heterologous (xenogeneic). Autologous skin grafts (autografts) come from the same individual. Homologous transplant (allograft) is a graft of skin transferred between different individuals of the same species. The heterologous skin transplants (xenografts) are taken from an individual of a different species (e.g., from pigs) (Hulín 2015).

Skin transplants are the most optimal form of covering superficial skin necrosis (e.g., in dialysis patients suffering from calciphylaxis) (Sprague 2014).

Definitive Skin Coverage by Free Skin Autografts

Free skin autograft is defined as a segment of the dermis and epidermis, which is completely separated from the vasculature in the donor site and is transferred to the recipient site on a different part of the body. When taking a free skin graft, blood, and lymph vessels are interrupted. Graft survival depends on the rapid restoration of blood supply to provide nutrition and removal of catabolites.

Graft survival depends on these factors:

1) Adequate nutrition of the transplant
2) Sufficient removal of catabolites from the graft.
3) Anatomical peculiarities of the donor and recipient sites.

4) Taxonomic and genetic relationship between the donor and recipient site.

Adequate and well-vascularized bed, adequate immobilization in the bed as prevention of interruption of newly-formed vessels and rapid vascularization from the recipient site are all important for the survival of the graft from a technical point of view.

Revascularization of the graft is the result of these three processes: 1. The connection between the arteries of the graft and bed (inoculation), 2. Ingrowth of vessels from the bed into the endothelial tubules of the transplant, 3. Overgrowth of blood vessels from the bed to the dermis of the transplant and the formation of new endothelial tubules. From the moment of placing the graft on the bed until its revascularization, the transplant cells use fluid from the bed for their nutrition. Although this nutrition is not sufficient, it temporarily helps them survive the first two days. Fluid gets through a number of lumens of blood and lymphatic vessels in between the graft and the bed, which is the same way in it enters the graft. During the first days, the fluid is absorbed from the bed and the graft swells. This is explained by the fact that the graft contains large amounts of osmotically active compounds in its intercellular spaces. After its removal, the transplant is chalky white, after 6 hours it starts to turn pink and its color is gradually intensified. This condition is caused by collapsed vessels of the graft and spastic vascular beds. After several hours, there is a release of the spasm, as well as the opening of the cut ends of the blood vessels in the graft. After 24 hours, the blood vessels endings are open and contain blood cells. After 48 hours, the transplant is already fixed to the bed by precipitated fibrin from plasma. On the fourth-fifth day of the transplantation, the transplant is engrafted. Its revascularization terminates on the 6th-7th day.

According to the thickness, free skin autografts are divided into two groups: full-thickness skin grafts and split-thickness skin grafts (Hulín 2015, Vidová Uğurbaş 2018).

Full-Thickness Free Skin Graft

The full-thickness skin graft contains the epidermis and dermis in full-thickness and therefore the sweat and sebaceous glands, hair follicles and capillaries. It is revascularized more slowly because of its thickness. For optimal revascularization, the transplant requires a good blood supply of the bed, perfect immobilization and removal of subcutaneous fat. It is mainly used to definitively cover defects in places with sufficient blood supply for the creation and growth of granulation tissue. The full-thickness skin graft is generally suitable to definitively cover defects on the face, to cover defects in the volar surface of the hand and fingers for its mechanical resistance and reinnervation. It is not suitable to cover the bone devoid of periosteum, cartilage devoid of perichondrium, tendon and nerve devoid of paratenon tissue and nerve devoid of perineural tissue. The advantages of full-thickness graft include a smaller tendency to contract after the engraftment and a smaller tendency to discoloration. Compared to a split-thickness skin graft it has a better cosmetic effect and is mechanically more resistant. A suitable place for harvesting the full-thickness graft is the front side of the wrist, the front side of the forearm, the supraclavicular area, groin, abdominal wall, thigh, inner arm, and prepuce (Hulín 2015).

The graft is harvested depending on the shape of the defect to be covered, using a blood imprint on wet sterile gauze. Transplant excision is done freehand with a scalpel. The fat layer is completely removed with sharp scissors to prevent damage to the base of the dermis by bruising. The donor site is closed by direct suture. Hemostasis is thoroughly reached in the bed (base of the defect), which is subsequently loaded with the graft. The graft is sewn into the bed while trying to precisely adapt to the edges in order to allow overgrowth of blood vessels horizontally. A pressure pad (made of cotton and gauze soaked in flavin) is applied to the graft. The pad is fixed by a few stitches on the surrounding skin, but it may also be fixed by long stitches by which graft has been sewn on (Figure 13, 14, 15). The pressure pad is used to create adequate pressure on the graft (to ensure optimal revascularization, the graft must be in all areas in contact with the base of the defect). The pressure pad is removed after five days (Vidová Ugurbas 2018).

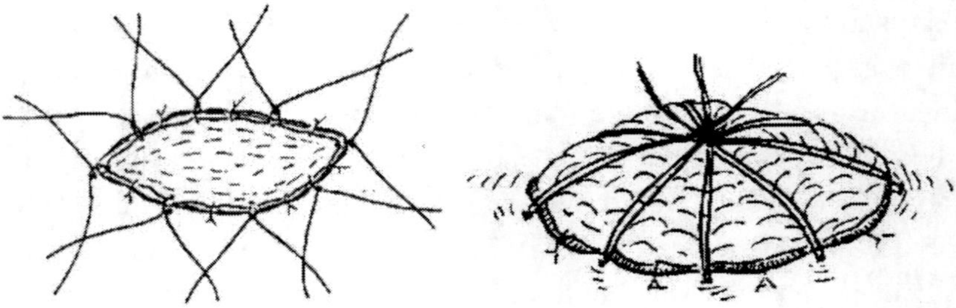

Figure 13. a, b - A free skin graft sewn into the defect and its fixation by a pressure pad.

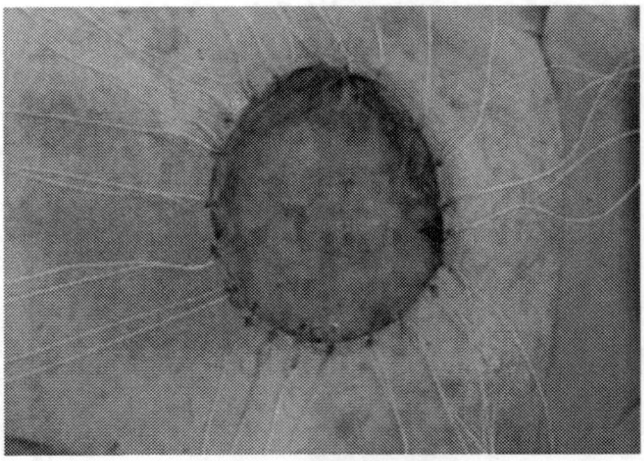

Source: Department of Plastic, Reconstructive and Aesthetic Surgery, Faculty of Medicine, Pavol Jozef Šafárik University in Košice and University Hospital, Košice.

Figure 14. Free skin graft sewn into the defect - long stitches are left in place to fix the pressure pad.

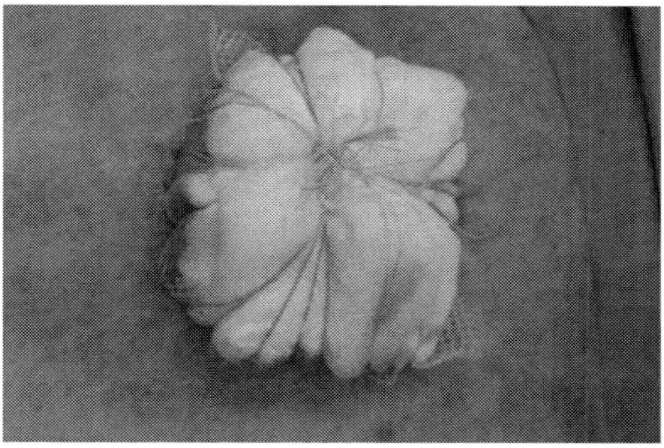

Figure 15. The pressure pad loaded on graft and fixed to the skin (Department of Plastic, Reconstructive and Aesthetic Surgery, Faculty of Medicine, Pavol Jozef Šafárik University in Košice and University Hospital, Košice).

Split Thickness Skin Graft – Dermo-Epidermal Autograft

The split-thickness skin graft is composed of epidermis and a small portion of the dermis. The use of a split graft is the most widespread method of skin transplantation. It may be used as definitive coverage of the defect, but also as a temporary cover. Dermo-epidermal grafts are classified according to their thickness into three groups: 1. Thin grafts containing up to 1/3 of the dermis, 2. Medium thickness grafts containing up to ½ of the dermis, 3. Thick transplants containing up to 3/4 of the dermis. The thin split graft is referred to as the Thiersch graft in the literature.

The use of a split-thickness transplant is recommended to cover a large skin defect, which is too large to be covered by a full-thickness transplant. The split transplant does not leave any defect at the donor site. The donor area can heal itself by secondary epithelization. In the absence of donor sites, when in need of covering several major areas, the area of the transplant may be increased by meshing at the ratio of 1: 1, 6: 1. Mesh grafts allow for better drainage of fluid from beneath the graft.

For split-thickness transplant harvesting, we use the Humby knife, drum dermatome, and electro-dermatomes (Brown dermatome, Padgett dermatome). Donor sites for harvesting the split transplant include the anterolateral part of the thigh, abdominal wall, the gluteal region, as well as the back.

The transplant is applied to a clean wound over the edges and is fixated by a few stitches. The suture of the graft to the bed is not necessary. Transplant is covered by a compression bandage, which is used to achieve the most intimate contact with the bed so as not to move or separate the transplant from the bed by hematoma or seroma. The compression bandage must not press the arterial supply and the venous drainage of the bed. After 48 hours, the graft is fixated to the bed using a fibrin network and revascularization begins. The donor site is treated by tulle gras (eventually in combination with Framykoin powder), wet and dry gauze, cotton, and elastic bandages. Tulle gras and gauze are left in place until their spontaneous separation. The donor site is healed by reepithelization within 10 days after the harvesting (Hulín 2015, Shimizu 2012).

Free split-thickness skin grafts can be stored. A simple and very effective method for storing of the skin graft is to return it to the donor site. The transplant can then be easily removed within 10 days without the use of anesthesia. After the 10th day, the removal of the stored transplant is harder and more painful. The split-thickness skin grafts may be cooled for up to 21 days in sterile conditions at a temperature of 4°C. The longer the transplant is stored, the lower the likelihood of successful revascularization after its insertion into the bed (Vidová Uğurbaş 2018).

Complications with the Use of Free Transplants

Free skin transplants are subject to contraction. The contraction may be primary and secondary. Skin defect covered by a free full-thickness skin graft or by a flap grows correspondingly as the rest of uninjured skin around. The split-thickness skin graft is also subject to contraction. Primary contraction is conditioned by the shortening of the elastic fibers of the skin graft immediately after its harvesting. This condition is solved by pulling the transplant at the moment of attaching it to the recipient site. Thick grafts with a thick layer of the dermis will contract more than thin grafts, because of the elastic fibers found in the dermis. The secondary contraction is caused by the maturation of scar tissue between the transplant and the bed after the revascularization of the transplant. Secondary contraction is much more important than the primary contraction. It starts around the 10th postoperative day and continues during the next six months. Secondary contraction is affected by the changes in the bed, not by the changes in the graft. The secondary contraction is influenced by the following factors: the thicker the graft and the more rigid the bed, the less is graft subject to the secondary contraction. Another complication is a color change. Since skin has differing colorization, the best option is to transplant full-thickness grafts and to use the skin from the surrounding area for the transplant. Split-thickness skin transplants, especially the Tiersch graft exhibit distinct color changes.

Factors leading to the transplant separation include hematoma, bleeding, wound infection and necrosis of the bed, which can be a result of placing the graft on the avascular region (the exposed tendon, cartilage, bone, or the avascular fat). The separation of the graft may also occur due to external mechanical factors, lack of limb immobilization, or improper use of the dressing on the area that is constantly in motion.

Besides autografts, epidermal substitutes, such as cultivated keratinocytes are used to permanently cover defects. Keratinocytes, epithelial cells of the patient are removed and cultivated for two to three weeks. Epithelial cells are vulnerable to mechanical influences and susceptible to bacterial infection. The defect onto which the cultured keratinocytes will be applied must be properly prepared (Hulín 2015, Vidová Uğurbaş 2018).

Temporary Cover of Skin Defect

To temporarily cover the defect it is possible to use biologic grafts (allografts, xenografts, fetal membranes, allogeneic acellular dermis, and cultivated allogeneic keratinocytes), biosynthetic and synthetic skin substitutes (Biobrane, Integra, Dermagraft, TransCyte, Apligraft).

Skin allografts represent the most suitable option of temporary skin substitutes, they prevent fluid loss and penetration of microorganisms. Same as autografts, allografts are also used meshed (cross-linked) or non-meshed. After the first placement, the transplant is rejected within 14 days, which is why they are removed at about 12 days after the placement. *Xenografts* support the migration of fibroblasts and the formation of granulation tissue. Their disadvantage is the hyperacute rejection, referred to by experimental studies, which takes place during the first few minutes to hours of placement. Allogeneic acellular dermis (acellular dermal allograft) comes from the cadaveric dermis. The dermis is devoid of all cellular components and thus antigenicity is significantly suppressed.

Biosynthetic and Synthetic Substitutes

The role of the biosynthetic skin substitutes is to ensure a similar structure and function of the skin. The double-layered appearance that mimics its structure and function is important. The function of biosynthetic and synthetic skin substitutes is to prevent fluid loss, prevent the penetration of microorganisms, support of mechanical integrity and support of autograft engraftment. They contain variously modified biologic material in combination with synthetic materials. Their main task is to replace the dermis. *Biobrane* is the biosynthetic non-resorbable membrane, made of a nylon net and a silicone membrane at the surface, which is covered with peptides derived from porcine collagen Type I. It is used for surface damage of the skin, where it is left to spontaneous epithelialization. After some time it has to be removed and replaced by a final cover (autografts or cultured keratinocytes). Another possibility is a biosynthetic skin substitute *Integra*, which is an analog of the dermis that consists of collagen fibers. Its surface is covered with a silicone membrane. It also serves as a template for neodermis formation. *Dermagraft* is a cryopreserved dermal analog with fibroblasts, which expand from the neonatal prepuces on a polyglactin mesh. *TransCyte* (formerly called Dermagraft -TC) provides a partial dermal matrix. It is made of silicone-coated nylon mesh and contains non-viable fibroblasts. *Apligraf* is one of the two-layer composite substitutes, the epidermal layer has the well-differentiated stratum corneum, the dermal layer is composed of human fibroblasts in a grid of bovine collagen type I. It is used for stimulating healing using growth factors that are produced by cultured cells (Hulín 2015).

Coverage by Tissue Expansion

Tissue expansion is a supplement to flap surgery as well as to other reconstruction surgeries. It facilitates closure of large defects that would otherwise require more complicated reconstruction techniques.

The expansion of the tissue is a mechanical process that increases the volume of the local tissue for reconstruction purposes. Expanders, which are used for tissue expansion, are silicone reservoirs with a valve, which are used to inject solutions (Figure 16). During expansion, the tissue expander is filled with a saline solution through a port (valve), which is incorporated in the expander, or it is connected to the expander via silicone tubing. Smooth or textured tissue expanders exist in various sizes and shapes (round, square, oblong, tubular). Textured (rough) expanders are less likely to migrate from the original site, the connective tissue fixates them more than the smooth expanders. Expanders are inserted into the formed cavity under the skin, under a muscle, blood vessels, nerves, etc.

The filling of the expander begins on the 7th to 10th day after its insertion, thereby initiating the expansion itself. The expander is filled in weekly – 10-day intervals, the tissue expansion occurs within 8 – 12 weeks. Gradually, the solution is injected in more stages, to form a sufficient amount of soft tissue above the expander, which is used to cover the defect. Subsequently, the expander is removed and the defect is covered by the expanded tissue. Selecting the location of the expansion should meet some basic requirements: it should have the same color and appearance as the affected area. Try to avoid places of previous scars or injuries.

The advantage of tissue expansion is that skin of quality and color matching the surrounding area is obtained, the donor site is not necessary, and the procedure is simple.

The disadvantage of tissue expansion is the length of treatment (several months).

A possible complication is an infection, which requires the removal of the expander, the expander extrusion, and wound dehiscence. Complications such as discomfort and pain are only temporary (Bauer 2007).

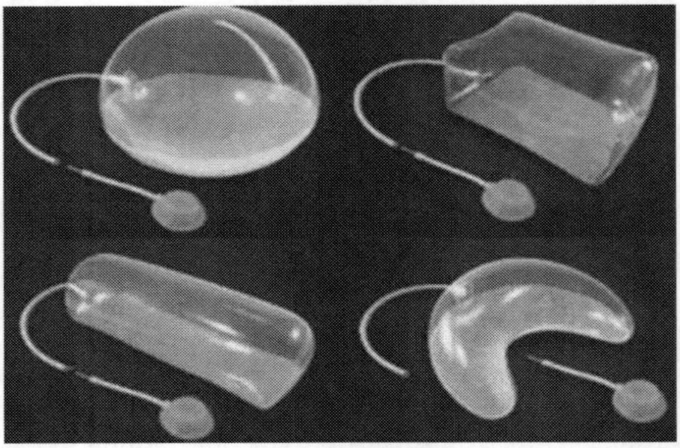

Figure 16. Tissue expanders (http://craniofacialteamtexas.com/pediatric-plastic-reconstructive-surgery/tissue-expansion/).

CONCLUSION

Hemodialysis accesses have a high incidence of complications. The most common complications in hemodialysis approaches include stenosis and thrombosis, Steal syndrome, infection, aneurysm, pseudoaneurysm, hyperfunction, venous hypertension, hand ischemia and subsequent skin defects (Bordils 2010)

Necrosis and bleeding are usually a result of repeated cannulation in single limited area of the arteriovenous angio-access. Skin necrosis overlying an arteriovenous fistula at the cannulation site is a common and potentially life-threatening problem. Skin necrosis generally requires by resection and repair with healthy tissue to closure of soft tissue and skin (Mallios 2018).

Flaps are used for coverage of defects of various differing etiology and composition. We can design the flap and adapt it accurately to fit the recipient site, according to the requirements and extent of the defect. The flap may comprise of a portion of skin with subcutaneous tissue, or with another tissue (fascia, muscles, bone), which are released from the donor site and transferred to the recipient site. For definitive coverage of skin defects of varying size and extent we can also use skin transplats. The skin can be transplanted as a whole (full-thickness) or in individual layers (split-thickness). Tissue expansion is a supplement to flap surgery as well as to other reconstruction surgeries.

Reconstruction of skin defects is needed wherever an extensive defect or loss of function is present. In the chapter we described all skin covering techniques with a description of their advantages and disadvantages.

REFERENCES

Bauer, B. S. 2007. "Tissue Expansion" in *Grabb and Smith's Plastic Surgery – 6th ed.* Edited by Charles Thorne, 84-90. Philadelphia: Lippincott Williams & Wilkins.

Bordils, G. A., Avendano, F., Gray, M. C., Arroyoet, C. C. 2010. Antebrachial Skin Necrosis after Reconstruction of an Arteriovenous Fistula in a Patient on Haemodialysis. *Nefrologia*. 30(4):0-486.

Chasmar, L. R. 2007. "The versatile rhomboid (Limberg) flap." *Canadian Journal of Plastic Surgery*. 15(15):67-71.

Frankovičová, M., Necpal, R., Patkaňová, L. (2015). Cievne prístupy. In: BREZA, J. – Haruštiak, S. – Kothaj, P. a kol. (ed.). *Princípy chirurgie IV*. Bratislava: SAP – Slovak Academic Press, 2015. s. 907-923. ISBN 978-80-89607-37-2.

Hulín, I. (ml). 2015. "Transplantácia kože." in *Princípy chirurgie IV*. edited by Breza J. et al., 1086-1094. Bratislava: SAP – Slovak

Academic Press. ["Skin transplantation in *Principles of Surgery IV.* edited by Breza J. et al., 1095-1102. Bratislava: SAP - Slovak Academic Press].

Lamberty, B. G., Cormack, G. C. 1990. "Progress in flap surgery: greater anatomical understanding and increased sophistication in application." *World Journal of Surgery* 14(6):776–785.

Mallios, A. et al. 2018. "Resection of Puncture Site Necrosis Over an Arteriovenous Fistula: Endoclamp Use for Preservation of Cannulation Sites." *Journal of Vascular Access* 19(3):316-318.

Marré, D., Jansen, L., Deo, S. 2020. Plastic Surgery Key. Fastest Plastic Surgery & Dermatology Insight Engine https://plasticsurgerykey.com/#.

Mathes, J. S., Levine, J. 2007. "Muscle Flaps and Their Blood Supply" in *Grabb and Smith's Plastic Surgery – 6th ed*. Edited by Charles Thorne, 84-90. Philadelphia: Lippincott Williams & Wilkins.

Osman, G. M. A., Al-shahat, O. A., Ayad, W. M. 2005. "Fasciocutaneous Flaps for Repair of Sacral Pressure Sores." *AAMJ* 3(2):19-29.

Palenčár, D. 2015. "Lalokové plastiky" in *Princípy chirurgie IV.* edited by Breza J. et al., 1095-1102. Bratislava: SAP – Slovak Academic Press. ["Flap plastic surgery" *In Principles of Surgery IV.* edited by Breza J. et al., 1095-1102. Bratislava: SAP - Slovak Academic Press].

Pirozzia, N. et al. 2013. "Limberg Skin Flap for Treatment of Necrosis and Bleeding at Haemodialysis Arteriovenous Angioaccess Puncture Sites." *European Journal of Vascular and Endovascular Surgery* 46(3):383-387.

Salam, G. A. et al. 2003. "The Basic Z-Plasty." *American Family Physician* 67(11): 2329-2332.

Shimizu, R., Kishi, K. 2012. "Skin Graft." *Plastic Surgery International* 2012: 563493.

Sprague, S. M. 2014. "Painful Skin Ulcers in a Hemodialysis Patient." *Clinical Journal of the American Society of Nephrology*. 9(1):166–173.

Thorne, CH. H. 2007. "Techniques and Principles in Plastic Surgery." in *Grabb and Smith's Plastic Surgery – 6th ed*. Edited by Charles Thorne, 84-90. Philadelphia: Lippincott Williams & Wilkins.

Vidová Uğurbaş, M. 2018. *Plastická chirurgia.* Košice: UNLP Košice. [*Plastic surgery*. Košice.: Louis Paster University Hospital].

In: Surgeon´s Perspective on Dialysis Patient ISBN: 978-1-53619-262-9
Editor: Maria Frankovicova

Chapter 12

KIDNEY TRANSPLANTATION

P. Zavacký*
Department of Surgery,
Medical Faculty of Pavol Jozef Safarik University
and University Hospital, Košice, Slovakia

ABSTRACT

Kidney transplantation is the treatment method that, from a medical point of view, most comprehensively replaces the function of the organ in the event of its irreversible failure. The first human kidney was unsuccessfully transplanted by Voronoy in Ukraine in 1933. The first kidney transplantation in former Czechoslovakia was performed in Hradec Králové in 1961. In general, organ transplants (Tx) require the technique of vascular anastomosis or surgical connection of vessels, which would allow flow from one vessel to another. Without such a connection, there is no hope of success.

Keywords: kidney transplantation, vascular anastomosis, rejection, HLA typing

* Corresponding Author's E-mail: peterzavacky963@gmail.com.

Abbreviations

ALPL	antilymphocyte antibodies
ATN	acute tubular necrosis
CM	crossmatch
CKD	chronic kidney disease
CT	computed tomography
DIC	disseminated intravascular coagulopathy
ESRD	end stage renal disease
HLA	human histocompatibility system
IKEM	Institute of Clinical and Experimental Medicine
KTx	kidney transplantation
PTA	percutaneous transluminal angioplasty
PTFE	polytetrafluorethylene
PSA	pseudoaneurysm
PTRA	percutaneous transluminal renal angioplasty
RAS	renal artery stenosis
RRT	renal replacement therapy
TRAS	transplant renal artery stenosis

Introduction

Kidney transplantation is the treatment method that, from a medical point of view, most comprehensively replaces the function of the organ in the event of its irreversible failure. In patients with kidney failure, transplantation provides the highest possible quality of life compared to other methods of kidney function replacement, and at the same time, from an economic point of view, this treatment modality is the cheapest way to treat kidney failure at its terminal stage.

The results of kidney transplantation vary depending on the experience of each transplant center. From a surgical point of view, these are mainly peri- and post-operative complications, including vascular etiology

(KDIGO, 2009; KDIGO, 2013). According to data from large workplaces with more than 50 operations carried out annually, kidney transplantation takes place with technical complications only in 5% of respondents per year. Adequate care for both the recipient as well as the donor, teamwork with clearly defined procedures, attention to detail all determine the problem-free course of the transplantation, a low number of complications and their fast resolution enables achieving positive results with one year and longer survival of the first kidney, which should be achieved in more than 95% of cases. Uncomplicated post-transplant course or rapid management of associated complications is a basic prerequisite for long-term stable function of the transplanted organ.

History of Kidney Transplantation

In general, organ transplants (Tx) require, in particular, the technique of vascular anastomosis or surgical connection of vessels, which would allow flow from one vessel to another. Without such a connection, there is no hope of success. Alexis Carrel and Charley Claude Guthrie were the most important figures in the development of these techniques. Carrel began working on the problem of vascular anastomoses in 1902. In 1905, he moved to Chicago, where he began working with Guthrie. They developed a method of fine continuous suture that penetrated all layers of the vessel wall and tested it on many tissue and organ transplants, including kidney transplants. Carrel and Guthrie performed the first heart transplant in a dog as early as 1905.

The first human kidney was unsuccessfully transplanted by Voronoy in Ukraine in 1933. The patient died after 48 hours. In 1933 and 1939, Voronoy performed six more kidney transplants, but all failed.

Another crucial milestone for the future of kidney transplantation was the research of N. Alwell in Sweden and W. J. Kolff in the Netherlands, who built the first dialysis machines. Later, dialysis was also undertaken in the United States, where they became part of standard ESRD (End-stage renal disease) treatment. The discovery of artificial kidney from the point of view of transplantation made it possible to stabilize the health status of patients by the so-called bridging before and after KTx (kidney transplantation), respectively, until the onset of the function of the transplanted kidney.

In 1951, David Hume, George Thorn, and Gustave Dammin, along with colleagues at Peter Bent Brigham Hospital in Boston, began a series of kidney transplants from a deceased donor. Their work proved that kidney function was good until rejection developed.

The first kidney transplantation in former Czechoslovakia was performed in Hradec Králové in 1961. A systematic kidney transplant program began 5 years later at the Institute of Clinical and Experimental Medicine (IKEM). In Slovakia, the first KTx was performed on June 16, 1972, at the Department of Urology, Faculty of Medicine, Comenius University in the Hospital of Academician L. Dérer in Bratislava (see Table 2.). It was performed by prof. MD. Zvara. It was a 48-year-old patient, a medical professional from the Slovak town of Vráble, who was treated for chronic renal insufficiency in the area of chronic glomerulonephritis for several months. The patient survived 8 years after the KTx and died of a cardiovascular disease, which he had been diagnosed with before the kidney transplantation.

After gaining the necessary experience, in 1978 a second transplant team led by MUDr. Rezníček has formed, but later also doc. MUDr. Breza (currently prof. MUDr. Ján Breza, DrSc. - Head of the Department of Urology, Faculty of Medicine, Comenius University in the Hospital with Medical Centre of L. Dérer in Bratislava since 1996) began to address the issue. In 1988, kidney transplants began to be carried out at the Surgical Department in Košice, followed by the Surgical Department of Roosevelt Hospital in Banská Bystrica in 1991.

Indications and Contraindications for Kidney Transplantation

Patients with chronic terminal kidney failure enrolled in a long-term dialysis program are placed on a waiting list for transplantation after completing basic examinations if they meet the required criteria. Candidates for kidney transplantation undergo a medical, social and psychological evaluation to assess factors that could influence successful post-transplant development. For the inclusion of a potential recipient, both expert opinion and the patient's consent are important, which the patient confirms with his signature. It expresses the attitude and responsibility to the risk associated with surgery and chronic immunosuppression. When selecting a patient for a kidney transplant, consideration should be given to whether the risk of surgery, general anesthesia, and long-term immunosuppression does not outweigh the benefit of the transplant to the health status of the potential recipient, the so-called "cost versus benefit".

Contraindications to kidney transplantation are classified as either absolute or relative (see Table 1.).

Absolute contraindications include malignant oncological diseases, where immunosuppression would significantly worsen the course of the malignancy, HIV positivity due to the fatal course of the underlying disease, liver cirrhosis, and viral hepatitis, where even liver failure and severe psychiatric illnesses may occur, for which regular use of immunosuppressants cannot be ensured.

Table 1. Contraindications of Kidney Tx

Contraindications of kidney Tx
Absolute: malignant oncological diseases
HIV positivity
liver cirrhosis and viral hepatitis
severe psychiatric illnesses
Relative: age of the recipient
renal disease with a risk of recurrence
infectious diseases
gastroduodenal disease
chronic pancreatitis
malnutrition or severe obesity
advanced atherosclerosis of the aortoiliac stage
non-compliant patients

Relative contraindications include the age of the recipient, kidney diseases at risk of recurrence, coexisting diseases causing a high risk of anesthesia, infectious diseases, gastroduodenal disease, chronic pancreatitis, malnutrition, and/or severe obesity, advanced aortoiliac atherosclerosis causing technical problems while inserting renal arteries of the graft. Non-compliant patients who are socially maladapted with a low presumption of adherence to the treatment regimen and cooperation with the attending physician are also a relative contraindication. The given respondents are always re-evaluated individually in cooperation between the dialysis nephrologist and the transplant nephrologist.

Compatibility in the major human histocompatibility system (HLA), which plays a crucial role in the risk of graft rejection, is important for the success of kidney transplantation.

The sensitization of HLA antigens and their compatibility is determined by the level of preformed anti-lymphocyte antibodies (ALPL). The degree of sensitization of the recipient to HLA antigens increases with repeated exposures to foreign antigens, such as repeated transfusions, or previous unsuccessful organ transplants. These antibodies may be of the IgG and IgM classes. After transplantation, IgG antibodies significantly contribute to chronic rejection - chronic graft dysfunction and significantly worsen the prognosis of the survival of the transplanted kidney.

After inclusion on the waiting list, the ALPL level in each patient is determined every three months. Prior to transplantation, a crossmatch (CM) of the recipient's serum with the donor's lymphocytes should always be performed. The crossmatch is performed before selecting a donor-recipient pair. In the microlymphotoxicity test, the reaction of the donor cells with the recipient's serum is examined. The serum must not be older than three months, but it is best to use the recipient's fresh serum. Its positive result indicates a high risk of hyperacute rejection and is a contraindication to transplantation.

A set of these immunological and immunogenetic tests determines the suitability of donor-recipient pairs and is a prerequisite for transplant success and long-term graft survival.

Vascular Graft in Transplant Surgery

In transplant surgery, there is often a need to elongate the vascular pedicle, because an insufficiently long vessel cannot be corrected. Various techniques for repairing a short or a damaged donor renal artery include end-to-end artery graft anastomosis, side-to-side branching artery anastomosis, and the use of an iliac arterial graft. The short donor renal vein can be corrected by transferring the recipient's external iliac vein after ligation of the internal iliac vein, extending the donor vein by renal hilar dissection, and using venous grafts.

Authors at the University of Oxford describe a case of 3 kidney transplants in which a polytetrafluorethylene (PTFE) vascular graft (Hybrid PTFE®, Atrium Medical Cooperation, Hudson, NH, USA) was inserted between the short renal and recipient vessels. Two of the kidneys described were allografts obtained from deceased donors and the third was a renal autograft. In the case of two grafts from deceased donors, donor iliac vascular grafts were obtained from the transplant team that performed a liver transplant and grafts from donor iliac vessels were not stored. The use of a saphenous vein graft for the potential need for coronary artery bypass graft surgery in these two transplant recipients was not preferred.

Poor vascular wall, intimal damage, media rupture, dissection, squeezing, and subintimal hematoma are indications of vascular resection. Autoarterial and autovenous autografts are the most suitable. Whether a vascular graft will be permeable depends essentially on the quality of the vascular connection. Well everted intima, average knot tension, not an extensive wall engagement, it all depends on the clinical experience of the surgeon and his surgical erudition. The quality of the vascular graft, its processing, method, and quality of collection and manipulation during suturing are all also particularly important.

Some papers also describe renal vessel reconstruction in kidney transplantation using a polytetrafluoroethylene (PTFE) vascular graft. One of them is a work published by authors at the University of Oxford in 2007, where they modified the short renal arteries of three renal grafts by inserting PTFE vascular grafts.

There are only a few published cases describing the use of PTFE grafts in the reconstruction of short or damaged renal vessels in kidney transplantation. Delphin described two cases in which PTFE grafts were successfully used to prolong short donor renal veins in two kidney grafts from deceased donors. In the Delphin study, PTFE grafts were permeable for at least 1and 2 years. In another case report, Blacklock described the reconstruction of a donor renal artery in a renal autograft using a PTFE graft.

Types of Adjustments

Damage to the arterial supply of a kidney from a deceased donor can occur at various levels and can affect any segment. Such damage, although severe, can usually be repaired with careful planning and microsurgical techniques.

Overview of the Techniques

Type 1

Iliac artery graft elongation - a transversely cut or shortened single renal artery can usually be reconstructed by an end-to-end anastomosis onto the recipient's iliac artery. Optionally, a free external or common iliac artery graft can be anastomosed with an end-to-end method to the damaged renal artery during final graft preparation. If the anastomosis is end-lateral to the external or common iliac artery, a free graft bifurcation may be formed to create a Carrel patch to facilitate the end-lateral anastomosis (see Figure 1). This is a particularly important option for elderly patients whose blood vessels are atherosclerotic.

Type 2

Revision of the aortic patch - This technique is useful in kidneys with dual blood supply, where there is an aortic injury between the outlets (a take-off of the renal arteries, or where the aortic outlet (take-off) between the two arteries is separated by more than 1 cm (see Figure 2). Be careful to avoid tightening or twisting the arteries or renal vein.

Type 3

Repairing damage to smaller arteries - damage to small upper polar arteries results in small infarctions, located at the upper pole of the graft, that are not harmful enough to require effort for vascular repair. Damage to the lower polar arteries is potentially more dangerous because the blood supply to the ureter of the graft can be compromised. The lower polar vessels are repaired either directly (see Figure 3a), by reimplantation into a larger renal vessel (see Figure 3b), or by using a side-to-side "connected" anastomosis to create a common orifice that could be anastomosed end-to-end to the hypogastric artery (see Figure 4a), or to the donor vascular graft (see Figure 4b). The combined technique is only possible when the vessels are long enough and similar in size.

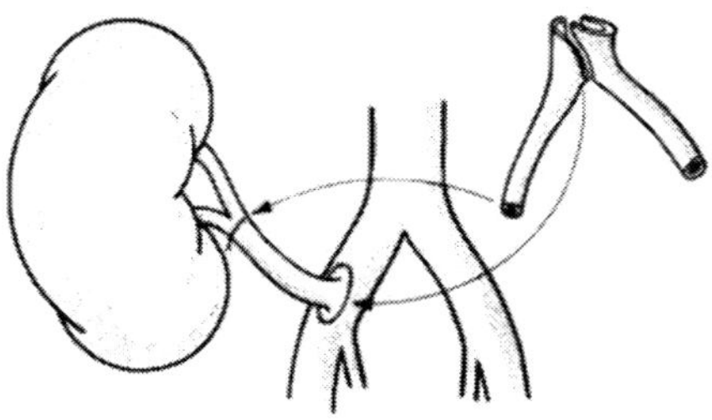

(Source: author)

Figure 1. Elongation of one renal artery using a donor external iliac graft.

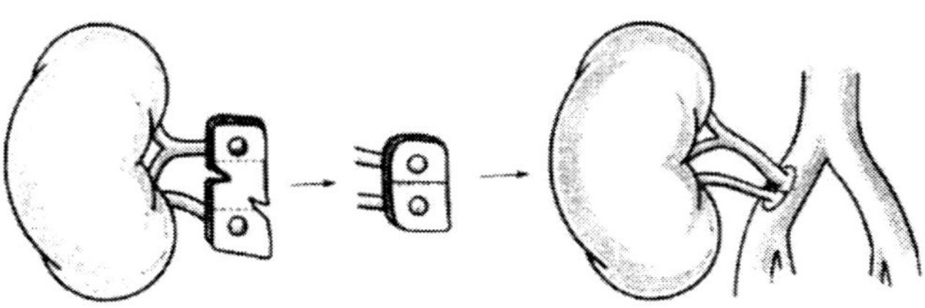

(Source: author)

Figure 2. Remodeling of the aortic patch in a double artery kidney.

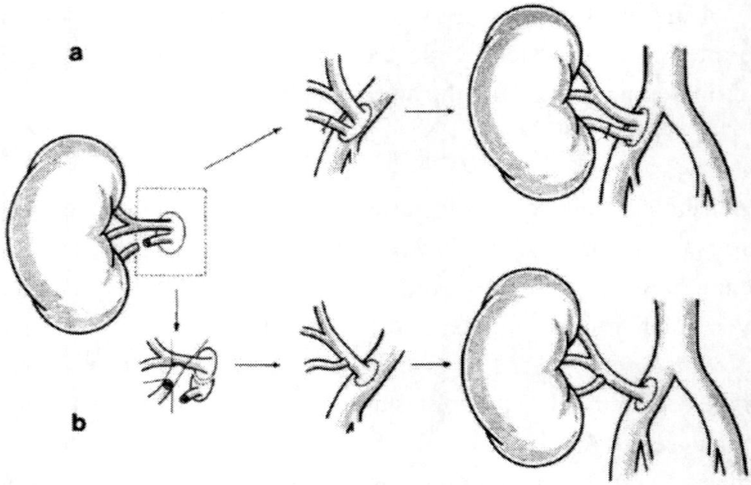

(Source: author)

Figure 3 a, b Repair of the damaged segmental artery a) direct repair, b) reimplantation into a larger renal vessel.

Type 4

Combination of types 1.-3.

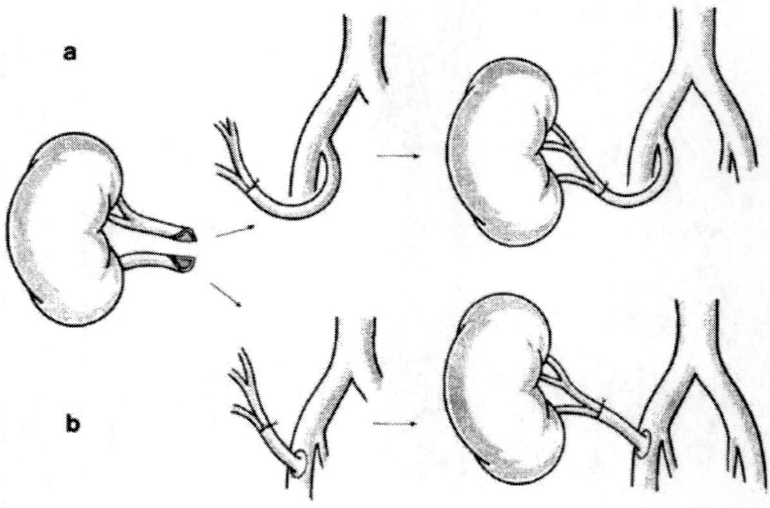

Figure 4. Combination of types 1.-3.

All of the basic techniques above can be used in combination (see Figure 4). This case was described by Professor Jafri of the Urological Clinic in Lahore in 2009.

KIDNEY TRANSPLANTATION

The surgical side of kidney transplantation has not changed significantly in recent decades, with the technique described in the 1950s by Professor Küss (1992) in use to this day. Kidney transplantation is an allotransplantation, i.e., the transfer of an organ between two individuals of the same species. Autotransplantation of the kidney means its transfer from the original position to the pelvis when the renal artery is affected or when the ureter is injured. Small differences in surgical techniques and tactics are due to the tradition and experience of a particular transplant center. During transplantation, the kidney is inserted extraperitoneally into the iliac fossa, its vessels are sutured to the iliac vessels.

An integral part of kidney transplantation is the reconstruction of the urinary tract. The goal of urinary tract reconstruction is to achieve optimal and socially acceptable drainage of urine from the transplanted kidney. Particular attention should be paid to the vascular anastomosis, as its reconstruction significantly affects not only the patient's quality of life after kidney transplantation but also the function and survival of the transplanted kidney as well as the patients themselves.

Operation Procedure

Introduce a urethral catheter of the largest possible diameter (22-24F) in the operating room and fill the bladder with a 10% Betadine solution. In heterotopic kidney transplantation, the right kidney is inserted extraperitoneally into the iliac fossa on the left side and, conversely, the left kidney into the iliac fossa on the right side (Figure 5). Most transplant centers prefer to place the right kidney on the left side and the left kidney on the right side. The reason is the need to maintain a parallel course of the artery and the renal vein.

Preparation of the Recipient's Vessels

After the overall preparation of the surgical field, make an oblique incision of the skin 2-3 cm above the inguinal ligament and the anterior superior iliac spine. In the line of incision, break the muscle layers up to the peritoneum. For better access to the bladder, interrupt and ligate the inferior epigastric vessels. In renal grafts with variant arterial anatomy, you can use the inferior epigastric artery to reconstruct the inferior renal polar artery. The spermatic duct should be discontinued only in indicated cases where it prevents the preparation of the bladder or could stenotize the ureter of the transplanted kidney and prevent their crossing. In such a procedure, the external iliac artery, as well as the renal artery, are placed ventrally and behind them, the external iliac vein and the renal vein are located. In pediatric transplants, especially in the case of placement of a vascular anastomosis of the kidney on the aorta and inferior vena cava, choose the incision on the right side. With this access, the preparation of the vena cava is easier.

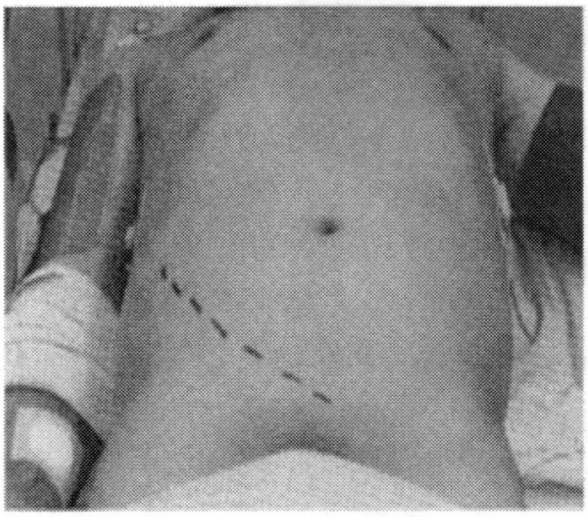

(Source: author)

Figure 5. Location of the incision in the Tx of the kidney.

Preparation of the Removed Kidney for Transplantation

Check and prepare the kidney for transplantation under sterile conditions in the operating room before the actual procedure. Leave the kidney immersed in crushed ice and work on a specially prepared instrumental table, the so-called back table. The anatomical structures of the kidney and the effectiveness of rinsing the kidney with preservative fluid during collection are checked. Properly washed kidney is homogeneously discolored, whitish in color. Its insufficient washing is evidenced by bluish marble stains most often located in the area of the upper or the lower pole. In case of insufficient washing, renal reperfusion is indicated. Start the preparation of the kidney by identifying vascular structures. Remove excess fat from the front and back surfaces and remains of the adrenal gland from the upper pole area. Leave the fat in the area of the golden triangle intact, which is the area between the lower pole, the ureter, and the hilum of the kidney. Here, arteries and veins arise from the renal vessels, supplying the ureter and pelvis. Disruption of these vessels results in urological complications after transplantation. Rotate the kidney by looking at its posterior surface and cleansing the renal artery from the aortic branch to the hilum. However, do not cut too deep into the hilum so as not to break the branching of the renal artery or the branch to the pelvis and the ureter. Always check the integrity of the arterial intima and the presence of accessory arteries that would require reconstruction. If the accessory arteries are undamaged and not too far from the stoma of the main artery, you can leave them on a common knob. If the distance is too great, leave them separately on aortic knobs. If the accessory arteries are ruptured or separated from the aortic knob, they can be sutured to the main artery end-to-side or reconstructed using vascular allografts obtained during collection from the donor, most often iliac vessels, or by means of autografts taken from the recipient, most often the inferior epigastric artery or the saphenous vein. For a kidney from a deceased donor, the short renal vein can be extended by various techniques using the inferior vena cava or the donor external iliac/lumbar vein (see Figure 7). The left kidney is preferred due to its longer renal vein rather than using a donor vena cava to extend the right renal vein in a kidney transplant from a deceased donor,

Reconstruction of small arteries is also necessary because the renal arteries are finite in the kidney. Ligature of such an artery leads to necrosis of the relevant part of the renal parenchyma, which can result in hematuria post-transplantation. Anomalies of the venous system are significantly rarer than those of the arterial system and occur more frequently in the right kidney. However, the problem is often a short renal vein on the right side. Especially in men and in obese patients, there are technical problems in suturing a venous anastomosis despite the release of the external iliac vein. In such cases, if a part of the inferior vena cava was left during procurement, you can create an auxiliary venous conduit from it. In this way, you can safely and effortlessly sew a venous anastomosis under any anatomical conditions in the recipient.

Do not dissect the ureter even if there is more fat around it, so as not to damage its vascular supply. It is better to remove excess fat only during transplantation after definitive verification of ureteral blood flow. The kidneys treated and prepared in this way are stored back in the solution with crushed ice until transplantation.

The kidney transplantation itself begins by creating access to the iliac vessels in the small pelvis. Choose the access from an oblique incision in the hypogastrium on the right or on the left side (Figure 5). Gradually intersect the aponeurosis of the external abdominal muscle, the external abdominal muscle and the transverse muscle, and finally the transverse fascia. Thus, you get to the peritoneum and proceed extraperitoneally in the iliac fossa. Intersect the inferior epigastric artery and the inferior epigastric vein, in men mobilize the spermatic cord and in women intersect the round ligament of uterus. In this way, you gradually get to the iliac vessels. The access is identical to that of vascular reconstructions in the iliac region. Dissect the external iliac artery and vein, or, if necessary, also the common or internal iliac artery and vein (see Figure 6). It is recommended that the accompanying lymphatic vessels are ligated to prevent the formation of a lymphocele. The anastomosis between the vessels begins with an end to the side connection of the vein of the transplanted kidney with the external iliac vein.

After finishing the anastomosis, put a clamp on the renal vein near the hilum of the kidney, restoring the blood flow to the external iliac vein, and check the anastomosis. This is followed by the connection of the artery of the transplanted kidney either end to end to the internal iliac artery after the artery is severed or end to the side to the external iliac artery. In recent years, the second method of arterial connection has been preferred, because, in end-to-end anastomoses, more frequent stenoses occur at the site of the anastomosis. In addition, an aortic knob to the renal artery can be used for deceased-donor kidney transplantation. The decision on the method of the anastomosis is also influenced by the quality of the wall of the iliac arteries. In sclerotic changes, the anastomosis is done where there are the smallest changes. If this is not possible, the pathologically altered intima must be removed in the given area together with the sclerotic plaque, i.e., first an endarterectomy must be performed and then an anastomosis must be performed. In repeated transplants in men, the internal iliac artery must be maintained at least on one side, otherwise, erectile dysfunction will occur. The anastomosis between the arteries is made by a continuous suture of non-absorbable material, preferably Prolen 5/0 or Vascufil 5/0 (Figure 7). After completing the anastomosis, place a clamp on the artery of the transplanted kidney at the hilum, release the flow through the iliac artery and verify the tightness of the anastomosis.

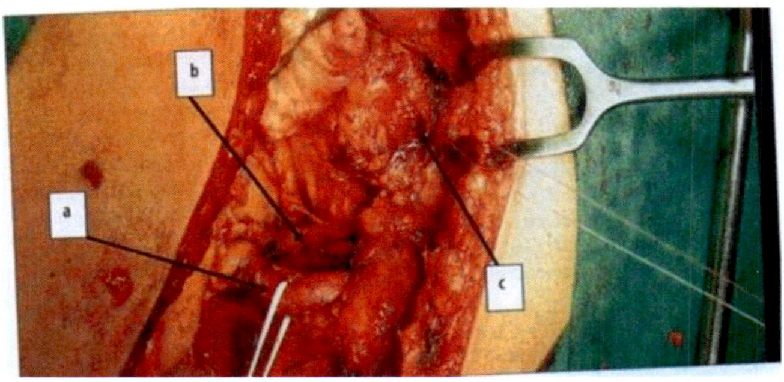

(Source: author)

Figure 6. Dissected external iliac vasa: a-iliac artery, b-iliac vein, c-bladder.

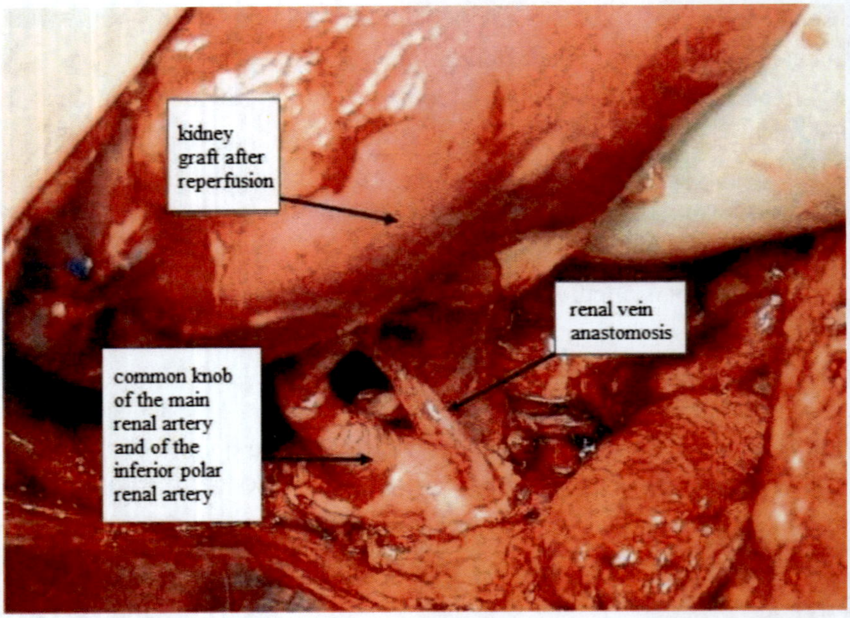

(Source: author)

Figure 7. Renal graft reperfusion - arterial and venous anastomosis.

After suturing both vascular anastomoses, proceed to the reperfusion of the kidney, release the clamps, first to the renal vein, and then to the renal artery. After the circulation has been restored, the transplanted kidney turns pink, slightly enlarges, and acquires its turgor (see Figure 11).

Postoperative Care and Immunosuppressive Treatment

Although much of the postoperative care of a patient after KTx is specialized, many aspects immediately after transplantation are identical to the management of a surgical patient. The first 24 hours are critical to ensure optimal conditions for the graft function.

KTx is a surgical intervention with a fresh surgical wound, therefore the need for postoperative analgesia is highly represented with a possible risk of developing hypotension, especially in the splanchnic area with centralized blood circulation, which is a risk factor (due to possible hypoperfusion) for the transplant itself. Monitoring of the recipient's basic vital signs, including renal parameters (such as hourly diuresis, laboratory parameters, and drainage of the drains) is a necessity in the early postoperative period. The optimal (early) onset of graft function cannot be achieved without adequate hydration of the patient. In the post-transplant period, the fluid intake is dependent on diuresis, clinical signs of the hydration status, and central venous pressure (CVP) value, which should be around 10 cm of H_2O. As part of hydration, the optimal composition of maintenance intravenous solutions is a combination of 0.9% saline and 5% glucose in a ratio of 2: 1, with the oral fluid intake being permitted from the first postoperative day onwards.

When administering transfusions to a patient after a kidney transplant, risks such as induction of antibody-mediated rejection or cytomegalovirus infection should be considered. Many patients with CKD (Chronic Kidney Disease) tolerate hemoglobin values around 80 g/l without significant symptomatology. If a blood transfusion is necessary, an erythrocyte mass without a "buffy coat", ideally leukoreduced, is preferred.

The urinary catheter is left for 7 days. Its task is the continuous derivation of urine, which prevents the possible decompression of the bladder and minimizes the risk of leakage at the site of a freshly sutured ureteroneocystostomy. On the other hand, the urinary catheter is also a potential risk factor as a gateway for infection. This is an important aspect when considering the iatrogenic suppression of the immunity of the patient. The introduction of a JJ stent should be standard, but antibiotic prophylaxis should not be forgotten. Its removal is carried out around 4 - 6 weeks after KTx, but the individual approach is also appropriate in this case.

The standard amount of waste in the drains after kidney transplantation is about 500 ml during the first 24 hours. A persistently high volume of serous stained fluid indicates the possibility of a urinary or lymphatic fistula. Determining which of the fistulas is can be done by running a simple biochemical analysis.

Table 2. Classification of immunosuppressive strategies

Classification of immunosuppressive strategies
induction of immunosuppression
maintenance immunosuppression
antirejection treatment

In the case of urinary fistula, the drainage contains a high concentration of creatinine, urea, and potassium and a low concentration of glucose; in the case of the lymphatic fistula, their concentrations are similar to serum values.

Early mobilization of the patient after kidney transplantation is just as desirable as after other types of surgery. Equally important is the care of pulmonary hygiene and of the surgical wound. The only difference compared to standard surgery is the use of immunosuppressive drugs, therefore, healing is slower, and stitches are extracted 14 to 21 days after the surgery.

The issue of immunosuppressive treatment is very extensive and beyond the scope of this work, therefore only the basic division is given. Each transplant center has its own dedicated protocol on the principles of initiation and saturation of immunosuppression, based on international nephrology recommendations ("NKF/KDOQITM, KDIGO Clinical Practice Guideline, ERBP"), fine-tuned according to the clinical experience of each center. Transplant center Košice (TC KE) is no exception. Today, this treatment is often individualized and "tailored" to the individual's clinical and laboratory needs. In principle, we distinguish 3 types of immunosuppressive strategies, which are listed in Table 2.

The induction of immunosuppression is based on the knowledge that relatively high perioperative and early postoperative immunosuppression can prevent the occurrence of acute rejection, or at least delay it or decrease its severity. Intense induction, e.g., using anti-lymphocyte antibodies, is particularly needed in sensitized patients at high risk of graft failure due to immunological causes, for example, immunized patients with repeatedly positive CM, after one and/or more KTxes in the past. Maintenance immunosuppression is a partial inhibition of the recipient's immune system and allows it to work with its basic defense system without attacking the transplanted organ. Anti-rejection treatment is intensive short-term immunosuppression, completely inhibiting the recipient's immune response directed not only to the allograft but also to all other foreign antigens. It must be time-limited, otherwise the risk of complications from immunodeficiency increases. Rejection is a complication of a sensitized respondent after KTx, or of non-saturation by immunosuppression, or otherwise induced decreased levels of an immunosuppressive drug, and should always be confirmed histologically after a KTx biopsy.

We recognize three basic types of rejection:

1. Hyperacute rejection is caused by pre-existing antibodies against AB0 antigens, or by antibodies established (due to pregnancy, transfusion, previous transplantation) against HLA antigens. These antibodies cause transplant vascular thrombosis immediately after graft reperfusion or during the first few hours. Hyperacute rejection can be prevented by respecting compatibility in the AB0 system and by performing a "cross match" before transplantation, possibly in case of transplantation with AB0 incompatibility, pre-transplant inhibition of AB0 antibody production is obligatory at the same time as their removal according to validated protocols. This type of rejection has a life-threatening course and most often ends in a graftectomy.
2. Acute rejection occurs when antibodies are produced at the instigation of incompatible transplant antigens, which causes necrosis of vascular cells, called acute vascular rejection. The vasculitis image is formed histologically in contrast to thrombosis in hyperacute rejection. Regarding the clinical aspect, it is divided into early and late acute rejection. Early acute rejection occurs during the first three months after transplantation, but most often on the 7th to 10th postoperative day.

3. Late acute rejection is defined as an acute rejection occurring after the third-month post KTx, independent of possible and/or present previous early acute rejection.
4. Chronic rejection, called chronic graft dysfunction, maybe a chronically delayed type of cellular response, or it may be a manifestation of undersized healing of acute rejection or rejection crises. A characteristic feature of the histological picture is vascular wall fibrosis, which leads to a decrease of its elasticity and consequently to the development of accelerated atherosclerosis and ischemic graft damage with progressive failure of function, ending in ESRD.

The treatment of all types of rejections always belongs to the hands of an experienced transplant nephrologist in cooperation with a specialized immunologist.

VASCULAR COMPLICATIONS AFTER KIDNEY TRANSPLANTATION

Vascular complications are among the most serious surgical problems after kidney transplantation. These complications impair the function of the transplanted kidney and can potentially lead to the loss of the graft, in some cases even endangering the patient's life. Vascular thrombosis or bleeding from anastomosis most often occurs in the early postoperative period, arterial stenosis and other vascular complications occur later in the period after kidney transplantation. In terms of time, we can classify vascular complications as either early or late. Early complications occur several hours to days after transplantation and are closely related to surgery and the body's immune response to foreign tissue. These include bleeding from anastomoses, kinking of the renal artery of the graft, and vascular thrombosis. Late vascular complications arise over time after transplantation and their progression is due to the progression of aortoiliac atherosclerosis, infection, technical errors in the construction of anastomoses, biopsy diagnostic interventions, rejection episodes in the transplanted kidney or chronic rejection (Table 3).

Early Vascular Complications

Early Thrombosis of the Renal Artery

Early arterial thrombosis is a serious postoperative complication that leads to graft loss and requires a graft nephrectomy. Its frequency is reported to be between 0.5-3.5%, with 80% of cases occurring in the first month after transplantation. Thrombosis is most common in multiple renal arteries, especially in the kidney, and in end-to-end anastomoses to the internal iliac artery. Risk factors include, in addition to activation of coagulation, graft hypoperfusion in systemic hypotension, dehydration, and severe acute tubular necrosis (ATN), kinking of too long renal artery of the graft, intimal damage in careless kidney explantation at procurement, and atherosclerosis of the donor and recipient. Arterial thrombosis can be the terminal event of hyperacute or reversible acute rejection.

Table 3. Vascular complications after kidney Tx

Vascular complications after kidney transplantation	
Early vascular complications:	early renal artery thrombosis renal venous thrombosis postoperative bleeding
Late vascular complications:	stenosis and late thrombosis of the renal artery renal vein stenosis and VIE isolated iliac artery aneurysm infectious aneurysm in the Tx area of the kidney lymphocele

Sudden graft anuria, swelling of the transplanted kidney, and pain in the wound dominate in the clinical image of early renal artery thrombosis of the Tx kidney. Diagnosis is based on an urgent USG examination which can be supplemented by CT angiography, DSA, or scintigraphic examination. Early renal artery thrombosis is almost always associated with the thrombosis of the entire graft and requires an urgent graftectomy because of the risk of developing disseminated intravascular coagulopathy (DIC).

Table 4. Causes of early thrombosis of the renal artery of the Tx kidney

Causes of early thrombosis of the renal artery of the Tx kidney
multiple renal arteries
kidneys from baby donors (< 5yrs old)
end to end anastomosis on the internal iliac artery
donor and recipient atherosclerosis
technical errors: kinking, damage to the intima, too "tight" anastomosis
graft hypoperfusion in systemic hypotension, severe acute tubular necrosis (ATN)
hyperacute or irreversible acute rejection

Thrombosis of the Renal Vein

This complication usually also leads to the loss of the graft. Occurrence is reported to be between 0.9-7.6%. It is manifested by painful graft enlargement, macroscopic hematuria, and subsequent anuria. The most common causes are anastomotic stenosis, venous compression by hematoma or by lymphocele, twisted vein, a transition of deep vein thrombosis into the renal vein, hypercoagulable states or reperfusion injury, diabetes, repeated transplantations, ATN (acute tubular necrosis), elderly recipient, coagulation disorders (V Leiden factor, antifungal or anticardiolipin antibodies). The diagnosis is based on the clinical image and may be supplemented by USG examination, CT angiography or graft scintigraphy may also be helpful. Renal vein thrombosis usually leads to the loss of the graft and a necessary graftectomy. With early diagnosis, thrombectomy can be attempted, and more rarely, heparin can be used to successfully treat a partial thrombosis. A small number of patients may develop deep vein iliofemoral thrombosis. The cause is not entirely clear, one of the causes may be swelling of the transplanted kidney, which compresses the external iliac vein. It is clinically manifested by swelling and pain in the ipsilateral limb and a decrease in the renal function of the transplanted kidney. If venous thrombosis is suspected, urgent thrombectomy is indicated, but in most patients, the graft cannot be rescued and urgent graftectomy is indicated for impending graft rupture. If a thrombectomy is performed within 1 hour of thrombosis formation, it is still possible to save the graft.

Postoperative Bleeding

Postoperative bleeding originates in the vascular anastomosis. The most common cause of early postoperative bleeding is small vessels in the hilum of the kidney, which were not apparent due to vasospasm before the closure of the surgical wound. Thorough intraoperative hemostasis reduces the risk of bleeding. Before the transplant, a detailed pharmacological history is important, specifically targeting the administration of long-acting antiplatelet agents (Acylpyrin, Anopyrin, Ticlid, Briligue, Clopidogrel and others), that affect primary hemostasis and, together with uremic thrombocytopathy, may contribute to diffuse bleeding. In the case of bleeding, blood clotting should be repeatedly tested, in order to rule out new-onset coagulopathy, as severe post-transplant complications such as peracute rejection may be associated with the development of disseminated intravascular coagulopathy (DIC). Postoperative bleeding is manifested by an increased amount of waste in the drains, and a decrease in hemoglobin as well as in blood pressure. If the loss is greater than 500-800 ml per hour, urgent surgical revision is indicated. A typical presentation is the development of a retroperitoneal hematoma, which stretches cranially along with the iliopsoas muscle, and many times the source of bleeding is not even found during revision. After removal of the hematoma and release of pressure in the retroperitoneum, the transplanted kidney is re-perfused.

Late Vascular Complications

Renal Artery Stenosis/RAS/

Renal artery stenosis is more common than thrombosis. The incidence of RAS is reported to be in the range of 1-23% and the number of positive diagnoses increases with the use of duplex sonography. Surgical or endovascular intervention is necessary for 1-3% of kidney transplant recipients. Stenosis can develop on the recipient's artery, the vascular anastomosis, and on the donor's artery. The causes of stenosis are documented in Table 5.

Table 5. Causes of renal artery stenosis of the Tx kidney

Causes of renal artery stenosis of the Tx kidney
Technical error
Arteriosclerosis of the donor and recipient vessels
Injury of vascular intima
Intimal hyperplasia
End to end anastomosis of the internal iliac artery
Kinking of the renal artery
Cytomegalovirus infection
Immunological causes

The presence of stenosis is indicated by persistent hypertension poorly controlled by treatment, graft dysfunction, polycythemia, and impaired renal function following the administration of angiotensin-converting enzyme inhibitors. The mechanism of the development of renovascular hypertension of the transplanted kidney is explained by the Goldblatt principle. Hypoperfusion in the transplanted kidney activates the renin-angiotensin-aldosterone system. The resulting effect is the extracellular retention of sodium and fluids. However, renovascular hypertension can also be caused by hemodynamically severe iliac stenosis proximal to the transplanted kidney. Hypertension, in this case, might be associated with symptoms of limb ischemia-claudication or trophic changes. Doppler ultrasonography is the first choice examination for suspected renal stenosis. Criteria of stenosis include an increase in maximum systolic velocity (V peak above 180-200 cm/s) and post-stenotic turbulence. If TRAS (Transplant Renal Artery Stenosis) is diagnosed in the early postoperative period, surgical revision with suturing of the arterial anastomosis is appropriate. For later stenoses, percutaneous transluminal renal angioplasty (PTRA) is the method of choice. Its technical success rate is 70-90% and has a low percentage of complications. Surgical treatment is reserved for lesions that are not accessible to percutaneous transluminal angioplasty (PTA) or to recurrences after PTA. There are several surgical options for renal artery reconstruction in the graft, although no technique has been shown to be the best. The clinical results of surgical treatment of renal artery stenosis are discussed by several authors who use arterial grafts with preserved, identical blood groups obtained from organs from deceased donors to reconstruct renal artery transplants in patients with specific lesions and subsequent unsuccessful PTA. There is also an interesting work published by authors from the University of Wisconsin in 2003, who dealt with the surgical treatment of renal artery stenosis of the transplant with preserved iliac artery grafts from deceased donors. Between 1991 and 2001, 21 patients underwent reconstruction of the allograft renal artery using a cadaveric iliac artery conduit at the transplant department of the Surgical Clinic. A successful intervention in preserved iliac artery grafts from deceased donors was defined as technical success as well as an increase in serum creatinine levels and/or blood pressure 6 weeks after surgery. The development of a hemodynamically significant lesion after renal artery reconstruction was considered a recurrence. Reconstruction using the cadaveric iliac artery was successful in 19 of 21 (90%) patients, and only one of these patients (4.8%) failed to relapse with a median follow-up of 42 months. Graft loss secondary to TRAS occurred in two patients. The authors did not find any long-lasting complications related to grafts of the cadaveric iliac artery, and most allografts continued to function well.

Surgical reconstruction of the renal artery graft with iliac artery grafts with the matching blood type should be considered as an option for a patient with specific anatomical lesions and for those in whom PTA was unsuccessful, as well as those with recurrence after PTA. Other surgical treatment options include revision and resection of the anastomosis, venous bypass with GSV, patch graft, or endarterectomy. The success rate of treatment is 63-92%, the risk of recurrence is 12%.

Reported success rates for PTA range from 70% to 90%, with a 20% to 40% incidence of recurrence. Interventional radiologists are trying to use metal endoprostheses capable of expanding to treat recurrent TRAS. This is based on the successful use of stents as PTA supplements in coronary, peripheral, and congenital renal vascular stenosis. The use of intra-arterial stents in TRAS has had modest clinical success in a small number of patients. The role of intra-arterial stents in the treatment of TRAS is currently unclear and requires larger studies with longer follow-ups. Several studies suggest that surgical revascularization should be considered suitable for recurrent TRAS after PTA.

PTA is a relatively non-invasive procedure and can be done with minimal morbidity and discomfort for the patient. In most patients, if they are correctly selected, the outcome will be successful after PTA. In patients who return or are unable to undergo PTA for technical reasons, a surgical adjustment should be considered. Primary surgical procedures are indicated for selected lesions, such as anastomosis or ostial stenosis and knobs in the renal artery. Under these circumstances, we prefer the use of an ABO-matched iliac artery graft from a deceased donor as a suitable arterial conduit for bypass or reconstruction of the renal artery allograft (Figure 8).

Late renal artery thrombosis is an uncommon complication, occurring several months after transplantation. It is most often associated with a rejection episode or with advanced renal artery stenosis. It can also arise as a complication of endovascular treatment for renal artery stenosis. In rare cases, graft artery thrombosis can also be combined with iliac artery thrombosis. Clinically, arterial thrombosis manifests itself by anuria and abdominal pain at the site of the transplanted kidney. If iliac artery thrombosis is also associated, the overall condition may be complicated by acute arterial occlusion of the ipsilateral lower limb. If thrombosis is diagnosed within 24 hours of the onset of clinical symptoms, intraarterial thrombolysis is the method of choice. After unperformed angiography, a 5 French catheter is inserted under X-ray control, the end of which is located 1 cm behind the anastomosis in the blood clot area. The success of the treatment is confirmed by angiography after the end of thrombolysis. Intraarterial thrombolysis is not recommended for the treatment of early renal artery thrombosis because fibrinolysis is potentially dangerous in patients shortly after surgery where there is a risk of hemorrhagic complications.

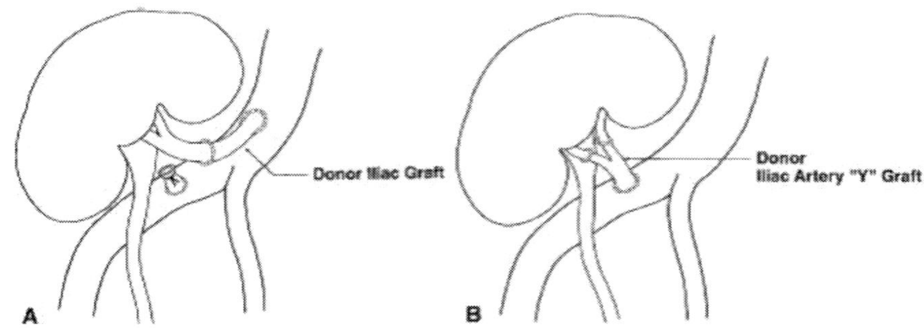

(Source: author)

Figure 8. Reconstruction of the renal artery using a conduit of the iliac artery from deceased donors. A. end to end anastomosis of the iliac artery conduit with the renal artery of the transplant. B. in patients with two renal graft arteries, iliac Y-graft was used to construct both vessels

Renal Venous Stenosis and External Iliac Vein

Venous stenosis is an uncommon vascular complication after kidney transplantation, most often occurring several months to years after transplantation. It is characterized by a short narrowing of the renal and pelvic vein at the graft site. The etiology of this complication includes perivascular fibrosis and compression by the surrounding perinephric fluid collection, which may be of infectious origin. The onset of stenosis is usually preceded by an episode of fever, and leukocytosis in the laboratory image. Radiological examination (sonography, CT) reveals the fluid collection around the transplanted graft and iliac vein. After the evacuation of this collection, the previous clinical symptoms subside. Over time, thrombophlebitis develops with perivascular fibrosis, which causes venous stenosis. Clinically, this stenosis manifests itself several months after the first attack with a progressive deterioration of renal function; in advanced stages, swelling of the ipsilateral limb may occur. The diagnosis is based on Doppler ultrasonography, which has a reduced color signal and increased velocities in the renal vein up to ten times (120-140 cm/s) compared to intraarterial veins (10 cm/s). The treatment of symptomatic renal and iliac vein stenosis is endovascular. PTA and possibly stent placement is recommended. Graftectomy is indicated in the case of progressive deterioration of renal function up to the stage of a functional graft. Kim et al. present a picture of a grafted kidney affected by parenchymal edema, microscopic findings show signs of venous congestion, inflammatory changes in the hilum, and vein thrombosis with inflammatory cellular infiltration of the venous wall comparable to thrombophlebitis.

Aneurysm of arterial anastomosis and infectious aneurysm in the area of the transplanted kidney

These are mostly pseudoaneurysms (PSA) caused by partial disruption of the arterial anastomosis. Some PSAs are also associated with local infection. Patients can often be asymptomatic. Hypotension and pain may not occur until rupture. Diagnosis is simple, verification by duplex ultrasonography sometimes requires angiographic examination. In a patient with a rupture, an urgent surgical solution is required, graftectomy and replacement of a damaged pelvic artery with an autologous venous graft is often the optimal solution. In the absence of infection and massive bleeding, the rescue of the graft is possible. The incidence of isolated iliac arteries is 0.003 to 0.17%, as part of the abdominal aortic aneurysm 2 to 7%. The incidence of isolated iliac arteries in men aged 65-75 years is 70 per 100,000, while in women the incidence is only 2 per 100,000. In the initial period of transplantations, infectious complications were relatively common, their treatment was complicated, infections resulted in the loss of the transplanted organ, sometimes resulting in the death of the recipient. The incidence of infectious complications in transplant patients has decreased significantly thanks to the preventive measures such as the gradual introduction of standard protocols in the collection program, the development of preservation methods and solutions, the modernization of immunosuppressive therapy, the standardization of surgical procedures, as well as to the targeted antibiotic prophylaxis. Nevertheless, if infections do occur, they pose a serious problem for patients with a transplanted organ. Graft infection before, during, or after a kidney transplant can cause serious complications, especially if it is a fungal infection. Infection can occur in several stages of the transplant process. (see Table 6.)

Table 6. Factors influencing the onset of infection during transplantation

Factors influencing the onset of infection during the transplant process
DONOR: with an open craniocerebral injury Hospitalized at ICU for more than 7 days
KIDNEY PROCUREMENT: multi-organ samples with intestinal or biliary tract opening
KIDNEY PRESERVATION AND IMPLANTATION: non-compliance with sterile precautions during explantation, packaging, transport, and transplantation

A patient after a kidney transplant is at increased risk of infectious complications due to immunosuppression. Approximately 50-74% of patients experience one or more episodes of bacterial infections and 30-75% of patients experience one or more episodes of symptomatic viral infections. The spectrum of pathogens is wide and infection with several agents is possible at the same time. Early intervention is important and, in the event of a severe course of an infection, reduction or even the omission of immunosuppression is necessary. Saving a life must take precedence over saving a kidney. An infectious aneurysm occurs in a transplanted patient when septic embolization into the vascular vasorum occurs. The source of septic emboli is the heart, the gateway to infection is transplantation, and the source of the infection itself is most often the organ donor and kidney transport. The most common pathogenic infectious aneurysms are Viridans streptococci (22%), Staphylococcus aureus (20%), Streptococcus faecalis (14%) and Staphylococcus epidermidis (11%). Aspergillus, Corynebacterium, Candida albicans, and Micrococcus are less common. Some importance in the development of infectious aneurysms is attributed to microbial arteritis in the field of atherosclerosis. Intima damaged by the AS process, which is normally highly resistant to infection, allows inoculation of pathogens into the vessel wall. The infection of the vessel wall can cause perforation and the development of a pseudoaneurysm. Patients on hemodialysis therapy for CKD (Chronic kidney disease) are highly vulnerable to staphylococcal bacteremia, which results in microbial arteritis. The most common pathogens that cause microbial arteritis are Escherichia coli, Salmonella, and Staphylococcus species, Bacteroides fragillis.

The clinical image varies depending on the size and location of the aneurysm, the time of transplantation, the age of the patient, the type of immunosuppression, and the bacterial agent. Clinical signs are abdominal pain (92%), fever (77%), leukocytosis (69%), positive blood culture (69%), deterioration of renal function (50%), palpable pulsating resistance in the hypogastrium (45%), and rupture of the aneurysm (30%). The diagnosis is confirmed based on clinical and laboratory examination and radiological imaging methods. In the laboratory picture, the levels of creatinine and urea increase, glomerular filtration is impaired, leukocytosis is present, and sedimentation is increased. Urinary obstruction and laboratory toxic levels of cyclosporine should be sonographically ruled out at this time in the patient. Some authors use indium 111-labeled leukocyte scintigraphy to determine infection, similar to prosthetic infections. When suspending an infectious aneurysm in a transplanted patient without a known agent, the administration of antibiotics is recommended, considering renal function, in principle graftectomy is always necessary.

Surgical treatment of an infectious aneurysm in the area of the transplanted kidney includes:

1. Bleeding control
2. Confirmation of the diagnosis, including a biopsy from the aneurysm wall for bacteriological examination
3. Surgical treatment of sepsis, which consists in resection of the aneurysm, ligature of the supplying artery, graftectomy of the Tx of the kidney and debridement of the surrounding tissues, drainage
4. Postoperative repetitive ligaments and debridement of necrotic masses
5. Arterial reconstruction of vital arteries after infection control so-called extra-anatomical bypass (for example, femoro-femoral cross over bypass graft) and intravenous antibiotic treatment)

Lymphocele

It is defined as the fluid collection of lymph around the transplanted kidney. It usually arises as a result of a technical error after the operation. Large lymphocele around the transplanted kidney can lead to obstruction of the iliac vein or to obstruction of the ureter by direct pressure or to dislocation of the bladder medially. Many times, we can think of it when the patient develops edema of the lower limb and at the same time, the renal function worsens. The incidence of lymphoceles is reported to be in the range of 1-40%. Most lymphoceles are asymptomatic. Clinically, 1-18% of lymphocele is manifested. It is necessary to rule out retroperitoneal urinoma during surgery.

Conclusion

Kidney transplantation is the treatment of choice in renal replacement therapy (RRT) for patients with end-stage renal disease (ESRD). Remarkable advances in surgical techniques have been reached in the last three decades. Standardization of surgical techniques, improvement of immunosuppressive therapy, organ preservation, and antimicrobial treatment significantly improved graft function, improved quality of life, and reduced the risk not only of morbidity but also of mortality of respondents.

However, grafts with anatomical variations are still kind of challenging for surgeons. Considering all these variations, the most common are multiple arteries, which can occur in up to one-third of potential kidney donors. The use of these grafts with multiple arteries has been a part of relative contraindications in the past, which may have led to an increased incidence of vascular and urological complications. However, there are now several surgical and microsurgical methods of intracorporeal and ex vivo surgery that are used to transplant grafts with multiple renal arteries. According to the available literature, there is a significantly higher percentage of graft survival and a lower incidence of complications in KTx if the vessels are adjusted to meet the criteria of quality vascular reconstruction.

REFERENCES

Abecassis, M., Bartlett, S. T., Collins, A. J., et al. (2008). "Kidney transplantation as primary therapy for end-stage renal disease: A National Kidney Foundation/Kidney Disease Outcomes Quality Initiative (NKF/KDOQITM) Conference." *Clin J Am Soc Nephrol*, *3*(2), 471-480.

Allen, R. D. M. & Chapman, J. R. (1994). "Early management of the uncomplicated transplant recipient." in *Manual of renal transplantation. 1st ed.* edited by Allen R.D.M. and Chapman, 111-127. J.R. Oxford: Oxford University Press.

Allen, R. D. M. & Chapman, J. R. Late renal transplant dysfunction and failure. in *Manual of renal transplantation. 1st ed.* edited by Allen R.D.M. and Chapman, 168-193. J.R. Oxford: Oxford University Press.

Allen, R. D. M. & Chapman, J. R. The surgical procedure. in *Manual of renal transplantation. 1st ed.* edited by Allen R.D.M. and Chapman, 68-89. J.R. Oxford: Oxford University Press.

Breza, J. ml., Žilinská, P., Buják, J. & Breza, st. (2009). "Urologické komplikácie po tranplantácii obličky." *Urol. List*, *7*(1), 38-48. ["Urological complications after kidney transplantation." *Urol. List*, *7* (1), 38-48.].

Brian, D., Shames, M. D., Jon, S., Odorico, M., D'alessandro, M. D., et al. (2003). "Surgical repair of transplant renal artery stenosis with preserved cadaveric iliac artery grafts." *Annals of Surgery*, *237*(1), 116-122.

Cecka, J. M., Cho, Y. W. & Terasaki, P. I. (1992). "Analyses of the UNOS Scientific Renal Transplant Registry at three years--early events affecting transplant success." *Trans-plantation*, *53*(1), 59-64.

Claas, F. H. & Rood, J. J. van. (1988). "The hyperimmunized patient: from sensitization toward transplantation." *Transpl. Int*, *1*(2), 53-7.

Colvin, R. B. (1991). The pathogenesis of vascular rejection. In *Transplant. Proc*, *23*(2), 2052-5.

Crain, M. R., et al. (2004). "Vascular complications of renal transplantation: angiographic diagnosis and intervention." *Semin. intervent. Radiol*, *9*(4), 235-245s.

Crumbly, A. J. & Sade, R. M. (1991). "The history of transplantation." *J. S. C. med. Assoc.*, *87*(6), 361.

Delphin, E. S. (1997). "Brief reports: successful extension of the transplant renal vein with and synthetic vascular graft." *Bol. Asoc. Med*, *89*, 206-207.

Frankovičová, M., Bober, J., Arendarčík, F., Martinček, M., Kubíková, M., Harbuľák, P. & Kriegerová, K. (1995). "Rekonštrukčné operácie v našom klinickom materiáli." *Bratislavské lekárske listy*, *96*(12), 658-660. ["Reconstructive surgeries in our clinical material." *Bratislava Medical Papers*, *96* (12), 658-660.].

Frauchiger, B., Bock, A., Spoendlin, M., et al. (1994). "Early renal transplant dysfunction due to arterial kinking stenosis." In *Nephrol. Dial. Transplant*, *9*(1), 76-9.

Grantnerová, B. (1998). *Včasná starostlivosť o pacienta s transplantovanou obličkou.* Banská Bystrica: Enterprise. [*Early care of a patient with a kidney transplant.* Banská Bystrica: Enterprise.].

Hammond, E. H., Ensley, R. D., Yowell, R. L., et al. (1991). "Vascular rejection of human cardiac allografts and the role of humoral immunity in chronic allograft rejection." *Transplant. Proc.*, *23*(2), 26-30.

Joseph, J. T., Kingsmore, D. B., Junor, B. J., Briggs, J. D., Mun Woo, Y., Jaques, B. C., Hamilton, D. N., Jardine, A. G. & Jindal, R. M. (2001). "The impact of late acute rejection after cadaveric kidney transplantation." *Clin Transplant*, *15*, 221-227.

Krylov, V. S., Stepanov, G. A., Acchurin, R. S., et al. (1983). "Autovenous plasty of vessels in emergency surgery." *Klin Khir*, 30-33.

Kuss, R. & Bourget, P. (1992). *An Illustrated History of Organ Transplantation. The Great Adventure of the Century.* Sandoz.

Kuviková, A. (1997). "Význam odtraňovania leukocytov z transfúznych prípravkov." *Slov. Lek.*, *7*(1), 27-29. ["The importance of removing leukocytes from transfusion products." *Slov. Lek.*, *7* (1), 27-29.].

Lacková, E. (1998). "Imunosupresívna terapia a pooperačná starostlivosť." in *Orgánové transplantácie: transplantácia obličiek. 1 vyd.* edited by LACA Ľ. et al., 86-136. Banská Bystrica: Dali. ["Immunosuppressive therapy and postoperative care." in *Organ transplants: kidney transplantation*. 1 ed. edited by LACA Ľ. et al., 86-136. Banská Bystrica: Dali.].

Lawrence, P. F., Lorenzo-Rivero, S. & Lyon, J. L. (2005). "The incidence of iliac, femoral, and popliteal artery aneurysms in hospitalized patients." *J. Vasc. Surg.*, *22*(4), 409-415.

Medricka, M., Janeckova, J., jarosciakova, J. & Bachleda, P. (2020). "Creation of arteriovenous fistula for hemodialysis in the older population." *Biomed Pap Med Fac Univ Palacky Olomouc Czech Repub* doi: 10.5507/bp.2020.013. Online ahead of print.

Mohamed, H., Anil, K., Ponusamy, A. T., David, M. H. & Hickey, P. (2007). *Renal vessel reconstruction in kidney transplantation using a polytetrafluoroethylene (PTFE) vascular graft, In Journal of surgical case reports*, Vo *22*(4), s1030-1032.

Naimark, D. M. J. & Cole, E. (1994). "Determinants of long-term renal allograft survival." *Transplant. Rev.*, *8*(1), 93.

Nargund, V. H. & Cranston, D. (1996). "Urological complications after renal transplantation." *Transplant. Rev.*, *10*(1), 24-33.

Pacovský, J. (2004). "Lymfokéla po transplantaci ledviny." *Urol. pro praxi*, *5*, 210. ["Lymphocele after a kidney transplant." *Urol. pro praxi*, *5*, 210.]

Patel, N. H., Jindal, R. M. & Wilkin, T. (2001). "Renal arterial stenosis in renal allografts: Retrospective study of predisposing factors and outcome after percutaneous transluminal angioplasty." *Radiology*, *201*(219), 663-667.

Port, F. K., Wolfe, R. A., Mauger, E. A., Berling, D. P. & Jiang, K. (1993). "Comparison of survival probabilities for dialysis patients vs cadaveric renal transplant recipients." *JAMA*, *270*(11), 1339-1343.

Rezníček, J., Zvara, V. & Breza, J. (1991). "Príbuzenské transplantácie obličiek." *Lek. Obz.*, *40*, 373-375s. ["Sibling kidney transplants." *Lek. Obz.*, *40*, 373-375s.].

Roberts, J. P., Ascher, N. L., Fryd, D. S., et al. (1999). "Transplant renal artery stenosis." *Transplantation*, *48*(4), 580-3.

Rosenthal, J. T. (1992). "The transplant operation and its surgical complications." In *Handbook of kidney transplantation*. 1st ed. edited by DANOVITCH, G. M. Boston: Little, Brown & Comp.

Sehgal, A. R. (2002): "What is the best treatment for end-stage renal disease?" *Am J Med*, *112*(9), 735-736.

Sis, B., Mengel, M., Haas, M., et al. (2010). "Banff '09 meeting report: Antibody-mediated graft deterioration and implementation of banff working groups." *Am J Transplant*, *10*(3), 464-471.

Sijpkens, Y. W. J., Doxiadis, I. I. N., Mallat, M. J. K., De Fijter, J. W., Bruin, J. A., Claas, F. H. J. & Paul, L. C. (2003). "Early versus late acute rejection episodes in renal transplantation." *Transplantation*, *75*, 204-208.

Slatinska, J., Honsova, E., Lyerova, L., Slavcev, A. & Viklicky, O. (2007). "Acute humoral rejection of renal transplant." *Vnitr. Lek.*, *53*(3), 249-252.

Suthanthiran, M. & Strom, T. B. (1994). "Renal transplantation." *N. Engl. J. Med*, *331*(6), 365-76.

Talbot-Wright, R., Carretero, P., Alcaraz, A., et al. (1991). "Bench surgery in renal transplantation." *Transplant. Proc.*, *23*(5), 2327.

Tilney, N. L., Whitley, W. D., Diamond, J. R., et al. (1991). "Chronic rejection--an undefined conundrum." *Transplantation*, *52*(3), 389-98.

Vammen, S., Lindholt, J., Henneberg, E. W., et al. (2000). "A comparative study of iliac and abdominal aortic aneurysms." *Int. Angiol*, *19*(2), 152-7.

Viklický, O., Janoušek, L., Baláž, P., et al. (2008). *Transplantace ledviny v klinické praxi.* Praha: Grada. [*Kidney transplantation in clinical practice.* Prague: Grada.].

Wolfe, R. A., Ashby, V. B., Milford, E. L., et al. (1999). "Comparison of mortality in all patients on dialysis, patients on dialysis awaiting transplantation, and recipients of a first cadaveric transplant." *N Engl J Med*, *341*(23), 1725-1730.

Zvara, V. & Řezníček, J. (1973). "Možnosti aktívnej liečby terminálneho štádia chronickej nedostatočnosti obličiek chronickou hemodialýzou a transplantáciou obličiek." *Lek Obzor*, *22*, 489. ["Options for active treatment of end-stage chronic renal failure by chronic hemodialysis and kidney transplantation." *Lek Obzor*, *22*, 489.]

In: Surgeon´s Perspective on Dialysis Patient ISBN: 978-1-53619-262-9
Editor: Maria Frankovicova

Chapter 13

VASCULAR ACCESSES AND POSSIBLE COMPLICATIONS FROM THE CARDIOLOGY POINT OF VIEW

D. Pella,[*] *MD*
1st Department of Cardiology VUSCH a.s, Faculty of Medicine, Pavol Jozef Šafárik University in Košice and University Hospital, Košice, Slovakia

ABSTRACT

Modern cardiology can be classified into two lines, namely invasive and non-invasive. Invasive (using blood) examination methods are used when a non-invasive examination procedure (such as non-invasive imaging tests) determines a diagnosis for which conservative treatment is not sufficient, or when, according to the latest recommendations by the European Society of Cardiology, it is necessary to choose an invasive cardiology procedure. Invasive examination methods are performed through various vascular accesses (for example, in selective coronarography access through the femoral artery or the radial artery is

[*] Corresponding Author's E-mail: dominik.pella@gmail.com.

used). In this case, a collision of cardiology, angiology, and vascular surgery occurs at the site of puncture, which may be complemented by various complications. Associated patient diagnoses, such as renal failure at various stages, including the need for dialysis or type 2 diabetes mellitus at the stage of chronic complications, may also be a complication itself. In the next chapter, we will mention two main examination methods, namely selective coronarography and CT angiography, however, invasive cardiology offers many more predominantly arrhythmology-related invasive examinations (invasive electrophysiological examinations, ablations of supraventricular tachycardias, atrial fibrillation ablation using cryo energy and the radiofrequency energy). All these examinations are performed through vascular accesses.

Keywords: selective coronarography, CT angiography

Abbreviations

ACS	acute coronary syndrome
CHD	coronary heart disease
MSCT	multislice computed tomography
PSA	pseudoaneurysm
ST	superficial thrombophlebitis

Selective Coronarography

Selective coronarography is an invasive cardiological examination that seeks to verify the presence of atherosclerosis progression in the coronary basin and to confirm or refute the presence of coronary heart disease. Coronary heart disease (CHD) is most often caused by the slow formation of one or more atherosclerotic plaques, which can then cause an obstruction in the basin of coronary arteries and can result in acute coronary syndrome (ACS). The plaque creation begins with the accumulation of lipoprotein elements in the intima of the artery, which mobilize macrophages and smooth muscle cells by activating cytokines.

They are accumulated in the given place - macrophages form foam cells by absorbing lipoproteins and together with migrating smooth muscle cells they form a fat-fibrotic lesion. Inflammatory mediators are also activated by various immune pathways with further accumulation of leukocytes and myocytes, with plaque enlargement increasingly narrowing the lumen of the artery. Using invasive measurements, selective coronarography quantifies the severity of stenoses in the coronary bloodstream. Selective coronarography consists of two stages, diagnostic and therapeutic. An iodinated contrast agent is injected into the coronary basin through a diagnostic catheter. The first stage aims to visualize coronary arteries and assess the presence of stenoses in the coronary bloodstream. Catheters are injected into the coronary artery through the sheath and placed in the artery using the Seldinger technique. The right or the left femoral artery or the right or the left radial artery are used to access the coronary bloodstream. In the case of the femoral access, the puncture is in the right or the left groin. In the case of radial access, it is a few centimeters above the wrist. The radial access has been preferred recently. The advantage of the radial access lies in the lower risk of local bleeding and vascular complications as well as faster mobilization of the patient after the procedure. A patient who undergoes selective coronarography via radial access can begin rehabilitation after only a few hours. The radial access is also more advantageous in terms of consequent home rehabilitation of the patient. A patient with radial access is instructed not to lift heavy items at home for at least seven days and not to wash hands in warm water. Despite several benefits mentioned above, the radial access may not be appropriate for each patient. In case of an acute coronary condition, where there is a vital indication of selective coronarography, we do not have the opportunity to assess the patient's clinical condition before examination thoroughly, taking their additional clinical diagnoses into account. In such a case, the invasive cardiologist makes decisions primarily based on anatomical conditions (for example, severe abdominal obesity can complicate the femoral access). In case of elective surgery in patients with other chronic diseases in addition to the ischemic heart disease, such as chronic heart failure with reduced left ventricular systolic function, renal insufficiency and type 2 diabetes mellitus at the stage of chronic complications, it is appropriate to choose the puncture site before the invasive examination itself. For patients with renal failure, selective coronarography is a risky examination. Iodinated contrast agent, eliminated from the body through kidneys, is used to show the coronary bloodstream. In patients with renal insufficiency, post-contrast nephropathy may occur, which may require dialysis. In patients with renal failure undergoing hemodialysis treatment, dialysis should be planned before and after the coronary arteries examination. The radial access can significantly complicate the formation of an AV fistula to start with the scheduled hemodialysis. Proper anatomical conditions, steady blood flow and mainly the maturation of the AV fistula (4 to 8 weeks) are all essential for the correct formation of the AV fistula. Selective coronarography through the radial access significantly complicates the maturation of the subsequent AV fistula, and therefore femoral access is suitable for patients with already planned hemodialysis treatment or if there is a risk that it might be needed. A thorough cardiological examination substantially helps the vascular surgeon to choose the appropriate access for hemodialysis. The coronarography finding itself may indicate the ischemic etiology of heart failure, which may be connected to reduced left ventricular systolic function. Severe left ventricular systolic dysfunction with an ejection fraction below 30% is a contraindication for the introduction of the AV fistula due to the inability of the heart to ensure sufficient cardiac output and quality blood flow through the AV fistula. The echocardiographic examination of the heart is an imaging examination of the first choice. With the help of echocardiography, we can comprehensively assess the morphology as well as the function of the heart as a pump. When planning the introduction of the AV fistula, it is especially important to assess the systolic function of the left ventricle in order to recognize all possible causes of heart failure (myocardial hypertrophy, heart valve disease, myocardial ischemia, structural myocardial damage). Chronic heart failure is a syndrome and can have both cardiac and extracardiac causes. Cardiac causes include ischemic heart disease, valve defects, hypertension, arrhythmias, cardiomyopathy, and more. Extracardiac causes include anemia, as well as renal, pulmonary, and endocrine diseases. The femoral access also has its advantages, such as lower technical complexity and easier access for the invasive cardiologist, as well as better maneuverability (for example, when displaying grafts after bypass surgery in the past and assessing their patency). Another advantage is the lower radiation exposure of the interventional cardiologist. The femoral access is more appropriate in patients with renal failure, where there is a higher risk of post-contrast nephropathy due to the possible planning of the AV fistula insertion. A disadvantage is a longer patient's rehabilitation period. The patient must stay in bed for at least 24 hours after the invasive procedure (this may vary depending on the closure of the arterial bed at the site of the puncture that was chosen by the invasive cardiologist). In terms of anatomical conditions, the femoral access is less advantageous than the radial access even in case of subsequent rehabilitation of the patient at home. Sitting and walking change the position of the puncture site, and if the puncture site is not healed sufficiently, damage to the vascular bed may occur. At the same time, it is not recommended to wash the puncture site after the invasive surgery with warm water or to imply various heparin products at the puncture site due to the risk of bleeding.

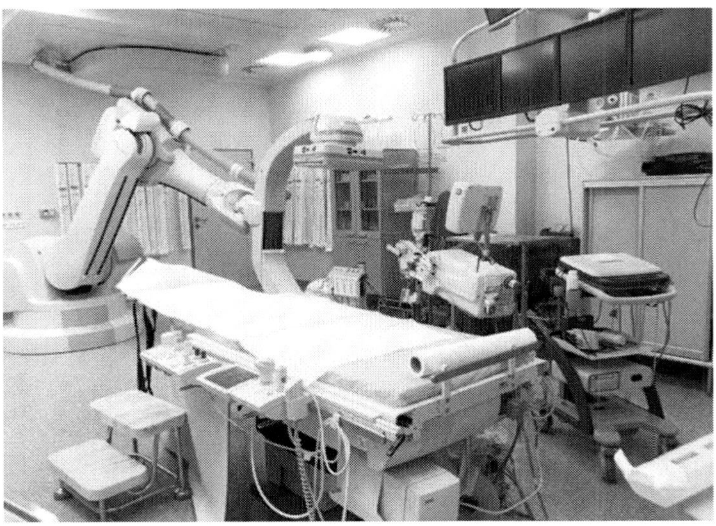

Figure 1. Catheterization hall (1st Department of Cardiology VUSCH a.s.).

Nowadays, we can consider selective coronarography a basic examination in modern cardiology. However, with the increasing number of surgeries, subsequent complications increase as well (in the coronary basin as well as at the site of the puncture). The most common complications include iatrogenic coronary artery damage (iatrogenic dissection, periprocedural myocardial infarction) as well as local complications at the site of the puncture, especially iatrogenic pseudoaneurysm (PSA). A pseudoaneurysm is a false aneurysm consisting of a sac and a neck. The sac is a blood-filled cavity of various shapes and volumes, which is surrounded only by the neighboring tissue, unlike the aneurysm, which is bounded by the artery's own wall. The neck is where the PSA is connected to the maternal artery. The prevalence of iatrogenic PSAs is in the range of 0.1-5.5%. Complications at the puncture site can be caused by inadequate puncture technique, the quality, and the length of the puncture site compression, antiaggregatory and anticoagulant treatment as well as the patient's discipline. Anatomical proportions of the puncture site are an equally significant factor in the risk of pseudoaneurysm creation. With obese patients (abdominal obesity), it is more suitable to choose radial access. With severe obesity, it can be difficult to perform the puncture with the subsequent invasive procedure and subsequent compression after the procedure. Patients with recorded severe aortic regurgitation have a greater risk of developing PSA due to the higher-pressure amplitude. The auscultation of the injection site before and after the selective coronarography is suitable for evaluating the presence of murmurs (turbulent flow in the artery). If we hear a murmur before an invasive procedure, it is highly probable that these are chronic changes and stable atherosclerotic plaques. If no systolic murmur was present before the examination and we hear it after the surgery, then there is a reasonable suspicion of a complication after the invasive procedure. The main symptoms of PSA include pain, hematoma, throbbing resistance, and a systolic murmur. The main diagnostic method is color duplex ultrasonography, which contains typical pendulum Doppler currents in the PSA neck and eddy currents in the PSA sac. Most iatrogenic PSAs are thrombosed spontaneously or by bandage compression. Rarely, surgical revision is required to prevent serious complications such as the rupture of a pseudoaneurysm.

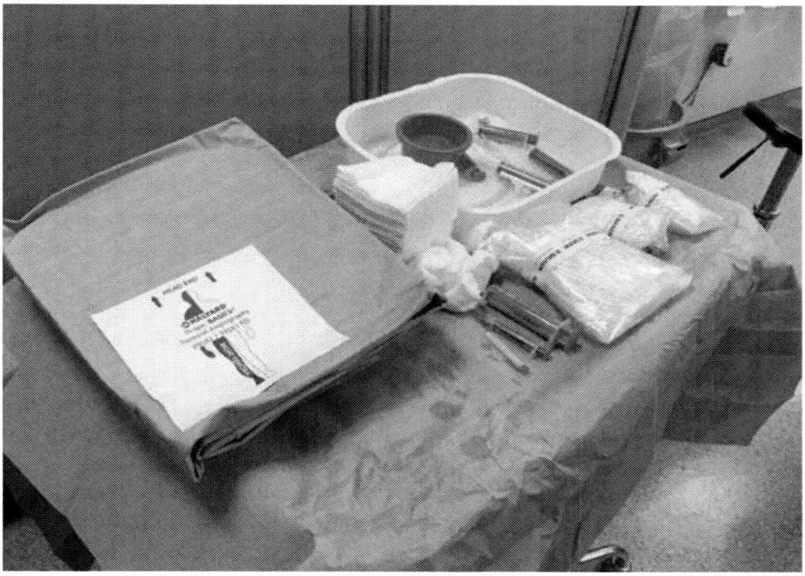

Figure 2. Preparation for selective coronarography (1st Department of Cardiology VUSCH a.s.).

In the treatment of post-catheterization PSAs, the first-line treatment (depending on the clinical finding at the injection site after selective coronarography) is a compression (with a pressure bandage or untargeted manual compression). Ultrasound-guided compression is significantly more efficient than untargeted compression. In patients receiving anticoagulation treatment, the efficiency of ultrasound-guided compression is lower than in patients without anticoagulation treatment. The basis of compression treatment is the compression of the PSA neck using an ultrasound probe with simultaneous control using color Doppler flow mapping. The aim is to interrupt the flow and further circulation in the PSA sac, which consequently thromboses. While compressing the PSA neck, it is necessary to check the patency of the femoral artery with ultrasound. Drawbacks of compression include time demands (sometimes compression of up to 30 minutes is required), other disadvantages include pain and necessary physical capabilities of the doctor. If manual compression is unsuccessful, it is possible to proceed with the percutaneous application of thrombin. Human thrombin is used during the procedure. Thrombin is slowly applied to the center of the pseudoaneurysm sac using a thin needle (22-gauge spinal needle), where it then triggers the coagulation cascade and then gradually the entire sac thromboses. The whole procedure is monitored by ultrasound and at the same time, the peripheral pulsations on the extremity are checked after the end of thrombin application. Following the procedure, the patient lies in the bed without a pressure bandage and maintains full bed rest for 6-8 hours. Then, in 24 hours, a control ultrasound examination is performed. Possible contraindications include the anatomical proportions of the PSA, namely short and wide PSA neck. This increases the risk of thrombus embolization into the arterial system of the lower extremity. In general, the smaller the PSA, the higher the probability of spontaneous thrombosis (PSA size less than 1 centimeter). If the pseudoaneurysm is larger than 6 centimeters, it is more appropriate to choose a surgical procedure (resection). In this case, the surgical procedure is more suitable due to possible compression of the femoral and nerve-vascular bundle by a pseudoaneurysm of larger dimensions in case of its thrombosis. The surgical procedure is the first choice of treatment also in cases when the patient has various skin excoriations above the sac (there is a risk of the PSA infection). Thrombin treatment may lead to thromboembolism of the lower extremity arterial system. This can be caused by a technical error during the procedure (the application of thrombin directly to the artery) or a false indication of the procedure (short and wide PSA neck mentioned). In some specialized centers, this method of thrombin application is preferred over manual compression, especially due to the duration of the procedures. Endovascular embolization of the PSA sac with a metal spiral is another treatment option (currently used less because of the procedure costs, the procedure length as well as the invasive nature of the procedure). The puncture of the bilateral femoral artery is required for endovascular embolization of the PSA sac with a metal spiral. This method is substituted by the application of thrombin. Surgical resection of the PSA (formerly a standard procedure for treating pseudoaneurysms) is now only used for the treatment of large and complicated PSAs that cannot be treated by manual compression or thrombin application, or in cases where there is an increased risk of infection over the sac or the compression of the femoral nerve and blood vessels. The disadvantage of the surgical procedure is the resulting long healing of a surgical wound due to the recurrent edematous overlap, bleeding into the surrounding tissues.

In connection with the technical improvement of medicine and invasive cardiology, catheterization instruments are more flexible, smaller in diameter and the radial access has been gaining prominence (via the radial artery). In addition, we have more options to close the arterial basin at the puncture site (e.g., Angio-Seal), where the lower incidence of iatrogenic vascular damages at the puncture site after selective coronarography is presumed.

Multislice Computed Angiography

Multislice computed tomography (MSCT) is used to identify or eliminate atherosclerotic stenoses in the coronary basin in symptomatic patients (the presence of typical pain behind the sternum) as well as in asymptomatic patients. Several studies suggest that MDCT examination may be beneficial in detecting the subclinical form of atherosclerosis and ascertaining coronary involvement.

The application of an iodinated contrast agent via the intravenous route is an essential component in the imaging of the vascular lumen, and at the same time, a certain level of plasma iodine concentration in the coronary basin is needed to assess their possible changes.

To perform the CT angiography, it is necessary to use a pressure injector which creates a high and uniform rate of contrast agent application with exact timing. Nowadays, two-piston systems are used where saline can be administered instantly after the administration of the contrast agent. Up to a third of the contrast agent can be saved in this way. The access for the administration of a contrast agent is most often via the superficial veins of the elbow pit or the back of the hand. The concentration, the volume and the rate of the contrast agent administration depend on several factors, including the equipment or the kind of treated area. The total volume of contrast agent administered and the correct timing of data acquisition always relate to the basic physiological parameters (the circulation time and the application site), the anatomical ratio (the location of the vessel in the circulation) and the total duration of the examination. The method of the contrast agent application has an important influence on the quality of imaging of vascular structures in CT angiography.

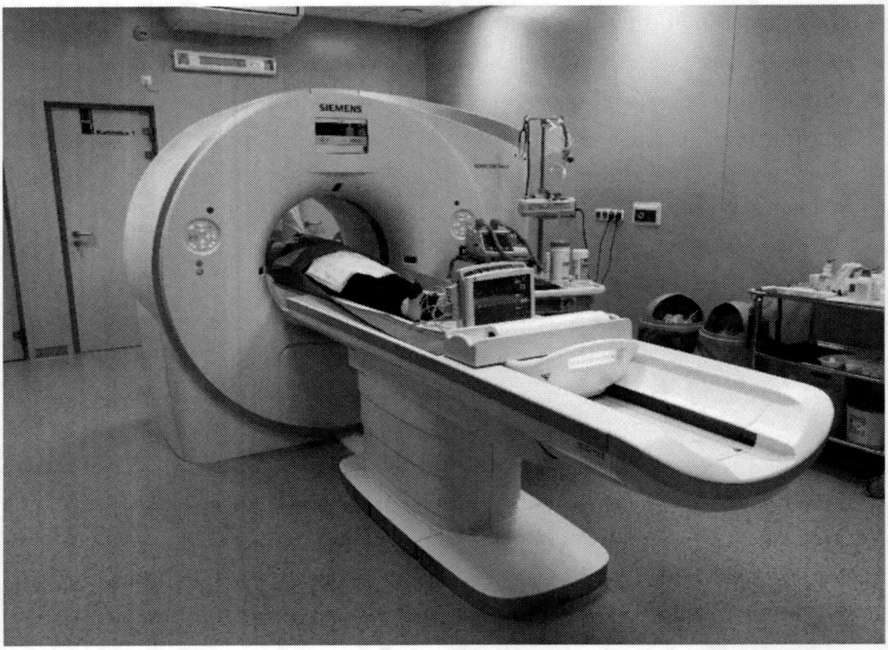

Figure 3. Multidetector CT device SOMATOM Force (1st Department of Cardiology VUSCH a.s.).

One of the most serious complications of the CT angiography is an acute allergic reaction to the contrast agent (occurring within 1 hour of the contrast agent administration). The treatment depends on the patient's clinical condition, which can range from an asymptomatic course to a serious, life-threatening condition requiring cardiopulmonary resuscitation.

A mild reaction is demonstrated by urticaria, bronchospasm, and a minor decrease in pressure. A severe allergic reaction to the contrast agent may lead to tachycardia, hypotension, bronchospasm, laryngeal edema, pulmonary edema and convulsions. Another complication is a chemotoxic reaction followed by contrast nephropathy.

The administration of the iodinated contrast agent via the intravenous route may also cause complications at the injection site. Most usually, these complications are associated with superficial thrombophlebitis. Superficial thrombophlebitis (ST) is an inflammation of the venous wall that is secondarily accompanied by the formation of a thrombus and its subsequent adherence to the vein wall, which is altered by ongoing inflammation. Hence, there is a risk of pulmonary embolization in superficial thrombophlebitis, but this risk is significantly lower compared to deep phlebothrombosis. Superficial thrombophlebitis mainly affects superficial veins. Superficial thrombophlebitis must be distinguished from thrombophlebitis which affects a healthy non-varicose vein. The cause of the ST is mechanical, microbial, or chemical damage to the vein. In the case of the coronary artery MSCT examination, iatrogenic damage may occur when the vein is punctured. The endothelium of the venous wall is damaged with a consequent formation of thrombi.

The main diagnostic methods of ST include the clinical examination of the patient. In the case of iatrogenic damage, the injection site may be painful, red, and hard to the touch. After that, the local symptoms of inflammation subside, the reddening of the skin changes to a brown pigmented band which disappears over time. The pain of the palpable hard band during the vein also disappears, but the painless harder band corresponding to the thrombosed vein persists for several months. Clinical examination is typically sufficient to determine a diagnosis. The treatment of superficial thrombophlebitis is founded on compression therapy. Anticoagulant treatment for superficial thrombophlebitis prevents the blood clot from expanding into deep veins. For cannula phlebitis on the forearm, which resolves spontaneously in a few days, local analgesic treatment is adequate. Surgical treatment is generally not necessary.

Cardiology, vascular surgery, and angiology overlap in several therapeutic disciplines. The patient should benefit as much as possible from each diagnostic or therapeutic examination procedure and, at the same time, there is also the lowest possible risk of potential complications. Hence, close communication between the cardiologist, the angiologist, and the vascular surgeon is especially important in determining the complex clinical condition of the patient. Therefore, in patients with renal insufficiency requiring hemodialysis, it is highly important for the cardiologist to perform comprehensive cardiological examinations (cardiac echocardiography, selective coronarography, laboratory tests, clinical examination, ECG), so that the vascular surgeon can properly indicate the hemodialysis access. At the same time, it is important to consider choosing the right approach for invasive cardiac examinations.

REFERENCES

Breza, J., Řezníček, J., Zvara, V. 1985. "Príprava krvného riečišťa pre hemodialýzu vytvorením fistuly medzi a. brachialis a do podkožia ramena transponovanou v. basilica." *Rozhl. Chir.* 64(11):708-712. ["Preparation of the bloodstream for hemodialysis by creating a fistula between the brachial artery and the subcutaneous are of the shoulder transposed by the basilic vein." *Rozhl. Chir.* 64 (11): 708-712.]

Cascardo, S., Acchiardo, S., Beven, E. G. 1970. "Proximal arteriovenous fistulae for hemodialysis when radial arteries are unavailable." *Proc. Eur. Dial. Transplant. Assoc.* 7:42-6.

Decousus H, Quéré I, Presles E et al., 2010. "Superficial Venous Thrombosis and Venous Thromboembolism. A Large, Prospective Epidemiologic Study." *Ann. Intern. Med.* 152: 218–224.

Decoususm H, Prandoni P, Mismetti et al., 2010. "Fondaparinux for the Treatment of Superficial-Vein Thrombosis in the legs." *N. Engl. J. Med.* 363:1222–1232.

Frank H, Werner D, Lorusso V, et al., 2003. "Simultaneous hemodialysis during coronary angiography fails to prevent radiocontrast-induced nephropathy in chronic renal failure." *Clin. Nephrol.* 60:176–182.

Franklin J A, Brigham D, Bogey W M et al., 2003. "Treatment of iatrogenic false aneurysms." *J. Am. Coll. Surg.* 197:293–301.

Frankovičová M. et al., 2018. *Cievna chirurgia*. Košice: Univerzita Pavla Jozefa Šafárika v Košiciach. [*Vascular Surgery*. Košice: Pavol Jozef Šafárik University in Košice].

Frankovičová, M. 2000. Chirurgia tepnožilových spojení pre potreby dlhodobej hemodialýzy. Bratislava: Herba. [*Surgery of arterio-venous junctions for the needs of long-term hemodialysis*. Bratislava: Herba.]

Gaudio C, Mirabelli F, Pelliccia F et al., 2009. "Early detection of coronary artery disease by 64-slice multidetector computed tomography in asymptomatic hypertensive high-risk patients." *Int. J. Cardiol.* 135(3):280–286.

Iłżecki M, Zubilewicz T, Przywara S. 2014. "Efficacy evaluation of bio trombina ® 400 in mini mall y invasive treatment of complications (pseudoaneurysms), after venipuncture for diagnostic purposes. Authors' own experience - case study of 38 patients." *Pol. Przegl. Chir.* 86(8):359-63.

Labounty T M, Gomez M J, Achenbach S, et al., 2013. "Body mass index and the prevalence, severity, and risk of coronary artery disease: an international multicentre study of 13 874 patients." *Eur. Heart. J. Cardiovasc. Imaging* 14:456-463.

Piedad B T, Kronzon I. 2003. "Iatrogenic femoral artery pseudoaneurysm." *Curr. Treat Options Cardiovasc.* Med 5:103–108.

Pohle K, Achenbach S, Macneill B et al., 2007. "Characterization of non-calcified coronary atherosclerotic plaque by multi-detector row CT: comparison to IVUS." *Atherosclerosis* 190:174–180.

Raupach J, Chovanec V, Lojík M, et al., 2003. "Léčba postkatetrizačních pseudoaneuryzmat: možnosti perkutánní aplikace trombinu jako nové metody." Čes Radiol 57:165–168. ["Treatment of postcatheterization pseudoaneurysms: possibilities of percutaneous application of thrombin as a new method." *Čes. Radiol.* 57: 165–168.]

Simon A, Chironi G, Levenson J. 2007. "Comparative performance of subclinical atherosclerosis tests in predicting coronary heart disease in asymptomatic individuals." *Eur. Heart. J.* 28:2967–2971.

Słonina J 1, Obremska M, Zaleska-Dorobisz U. 2010. "Personal experiences in direct ultrasound-guided injection of thrombin into the lumen of pseudoaneurysm as a method of treatment in case of iatrogenic femoral artery damage." *Pol. J. Radiol.* 75(2):33-7.

Svojanovský J, Ševela K, Souček M. 2011 "Kontrastní látkou indukovaná nefropatie." *Interní. Med.* 13(5):205–208. ["Contrast-induced nephropathy." *Interní. Med.* 13 (5): 205–208.]

Tuna M, Raupach J, Chovanec V et al., 2004. "Léčba postkatetrizačních pseudoaneuryzmat pomocí perkutánní aplikace trombinu." Supplementum Cor Vasa 46(4): 99. ["Treatment of post-catheterization pseudoaneurysms by percutaneous application of thrombin." *Supplement Cor. Vasa* 46(4):99.]

Weinmann E E, Chayen D, Kobzantzev ZV et al., 2002. "Treatment of postcatheterisation false aneurysms: ultrasound-guided compression vs ultrasound- guided thrombin injection." *Eur. J. Vasc. Endovasc. Surg.* 23: 68–72.

In: Surgeon´s Perspective on Dialysis Patient ISBN: 978-1-53619-262-9
Editor: Maria Frankovicova

Chapter 14

Case Studies of Patients at the Department of Vascular Surgery

Jana Pobehová*, MD
Department of Vascular Surgery,
East Slovak Institute of Cardiovascular Diseases, Košice, Slovakia

Abstract

We present five interesting case reports from our department concerning vascular accesses and their complications.

Keywords: vascular access, complication, hemodialysis

Abbreviations

ACC	common carotid artery
AFC	common femoral artery

* Corresponding Author's E-mail: jana.pastvova@post.cz.

AFP	deep femoral artery
AFS	superficial femoral artery
AIE	external iliac artery
APo	popliteal artery
AVF	arteriovenous fistula
CRP	C-reactive protein
CTAG	computed tomography - angiography
CT	computed tomography
DSA	digital subtraction angiography
IJV	internal jugular vein
LMWH	low-molecular-weight-heparin
MRSA	methicillin-resistant Staphylococcus aureus
p.p.i.	per primam intentionem (by first intention)
PTA	percutaneous transluminal angioplasty
VUSCH	East Slovak Institute of Cardiovascular Diseases.

CASE STUDY NO. 1

A 59-year-old male I. K., after a kidney transplant 10 years ago, was sent to our department for hospitalization for the removal of arteriovenous fistula (AVF) on the left wrist, which had been established 19 years ago, before the dialysis process began. Besides renal dysfunction and status post kidney transplantation, the medical history contained only arterial hypertension. In the past, the patient overcame recurrent inflammations at the site of the dilated AV fistula. The ultrasonographic finding described a transient brachial artery but dilated to a thickness of about 1 cm, as well as the radial artery measuring 0.6 cm and the ulnar artery that had not been dilated. AVF thrombotic throughout the whole course with a soft thrombus.

After completing the required preoperative examinations, the patient underwent surgery at our department: during the surgical revision, the dilated AVF on the left wrist was resected to about 8 cm. However, the wall of the vein and artery was inferior after the removal of AVF, evaluated peri-operatively as an inverted pseudoaneurysm. With regard to the diameter of the inlet and outlet part of the radial artery, which had to be replaced, we decided to replace it with an interposition graft of the great saphenous vein (taken from the ankle on the lower limb), which was sutured on both sides of the artery using an end-to-end anastomosis. Postoperatively patient medicated with LMWH, antibiotics in a prophylactic dose. The patient was released into home care on the third-day post-op, stable, with the wound healing p.p.i. (per primam intentionem).

One month after the operation, the patient is stabilized and compensated, and the left upper limb is congested, the wounds are calm and healed, the pulsations on the brachial, radial, and ulnar arteries on the left are well palpable.

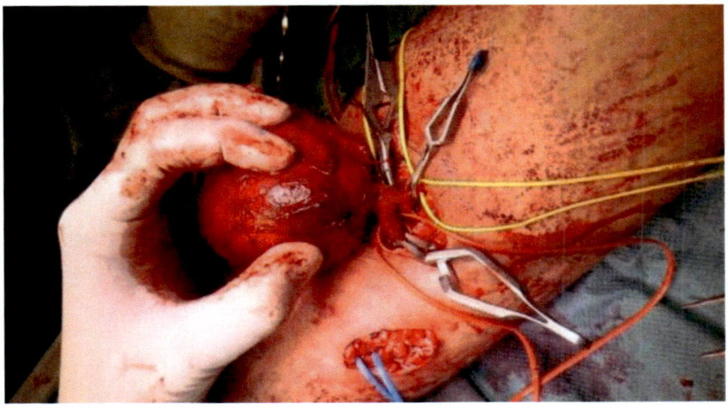

Source: Department of Vascular Surgery, VÚSCH, a.s.

Figure 1. Dilated cephalic vein on the left, the inlet and outlet part of the artery on the rubber bands.

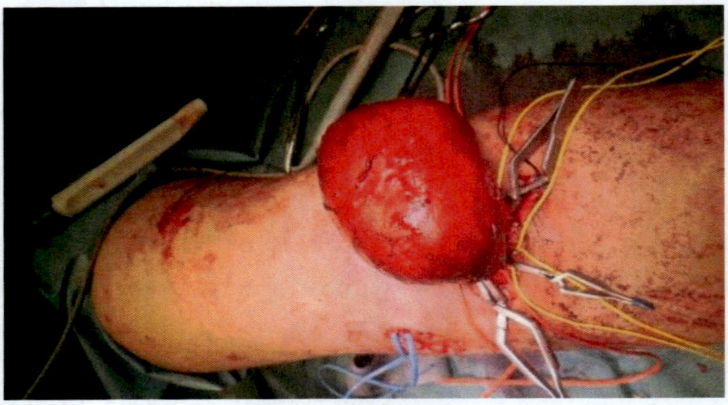

Source: Department of Vascular Surgery, VÚSCH, a.s.

Figure 2. Superior view of the dilated part of the cephalic vein.

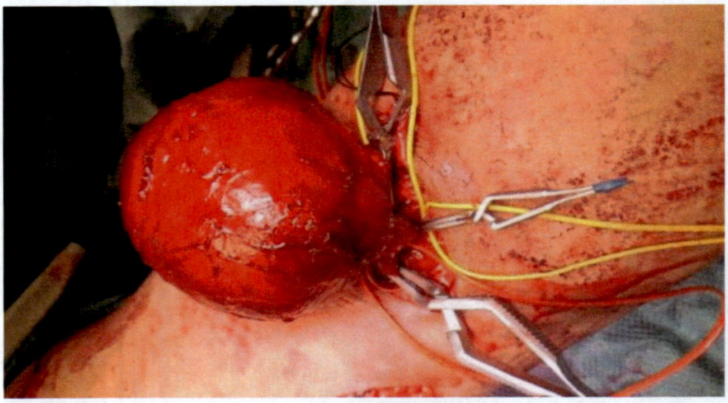

Source: Department of Vascular Surgery, VÚSCH, a.s.

Figure 3. Dilated cephalic vein of drainage AVF on the left.

Case Study No. 2

A 49-year-old male M. D., enrolled in a dialysis program, had an AV fistula on the left wrist since 2011, which became infected after repeat injections, the patient was acutely admitted initially for a spontaneously formed hematoma of the right thigh with CTAG-verified pseudoaneurysm on the deep femoral artery, with marked anemia and hemorrhagic shock, manifested as sudden pain and swelling of the left thigh for 48 hours. The patient was dialyzed using a permanent catheter inserted into v. jugularis interna on the right side. Previously hospitalized in the catchment internal medicine department with a febrile condition and anemia. For the persistence of temperatures, a dual combination of antibiotics, positive inflammatory parameters (leukocytes, CRP, procalcitonin), and blood culture on MRSA were used.

In addition to nephrotic syndrome, arterial hypertension, chronic hepatitis B, lung fibrosis, and polyneuropathy are present in the patient's medical history.

Acute stage erythrocyte masses, fresh frozen plasma for hemoglobin values 54 mmol/l, increase to 92 mmol/l after administration.

During the initial objective examination, massive solid edema present on the right thigh in the proximal and middle part, painful to touch, acral parts bilaterally warm, without deficits.

Ultrasonographically, the patency of the arterial and venous vessels of the right lower limb confirmed, up to the periphery, in the right thigh large hematomas, indistinctly bounded, with more fluid and dense parts, collections cannot be measured more accurately due to large size - practically up to 15 cm wide, 8-9 cm thick, length more than 10 cm!

In the depth of the proximal third of the thigh, there is a cavity with possible active extravasation of about 1.5 cm, but the finding is not unequivocal - the patient is restless, the examination with a probe causes pain, the connection with AFP cannot be assessed.

The patient was admitted to our Department for an urgent surgical solution and was acutely operated on; an extensive hematoma was removed, AFP at the depth on its third branch ligated for aneurysmal enlargement and rupture. The area was drained. The critically ill patient was transferred to the Department of Anesthesiology and Intensive Care to monitor vital signs and stabilize the condition. After stabilization and transfer of the patient to the department with a time interval of 14 days, the removal of aneurysmally dilated and infected AVF was planned on the left forearm under general anesthesia. The radial artery on the left reconstructed by venous plastic, the dilated and partially dethrombotized drainage cephalic vein of AVF extirpated from the auxiliary incisions on the forearm. Postoperatively, the patient was stable, then dialyzed through a permanent catheter, wounds on the upper and lower limbs heal primarily, limb circulation normal, limbs functional and without deficits. The patient was released to home care after 22 days of hospitalization.

During repeated outpatient check-ups, the patient feels good, the pain of lower or upper limbs is not reported, the right lower limb warm to the periphery without deficit, the upper limbs warm also without deficit, wounds calm, sutures firm without hematomas. A permcath implanted in the right IJV. The patient continues in the dialysis program and chronic medication according to an internist and a nephrologist.

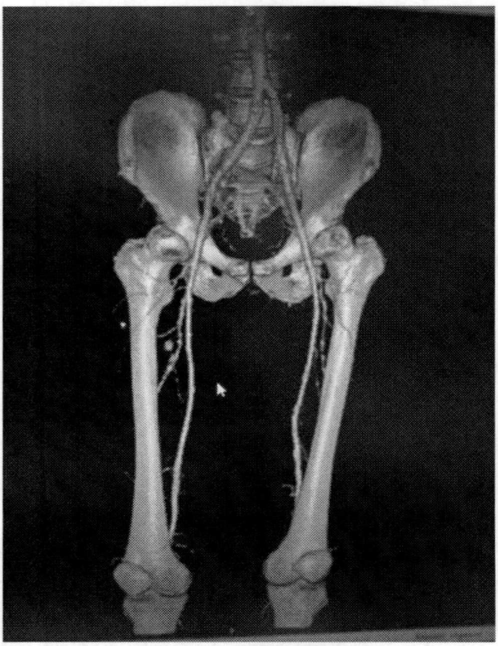

Source: Department of Vascular Surgery, VÚSCH, a.s.

Figure 4. 3D reconstruction of the patient's arteries.

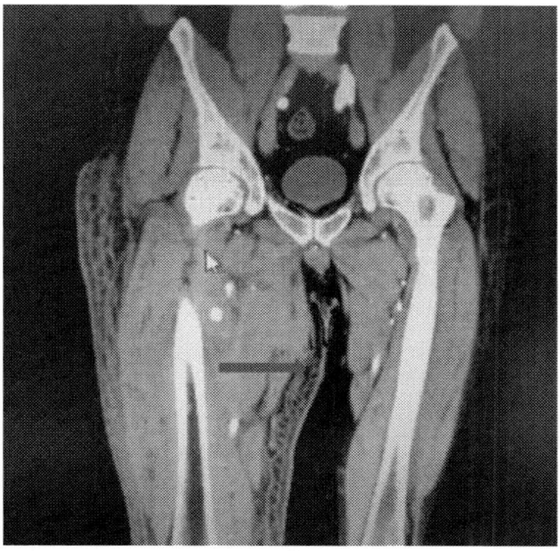

Source: Department of Vascular Surgery, VÚSCH, a.s.

Figure 5. Sagittal section (arrow shows enlarged deep femoral artery on the right side).

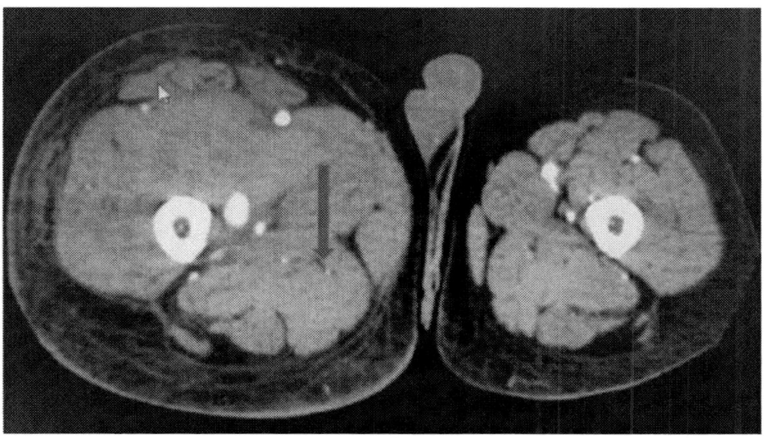

Source: Department of Vascular Surgery, VÚSCH, a.s.

Figure 6. Coronal section, shows AFP aneurysm on the right side (see the arrow).

Case Study No. 3

An 18-year-old male admitted to our Department to establish an AV fistula for long-term hemodialysis. The patient monitored by a nephrologist for hereditary nephritis, gradual deterioration of renal parameters in the terminal stage. In the first session, the AV fistula was sutured on the left wrist in the fossa Tabatière, which was dysfunctional in the early postoperative period due to the gracile venous system on the left upper limb.

Therefore, we tried to establish the fistula on the left upper limb more proximally on the forearm, but the veins were also gracile, non-graftable in the given section. Subsequently, the AV fistula was sutured only in the area of the left cubital fossa: brachio-cephalic, which was functional, usable for long-term hemodialysis after maturation. However, over the next 12 months, the course of dialysis worsened due to stenosis in the venous segment of the fistula.

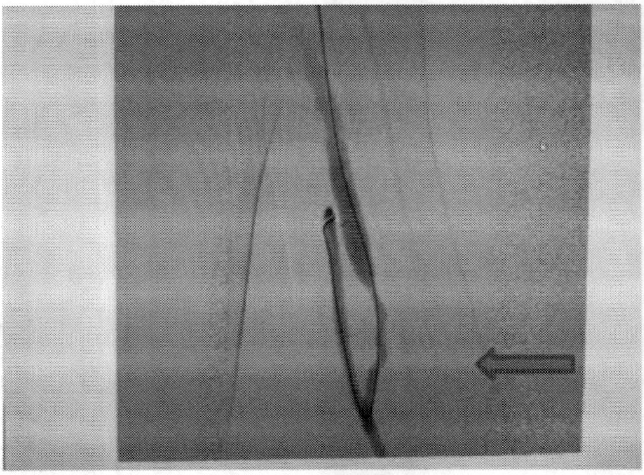

Source: Department of Vascular Surgery, VÚSCH, a.s.

Figure 7. PTA of the stenosis of the cephalic vein on the right side (marked with an arrow).

Therefore, the injection and DSA of the AV fistula, the supply artery, and the drainage stream were realized, where two hemodynamically severe stenoses in the drainage part in the cephalic vein are confirmed on the left shoulder. These were treated with PTA, with good effect.

Subsequently, over the next half-year, there is a significant dilatation of the draining venous part, which must be solved angiosurgically: banding of the AV fistula using Provena and suturing the original anastomosis.

The cephalic vein was significantly dilated to about 7 cm proximal to the anastomosis, cut longitudinally in the given section, sutured to reduce its dilatation, then de novo sutured AV anastomosis, reduced, which was finally strengthened by winding the Provena system. At the same time, the thrombectomy of the inlet and outlet parts of the fistula was necessary to see if there was closure with thrombi.

The patient continues with long-term hemodialysis, goes for regular check-ups, and is included in the transplant program.

Case Study No. 4

The 62-year-old female patient was transferred to the Department of Vascular Surgery VÚSCH, a.s. in an acute condition from the catchment dialysis center after an unsuccessful attempt to insert a central venous catheter - permcath into the internal jugular vein (VJI on the right) in a puncture manner (Figure 8). The catheter was punctured into the right carotid artery (ACC l.dx.). Due to the clinical symptoms (impaired consciousness) of the patient, an accelerated diagnosis was made first: CTAG examination, which confirmed implantation into ACC l.dx., obstruction of inflow into the area of the right cerebral hemisphere and partial thrombosis of the artery at the site of insertion.

Immediately after transport, the patient was transported to the operating room, where under general anesthesia, there was a surgical revision of the neck on the right, by a classic longitudinal incision, by first preparing IJV l.dx. positioned ventrolaterally. ACC l.dx and its branches were prepared. The place of entry of the catheter was sewn with the so-called tobacco suture, and the catheter was extracted. Due to the possibility of thrombosis in the surrounding area, an ACC l.dx thromboembolectomy was performed - proximally and distally, smaller fresh thrombi were removed. The patient was hospitalized at the Department of Anesthesiology and Intensive Care of VÚSCH, a.s. CT of the brain was performed to check the status, where no fresh focal ischemic changes from partial cerebral hemorrhage were demonstrated. After extubation, the patient had no symptoms of impaired consciousness or neurological deficit. After stabilization and hemodialysis, the patient was transferred to a catchment surgical ward. Subsequently, during the next month (after the surgical wound healed), an arteriovenous fistula for dialysis was sutured onto the patient, the fistula is fully functional after maturation and is used in her dialysis program.

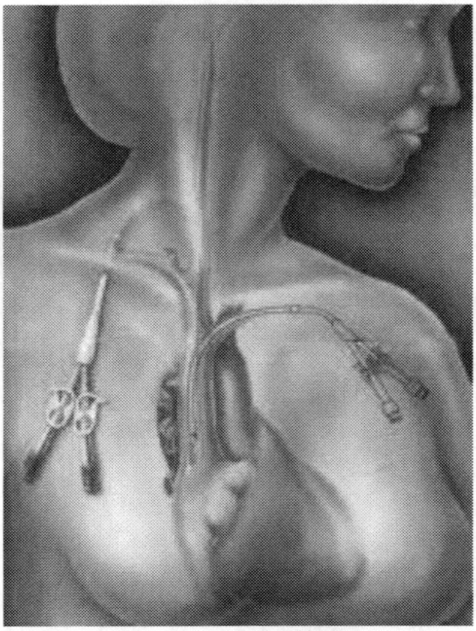

Source: author.

Figure 8. Scheme of permanent catheter insertion.

CASE STUDY NO. 5

42-year-old female, cardiac, type I diabetes- compensated with insulin, with autoimmune thyroid disease, in corticoid therapy, after repeated failed attempts to form an AV anastomosis (first attempt- radiocephalic on the upper left limb, then brachiocephalic one), dialyzed through a permanent catheter in the IJV l.dx., after repeated cardiac catheterizations and interventions on the arteries of lower limbs (Figure 12), was transplanted a kidney from a deceased donor in June 2019 (Figure 9, 10). The kidney was sutured with an end to side anastomosis on the external iliac artery on the right. Two hours after the transplantation, there is a significant deterioration of the clinical picture on the right lower limb, on which a PTA stent PTA recanalization AIC l. sin + PTA AII l., sin had been implanted in the past in 2014, and in 2018 angioplasty was realized with the implantation of two drug-releasing stents into the AFS l. dx., and balloon angioplasty APo l. dx. for the development of critical limb ischemia.

A vascular surgeon was called to the operating room, based on an urgently performed USG of the pelvic arteries and the arteries of the lower limb on the right, where an artery occlusion was present under the sutured kidney and distally towards the femoral area. Therefore, the right groin was initially open, common femoral artery (AFC), superficial femoral artery (AFS) and deep femoral artery (AFP) were dissected. No palpable pulsations, with severe atherosclerotic changes in the entire dissected section of the arteries, were present. After heparinization and arteriotomy, we found a dissected plaque present proximally and closing the AFP gap. Therefore, we open the original wound in the lower abdomen after transplantation on the right (Figure 11), revise the graft, whose vessels are functional, but distal AIE pulsations are absent, an atherosclerotic plaque from the arteriotomy on the artery is extracted, distal to AFC, inflow from the proximal part is sufficient, while the graft function is preserved. Arteries closed for sufficient width after endarterectomy by primary suture with non-absorbable fiber. However, AFS is chronically closed from the offset.

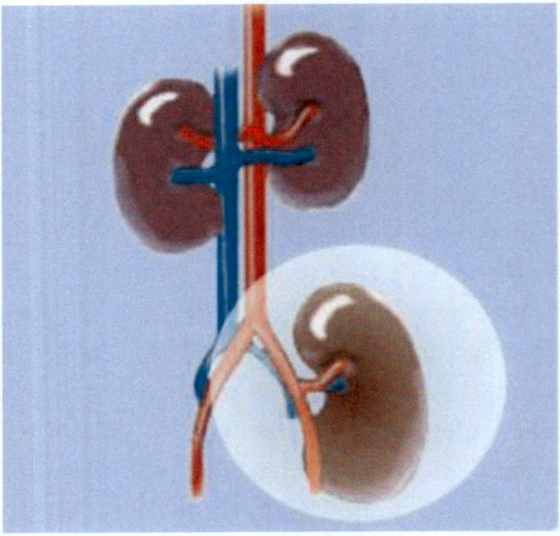

Source: author.

Figure 9. Kidney transplantation scheme.

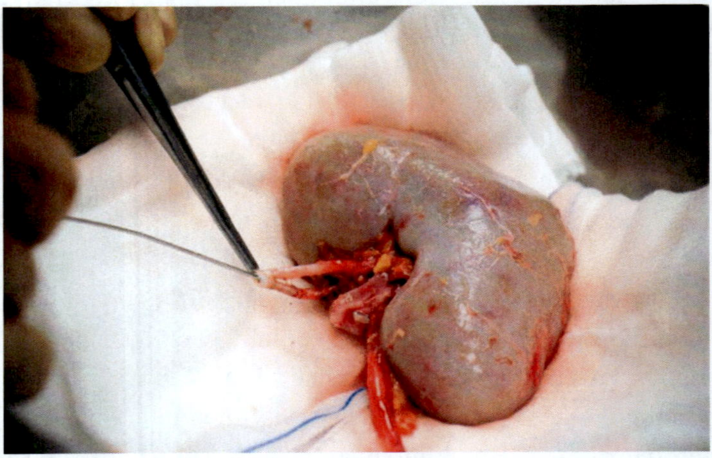

Source: author.

Figure 10. Kidney from a donor.

After the end of the operation, the patient was monitored at the ICU of the Transplant Department, where repeated control sonographic examinations confirm the flows into the graft and arteries of the right lower limb. However, the patient's condition on the 2nd postoperative day is complicated by cardiorespiratory failure, after which she was connected to artificial lung ventilation. Hospitalized in the Department of Anesthesiology and Resuscitation, where there is a gradual development of the patient's septic state, an increase in inflammatory laboratory parameters, and subsequently hypofunction, eventually dysfunction of the transplanted kidney. The flow to the right lower limb is still maintained, so after the consultation of experts in nephrology, transplantology, vascular surgery, and angiology, surgeons perform reoperation and evacuation of the graft, which is dysfunctional and is a likely source of the infection and of the failure of vital functions of the patient. Postoperatively, the condition gradually improves, both laboratory and clinically, the patient is disconnected from artificial lung ventilation, transferred to the inpatient transplant department. The patient gradually rehabilitates and is verticalized. wounds heal primarily. During a control ultrasound examination of the arteries and veins of the right upper limb, edema is present, and a permanent catheter is inserted in the IJV l.dx. an angiologist documents a clinically asymptomatic short embolus in the subclavian artery on the right, the flow is preserved distally to the arteries of the upper right limb. Therefore, due to the overall condition of the patient and the asymptomatic short closure, we withdraw from embolectomy and vascular reconstruction on the arteries of the upper right limb. The patient was instructed that in the manifestations of upper right limb ischemia, intervention in the arterial system is necessary. After 40 days of hospitalization in a hospital facility, the patient was discharged home with the dispensary care of a nephrologist, an angiologist, a cardiologist, and a vascular surgeon.

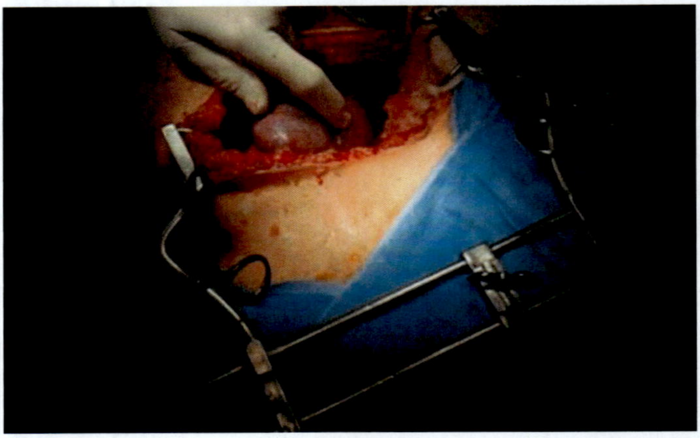

Source: author.

Figure 11. *In situ* surgical wound.

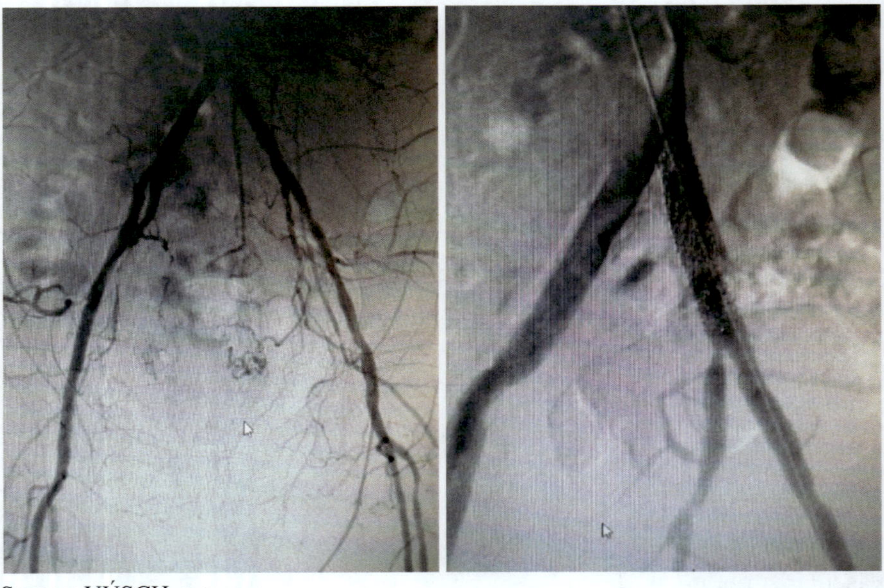

Source: VÚSCH, a.s.

Figure 12. a, b - Clear angiography and stent + PTA common iliac artery on the left.

In: Surgeon´s Perspective on Dialysis Patient ISBN: 978-1-53619-262-9
Editor: Maria Frankovicova

Chapter 15

Thoracosurgical Complications in Dialysis Patients

J. Belák*, MD
2nd department of Surgery,
Faculty of Medicine, Pavol Jozef Šafárik University in Košice and University Hospital, Košice, Slovakia

Abstract

In this part of the publication, the author wants to draw attention to possible complications in dialysis patients from the point of view of a thoracic surgeon. It deals with the possible consequences of the cannulation of large veins, pleural tap, inflammatory complications in the pleural cavity. In individual subchapters he deals with pneumothorax, hemothorax, pleural effusion, thoracic empyema, and fibrothorax. He describes their clinical symptoms, diagnostic possibilities, and the treatment itself.

Keywords: pleural effusion, pneumothorax, hemothorax, fibrothorax

---

* Corresponding Author's E-mail: jozef.belak@upjs.sk.

Abbreviations

CT	computed tomography
LDH	lactate dehydrogenase
NMR	nuclear magnetic resonance
VATS	video-assisted thoracoscopic surgery

Introduction

Hemodialysis as a process replacing kidney function in a patient with acute or chronic kidney disease also brings complications that require intervention of a thoracic surgeon. These complications are mainly pneumothorax, which may occur after central venous catheter insertion, hemothorax which may occur after central venous cannulation or after a pleural tap, pleural effusion, which persists even after repeated pleural taps, empyema of the chest after infections in the pleural cavity, bounded fluid collections in the pleural space affected by fibrothorax, which all significantly reduce respiratory volumes and lead to respiratory failure.

Pleura

The pleura is formed by two serous membranes with a soft, moist surface, one covering the lungs and the other the inner surface of the chest wall. During embryonic development, the two pleural cavities separate from the centrally located pericardial cavity by the formation of a pleuropericardial membrane. Topographically, the individual parts of the parietal pleura meet in sharp folds. The vascular supply of the visceral pleura comes from both the bronchial and pulmonary artery systems. Venous drainage is collected in the pulmonary veins. The parietal pleura supplies exclusively from the systemic arteries of the thoracic wall, diaphragm, and mediastinum, and the cervical pleura from the branches of the subclavian artery. Venous drainage leads through the corresponding veins into the superior vena cava. Lymphatic drainage of the pleural space is provided by special structures: in some small areas of the parietal pleura on the anterior wall of the chest, mediastinum, and diaphragm are located small ovoid openings, often in groups that form a direct connection of the pleural space with an extensive network of lymphatic channels. Their size is up to 2μm and they are predominantly in the lower parts. The lymphatic network is drained regionally, into the intercostal and substernal nodes, part of the mediastinal pleura even directly into the mediastinal nodes. Some lymphatic channels also lead to the axilla. Transdiaphragmatic anastomoses allow the passage of fluid from the peritoneal cavity into the pleural cavity. Lymphatic drainage of the visceral pleura leads directly to the deep plexuses in the interlobular and peribronchial cavity, but in approximately 20% of cases, direct connections to the mediastinal nodes were observed, which occur more frequently in the upper lobes as opposed to the lower lobes of the lungs. Although the lymphatic network under the visceral pleura is rich, we almost never see subpleural lymph nodes. The innervation of the parietal pleura is ensured by a rich network of somatic, sympathetic, and parasympathetic fibers. On the costal pleura, these fibers pass through the intercostal nerves. The diaphragmatic pleura is innervated via the phrenic nerves. The visceral pleura is without innervation. The formation of fluid in the pleural cavity is ensured by the constant secretion of pleural fluid, originating mainly from the capillaries of the parietal pleura. Quantitative determination is very problematic, but it is estimated that under normal circumstances, the volume of fluid in the pleural cavity is approximately 1 ml. It is regulated by the relationship between hydrostatic pressure, osmotic pressure, and lymphatic drainage of the pleura. Excess fluid, even some small particles and cells are removed from the pleural cavity by breathing movements through preformed openings into the lymphatic vessels. However, under pathological conditions, fluid may also originate from other sources: in pulmonary edema, it is filtered directly from the pulmonary interstitium into the pleural space through the semipermeable visceral pleura. Peritoneal fluid may enter the chest through crevices in the diaphragm in ascites patients, or in peritoneal dialysis.

PNEUMOTHORAX

Pneumothorax is a pathological accumulation of air in the pleural cavity. In a dialyzed patient, it can occur while inserting a catheter into the subclavian or jugular vein, or during a pleural or pulmonary biopsy. Under normal circumstances, intrapleural pressure fluctuates between -8 and -9 mmHg during inspiration and -3 and -6 mmHg during expiration. Negative intrapleural pressure is maintained by continuous absorption of fluid from the intrapleural space through the pleural capillaries. Due to the elasticity of the lungs, the intrabronchial pressure in the lungs is greater than the intrapleural pressure. Intrabronchial pressure fluctuates during the respiratory cycle in the range of -1 to -3 mmHg during inspiration and at +1 to +5 mmHg at expiration. Equilibrium of the pressure gradient may occur due to disruption of the continuity of the parietal pleura or visceral pleura. Valve mechanism in the area of injured lungs can cause accumulation of air in the pleural cavity and may lead to the development of tension pneumothorax. The pathophysiological consequences of pneumothorax depend on the extent of pneumothorax, its tension, and the condition of the affected lungs. Patients with advanced pulmonary disease that results in decreased lung elasticity have a small transpulmonary pressure. Under these circumstances, the collapse of the lung parenchyma is slow and less extensive. However, even a small reduction in vital capacity in these patients may result in increased respiratory effort and may cause respiratory failure. This may also apply to dialysis patients. The severity of clinical signs depends on the extent of pulmonary parenchyma collapse, the concomitant pulmonary disease, and the rate of volume change in the development of pneumothorax. The asymptomatic course is usually in small-scale pneumothoraxes and pneumothorax appears only by routine X-ray of the lungs. In 80% of patients, symptoms appear at rest or during normal physical activity. Chest pain is the most common symptom, and if pneumothorax is small, it may be the only symptom. The pain is sharp at first, pleuritic, then dull, persistent. However, it can escalate, radiate into the epigastrium, and simulate acute abdomen. Shortness of breath is the second most common symptom. It occurs in large pneumothoraxes and in the accompanying pulmonary diseases. Severe dyspnea with circulatory failure is an associated symptom of tension pneumothorax. Nonproductive cough, hemoptysis and cyanosis are less common symptoms. Reduced motion of the chest wall on the affected side also occurs. The percussion is hyperresonant, sometimes even tympanitic. Tactile fremitus is reduced, sometimes absent. On the affected side, the breathing is weakened, at times absent. A characteristic physical finding only appears when the lung collapse exceeds 25%. The diagnosis is made based on an X-ray of the lungs. At the periphery of the hemithorax, the lung markings are absent. Compared to the contralateral side, the lung field is clearer, the visceral pleura appears as a thin white line delimiting the lungs in the intrapleural space (Figure 1).

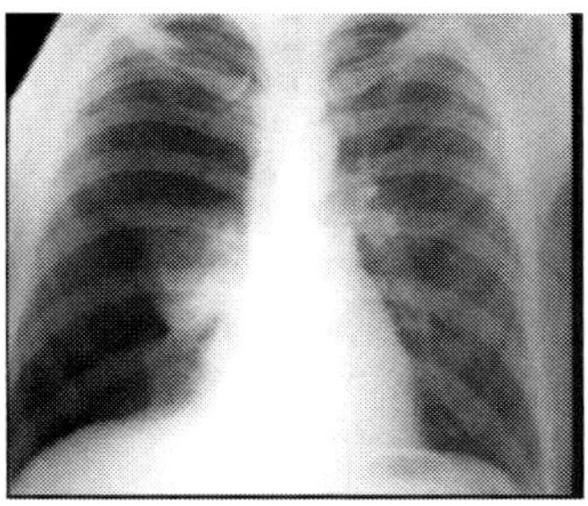

Figure 1. X-ray showing pneumothorax in the right pleural cavity.

Sometimes the diagnosis is clarified by a CT scan. The most common differential diagnostic problem is a large bullous emphysema. In these cases, CT scan is appropriate. One of the complications is pleural effusion of varying magnitude and occurs in approximately 20% of patients. In its simple form, it does not pose a significant risk. Hemothorax occurs in only 3% of the cases, but it significantly increases mortality. Respiratory failure is particularly common in the elderly. Empyema is a rare complication. Tension pneumothorax is characterized by an ever-increasing volume of intrapleurally accumulated air. A valve mechanism may form in the chest wall after its injury or at the site of a lung lesion. Progressive accumulation of air causes the mediastinum to move to the healthy side, compression of the superior vena cava, angulation in the area of the cavoatrial junction, which results in impaired filling of the heart and a reduction in its stroke volume. In addition, lung compression occurs on the healthy side, resulting in a pulmonary short circuit through the unventilated alveoli. The critical overpressure value is 15 to 20 cm H_2O. Evolving hypoxia, acidosis, and circulatory failure have fatal consequences. The clinical picture is usually alarming. Patients are restless, anxious, dyspneic. Cold sweat and cyanosis appear as well. They suffer tachypnea, tachycardia, and hypotension. The affected half of the chest is expanded, the intercostal spaces and the supraclavicular fossa are filled. Percussion over the pneumothorax is hyperresonant, auscultation detects absent breath sounds. Tense pneumothorax signals the overall clinical picture, tracheal deviation and the shift of the apex beat to the healthy side. The diagnosis is confirmed by an X-ray of the chest, which shows the collapse of the lungs and the mediastinal shift to the contralateral side. In an emergency, treatment cannot be delayed by a radiographic examination. A simple proof is provided by inserting a thin needle into the chest in the second intercostal space in the midclavicular line. The needle is connected to an open syringe filled with normal saline. An urgent therapeutic procedure is the decompression of the affected hemithorax with a thicker needle and keeping the needle in place until final treatment by a chest tube or surgical revision.

Apart from a small amount of stabilized mantle pneumothoraces, i.e., an air volume of less than 25% of the thoracic cavity volume, which can be treated by only monitoring, since approximately 1.25% of the intrapleural air is absorbed daily, pneumothorax treatment is surgical. The aim of surgical treatment is to restore the full lung capacity and at the same time to prevent the continued escape of air from the visceral pleural defect. The following procedures are available: pleural tap, chest drainage, videothoracoscopic and video-assisted procedures, treatment of pneumothorax from classic thoracotomy. The basic precondition for the success of decompressive treatment of pneumothorax is a closed defect in the visceral pleura, in which, after evacuation of pathologically accumulated air, the lung can expand. The essence of the method is a single or continuous aspiration of intrapleural air and restoration of physiological pressure conditions. In the case of a tension-type pneumothorax, pleural tap is a life-saving procedure. This is especially true for field treatments, where there often is not time or sufficient equipment to perform a standard chest drainage (chest tube). Patients with tension pneumothorax are in immediate danger of death and it is necessary to immediately release the overpressure in the pleural cavity. At this point, pleural tap is a simpler procedure and thus easier to perform even for doctors without sufficient erudition than conventional chest drainage. The decisive fact for the patient's survival at a given moment is the speed and success of the procedure. Moreover, its purpose in this case is not to expand the lung, but only to reduce intrapleural pressure. Therefore, by inserting a needle into the pleural cavity, it is sufficient to substantially convert the tension-closed pneumothorax to an open one, which no longer acutely endangers the patient. The technique of inserting a needle into the pleural cavity itself is not a big problem and is generally known. The essence of the tap is a single or continuous aspiration of pathologically accumulated intrapleural air. The actual decompression is performed after premedication of the patient under local infiltration anesthesia of the entire thickness of the chest wall, most often in the second or third intercostal space of the midclavicular or anterior axillary line of the respective hemithorax.

Chest drain is the gold standard treatment of pneumothorax. The purpose of drainage is to restore physiological pressure conditions in the pleural cavity and thus allow the lungs to expand normally. There is no absolute contraindication to chest drain, a relative contraindication is the current presence of coagulopathy. Active drainage is the most common therapeutic procedure in pneumothorax. It can be used to achieve lung re-expansion even in the case of continuous air leakage from the lungs. Active drainage is necessary until the bubbling in the collection bottle stops. The drainage can then be changed to passive (according to Bülau) or the drain can be closed for 24 hours. If complete re-expansion of the lungs remains after X-ray examination, the drain can be removed. There are several aspects to choosing where the drain is inserted through the chest wall into the pleural cavity. It follows the general recommendations of renowned authors or workplace practices or is modified by the type and location of pneumothorax. Either the drain is introduced in the second or third intercostal space in the respective midclavicular line, or the drainage is inserted in either the anterior or midaxillary line, at one of the intercoastal spaces, ranging from the third to the sixth. Chest drains should meet these criteria, should be flexible and resilient, should be strong enough to withstand the pressure of the chest wall, must have a non-wetting inner surface and must be made of materials that do not cause adverse reactions in the pleural cavity. Chest drainage is performed under local anesthesia in the appropriate intercostal space. Drainage systems are used to return physiological conditions in the pleural cavity after chest drainage. Depending on the situation in the pleural cavity, we can use several drainage systems, passive drainage systems, active drainage systems and a balanced drainage system. In the case of passive systems, it is a one-way drainage of air from the chest during expiration which causes the intrapleural pressure to increase. At the same time, the return of air to the pleural cavity is prevented due to the water valve or the nature of the construction of the Heimlich valve. They are called passive drainage because no active source of vacuum is used to aspirate the pathological contents from the pleural cavity. One option is to use a single-bottle drainage system. In the literature, this system is called Bülau-drain. This system combines both respiratory mechanics and gravity. It consists of one bottle in which there are two tubes (Figure 2). The bottle serves as a collection container and at the same time as a water valve. The longer tube is immersed 2 cm below the surface of the sterile fluid, the other is above the surface and interacts with the surrounding space. The principle of this system is simple, if during expiration an overpressure develops in the chest and is transferred to the drain, then at a pressure higher than 2 cm of water column air escapes into the bottle and through the short tube into the surrounding environment. During inspiration, the sterile fluid being drawn in prevents the air to flow back into the pleural cavity. This drainage system is ideal for the treatment of an uncomplicated pneumothorax. The second type of passive chest drainage is the Heimlich valve as an alternative to a single-bottle drainage system (Figure 3). It is a one-way valve consisting of a clear solid plastic tube, inside which is a rubber flap functioning as a one-way valve. This allows air to escape from the pleural cavity but prevents air from being sucked back through the chest drain. The flap is connected to the chest drain facing away from the patient. Its use also enables outpatient treatment.

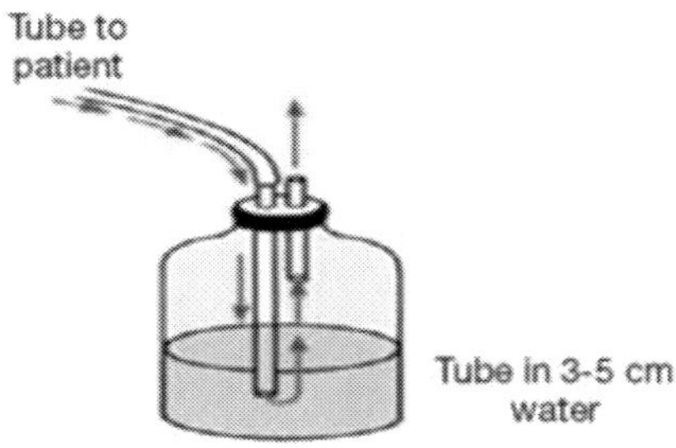

Figure 2. Bülau drain.

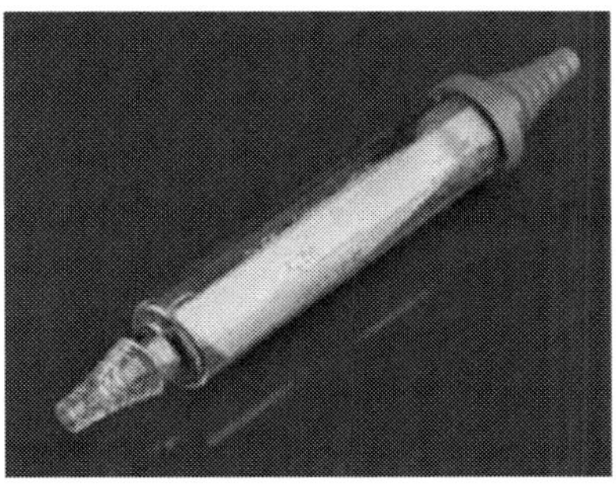

Figure 3. Heimlich valve.

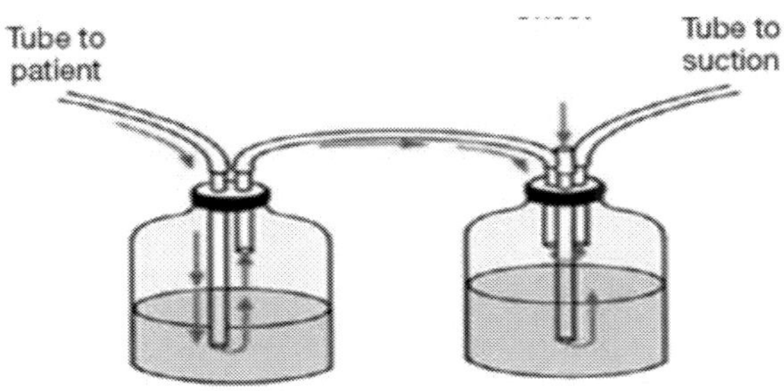

Figure 4. Two-bottle drainage system.

Active drainage systems must be used to ensure complete lung re-expansion. They are called active because a mechanical device must be used to create a vacuum. Depending on how they are arranged, we can speak of a two-bottle or three-bottle system. The two-bottle system consists of two glass bottles (Figure 4). The first bottle is connected to the drain from the patient and serves as a collection bottle. The second bottle is a vacuum regulator. The vacuum level should be between -10 and -20 cm H_2O. In case of significant air leakage from the lung parenchyma, it is recommended to reduce the active vacuum in the drainage system to -5 cm H_2O in developed lungs, to avoid suction of air from the lung parenchyma into the drainage system. In the case of a three-bottle system, an additional bottle is added, which is used to collect fluid from the pleural cavity, the second bottle has a water valve, and the third bottle regulates the vacuum. In addition to these bottle systems, it is also possible to use disposable plastic three-bottle systems, which are becoming a common part of treatment. It is a combination of three bottles into one simple and mobile module. They consist of a collecting part, a part with a water valve and a part for regulate the vacuum. Their advantage, unlike bottle systems, is their ease of use and operation (Stolz, 2010).

In cases of continued air leakage from the drain and after CT documentation of severe concomitant lung disease, surgical treatment of pneumothorax is indicated either by videothoracoscopy or by thoracotomy. Such concomitant lung diseases can be bullous emphysema. The aim of the operation is to treat the site of air leakage from the lungs by wedge-shaped or tangential resection of the lungs and then to take measures to prevent lung collapse in the future. By default, a partial pleurectomy is performed in the upper tertiary of the pleural cavity, and a pleural abrasion is performed more distally.

Hemothorax

Hemothorax is another possible complication after a thoracocentesis or cannulation of large veins. Hemothorax is a pathological accumulation of blood in the pleural cavity. Depending on the amount of blood, the hemothorax is divided into small - less than 400 ml of blood, medium - 500 to 1500 ml of blood and large - over 1500 ml of blood. Blood that enters the pleural cavity coagulates rapidly, but due to the movement of the lungs and heart, it defibrinates, becomes fluid, and is not radiographically recognizable from pleural effusion. If no infection is present, smaller hemorrhagic effusions are absorbed in most patients. In larger hemorrhages, defibrination is imperfect, with clots remaining that are not accessible by evacuation or chest drainage. Bacterial contamination supports this process. A sealed fibrin sac is formed that contains serum and coagulated blood elements. Due to the osmotic forces during the breakdown of blood elements, fluid can be sucked into the formed sac, which enlarges and compresses the lungs. Eventually, a solid fibrothorax is formed. The large loss of circulating blood volume causes symptoms of hypovolemia and, in addition, its pressure on the venae cavae adversely affects the filling of the heart and its stroke volume. The clinical manifestations of bleeding into the pleural cavity depend on the rate and amount of blood loss and the concomitant disease. Small bleeding up to 400 ml has an asymptomatic course. Physical examination does not detect more noticeable pathological changes. Symptoms of hypovolemia such as restlessness, cold sweat, tachycardia, hypotension, acrohypothermia, oliguria, appear in blood loss over 1000ml. Shortness of breath, chest pain, cyanosis are symptoms of increased pressure on the lung parenchyma. Physical examination determines the collection in the thoracic cavity: basally suppressed percussion, weakened tactile fremitus, impaired breathing. As part of the diagnosis, an X-ray image of the chest confirms the fluidothorax, i.e., we see an opacification of the costophrenic angle that proceeds in the proximal direction. Bleeding less than 250 ml may not appear radiologically. Heavy bleeding causes opacification of the entire hemithorax and transfer of the mediastinum to the contralateral side. However, only a diagnostic thoracentesis in the context of clinical signs makes for a convincing diagnosis. A CT scan is used to assess the amount of blood in the thoracic cavity and to distinguish it from the blood clot (Figures 5, 6).

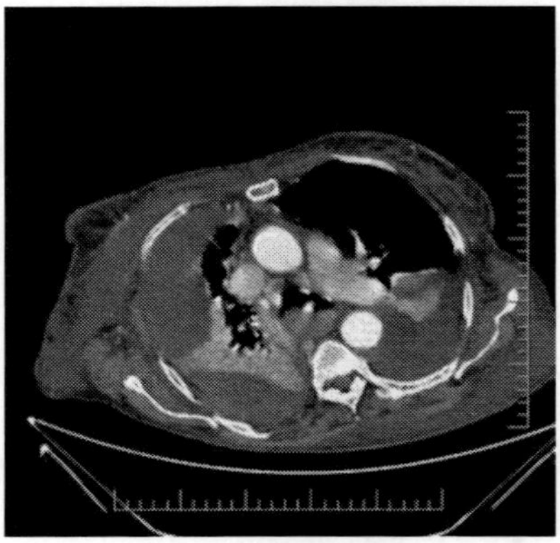

Figure 5. CT of a hemothorax (axial projection).

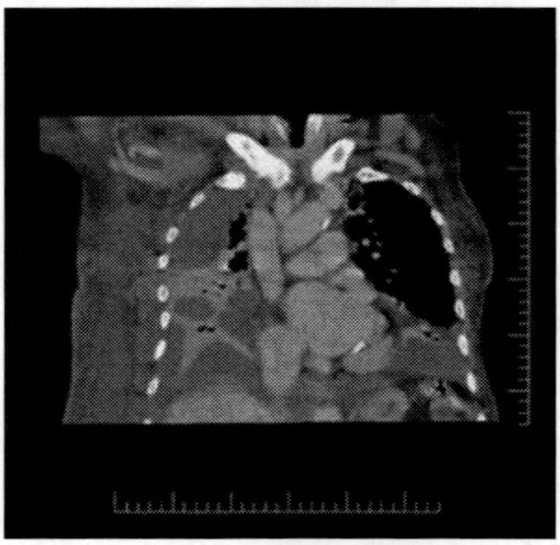

Figure 6. CT of a hemothorax (coronal plane).

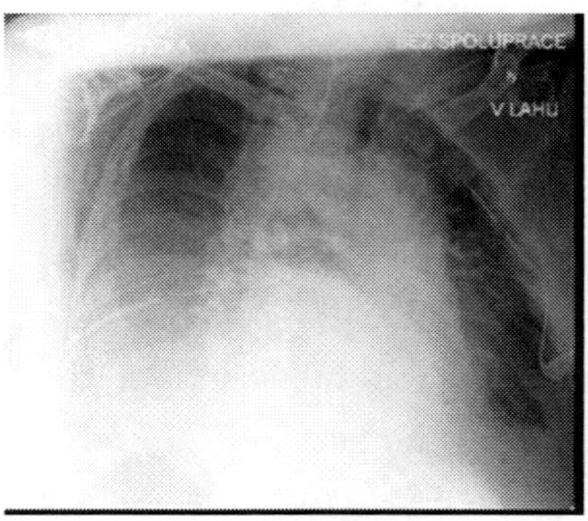

Figure 7. Chest x-ray after the evacuation of a hemothorax via drainage.

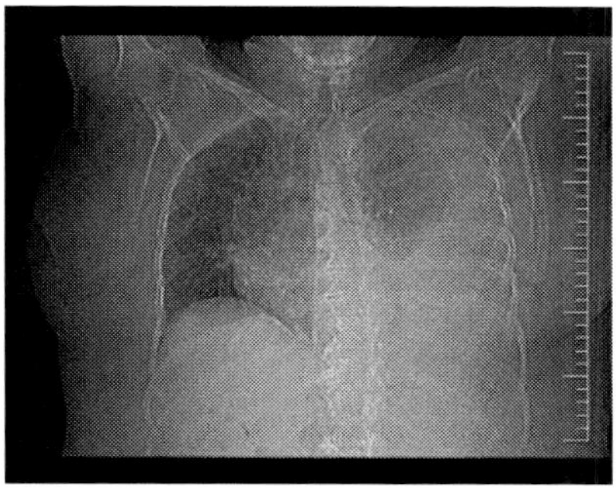

Figure 8. CT of a pleural effusion in the left pleural cavity.

Regardless of its etiology, the treatment of hemothorax should be active. The course of treatment depends on the amount of blood loss, the symptoms of active bleeding and the accompanying pathology. A small hemothorax, which is not associated with another serious disease, requires only a needle decompression, which takes place at the same time as diagnostic thoracentesis of the pleural cavity. The most suitable place for diagnostic and at the same time evacuation of the chest puncture is the sixth intercostal space in the posterior axillary line. In case the test is positive, defibrinated blood is obtained, which differs in color and consistency from intravascular blood. If blood clots, this is evidence that extravascular blood is not evacuated, but the liver or spleen may have been hit by the needle. With repeated accumulation of blood in the pleural cavity, drainage of the pleural cavity is more appropriate than repeated punctures. The middle-level (500-1500 ml of blood in the chest cavity) hemothorax on a chest X-ray causes opacification a quarter to a half of the hemithorax. It requires a more proactive approach. It is better to drain the thoracic cavity immediately than to attempt a needle decompression. (Figure 8). The chest drain also removes smaller clots that would clog the needle and allows us to continuously monitor continued bleeding. The optimal site for chest drainage in cases of hemothorax is the fifth or sixth intercostal space in the midaxillary line. Placing the chest drain lower is not recommended due to the risk of injury to the diaphragm and abdominal organs. There are several recommendations on how to proceed with further treatment of hemothorax. Practical experience has shown that the rapid evacuation of 500 to 1500 ml of blood immediately after drainage does not mean that it is a fresh, ongoing bleeding. If the additional blood loss is less than 200 ml per hour, it is hoped that the bleeding may stop spontaneously. However, the condition is an evacuated chest cavity confirmed by x-ray. Indications for thoracotomy due to surgical hemostasis are bleeding from the drain which exceeds 300 ml per hour for three hours, blood loss of about 200 ml per hour, but persists unchanged for five hours, increased opacification on a chest X-ray at the above-mentioned blood loss values, persistence of hypotension and symptoms of hypovolemia with adequate treatment of blood loss. A large hemothorax is associated with a critical condition of the patient, the mortality reaches 50-75%. The symptoms of hemorrhagic shock and hypoxia are significant; therefore, a comprehensive therapeutic procedure is needed. That is, chest drainage with active suction, intubation and controlled ventilation, transfusion for blood loss and circulating blood volume, early thoracotomy for the purpose of surgical hemostasis. At times thoracotomy may be avoided if, after draining the blood in the chest cavity using a chest drain, the patient's overall condition is significantly improved, the patient responds well to the blood transfusion, the chest drain draws less than 200 ml per hour for the first two hours, and a chest X-ray shows expansion of pulmonary parenchyma. It is not acceptable to delay a thoracotomy with continued significant blood loss present, as well as wait for the hemorrhagic shock to resolve on its own. Surgical treatment of the source of bleeding is the best way to prevent the deepening of hemorrhagic shock.

A clotted hemothorax cannot be removed by simple drainage of the chest cavity. The drains become clogged with clots and replacing them will not help. If chest drainage is unsuccessful and a massive opacification on the chest x-ray remains, thoracotomy is performed to evacuate the clots from the pleural cavity. This achieves immediate lung re-expansion and avoids complications in the form of empyema or fibrothorax.

PLEURAL EFFUSION

Pleural effusion is the accumulation of fluid in the pleural cavity due to excessive transudation or exudation of interstitial fluid from the pleural surface (Figures 9, 10). This also occurs in dialysis patients. Pleural effusion is not a separate disease entity, but only a clinical manifestation of systemic or pleural disease. The etiology of pleural effusions is diverse. The passage of fluids through pleural membranes depends on hydrostatic and colloid osmotic pressure. The pressure difference between the systemic and pulmonary circulation causes a massive transport of fluids through the pleural space, it is 5000 to 10000 ml in 24 hours. The second important mechanism of fluid transport from the pleural space is lymphatic drainage. It is not so significant in volume, it is 150 to 500 ml in 24 hours, but its importance lies in the absorption of proteins from the pleural cavity. The mechanisms of abnormal fluid accumulation in the pleural cavity are the following: increase in hydrostatic pressure, increase in capillary permeability, decrease in colloid osmotic pressure, increase in intrapleural negative pressure, and damage to the lymphatic drainage. Pleural effusions are divided into transudates and exudates. Transudate occurs when systemic factors that affect the production and absorption of pleural effusion are disrupted. Examples are a decrease in plasma colloid osmotic pressure and an increase in hydrostatic pressure in the systemic or pulmonary circulation. In this case, the primary process does not involve the pleura. In contrast, exudate results from pathological damage to the pleura or pleural lymphatic system. Small pleural effusions may be asymptomatic. On the other hand, a developing pleural effusion induced by pleural inflammation may be manifested by a sharp, stabbing pleuritic pain. Shortness of breath is caused by alterations in pulmonary function due to high mechanical pressure. Its extent also depends on the underlying disease that caused the pleural effusion. Compressed lung parenchyma predisposes to atelectases and intercurrent lung infections, which may alter the original clinical picture. The complex clinical picture is further altered by specific clinical signs of the underlying disease. Physical examination will alert you to fluid in the pleural cavity: basally suppressed percussion, weakened tactile fremitus, impaired breathing, and tubular breath sounds above the effusion. The physical finding depends on the amount of fluid and location of the effusion. According to the amount of fluid, we distinguish small (200-300 ml), medium-sized (800-1000 ml) and large exudates, which fill the entire pleural cavity, compress the lungs, and shift the mediastinum to the healthy side. X-ray examination is the first test used to detect pleural effusion. In the standard lung image, the pleural effusion manifests as a opacification over the diaphragm with a concave contour in the area of the costophrenic angle and its gradual disappearance proximally. About 250 ml of pleural effusion already causes obvious obliteration of the costophrenic angle. As a result of adhesions in the pleural cavity, encapsulated effusions can be formed, which present variously on x-ray. Pleural tap and laboratory tests are essential in the differentiation of pleural effusions. The assessment of the amount of effusion already has a certain significance, because up to 70% of massive effusions occupying the entire hemithorax are caused by malignant pleural disease. An ultrasonographic examination of the chest, which will show a collection of pleural fluid, possibly also with an adjacent involvement of the lung parenchyma or the chest wall, can be helpful. It can also be a guide for a targeted thoracentesis. A CT scan, which identifies pleural fluid and diseases of the parenchyma with high accuracy and by assessing fluid density can serve as an important factor in planning further procedures. At present, the routine technique of CT guided thoracentesis is highly accurate and safe. However, the pleural tap will make the final diagnosis. First, it is necessary to assess the appearance of the obtained fluid, possibly its odor, to examine it biochemically (glucose, amylase, LDH, protein levels), to make a differential diagnosis of cellular elements, to examine it microbiologically and cytologically. If the pleural fluid has a putrid odor, the patient is likely to have an anaerobic infection in the pleural cavity. If the effusion is bloody, its hematocrit should be examined. If the effusion hematocrit is greater than 50% of the peripheral blood hematocrit, the patient is suffering from a hemothorax. If the pleural effusion is rocky, milky, it is advisable to examine the supernatant after centrifugation. Differentiation of blood elements is also important. More than 10,000 elements/μl is most common in parapneumonic effusions, but it can also be present in pancreatitis, pulmonary embolism, collagenosis, malignancy, and tuberculosis. A differential count is better than the total count. If there are predominantly polymorphonuclear leukocytes in the pleural effusion, it is most likely an acute process (pneumonia, pancreatitis with pulmonary involvement, intraperitoneal abscess). If mononuclear elements are dominant in the effusion, it is probably a malignancy. The predominance of lymphocytes supports the suspicion that the patient has a malignancy or tuberculosis. The presence of a reduced glucose level below 40 mg/dl should be an indication for drainage, as it is present in empyema, malignancy, tuberculosis, rheumatoid effusions or even in hemothorax. Abnormal levels of amylase in the pleural effusion indicate esophageal rupture, pancreatopathy, or malignancy. In each case of pleural effusion tap, the LDH level should be measured, which is a very good indicator of the degree of inflammation in the pleural cavity. If LDH levels rise during repeated taps, it means that the inflammation is getting worse and treatments need to be stepped up. Conversely, if LDH levels show a declining trend in a series of thoracenteses, this signals improvement, a healing of the inflammation. Cytological examination can help diagnose malignant pleural effusion, but it is not always reliable. The diagnostic yield is reported to be about 60%. It is important for the physician to properly diagnose the nature of pleural effusion before deciding on further treatment. Invasive examination procedures are the method of choice: needle biopsy of the pleura, thoracoscopy, thoracotomy. If the patient also has documented changes in the pulmonary parenchyma on CT or is presenting with massive hemoptysis, a bronchoscopy should be performed as well. Small pleural samples can be obtained via needle biopsy. The sovereign method of choice is currently videothoracoscopic biopsy, in which the entire surface of the pleura in the examined hemithorax can be directly visualized by a camera inserted through a small incision. The diagnostic accuracy of videothoracoscopic samples is more than 95% with minimal morbidity and no mortality. Videothoracoscopy virtually made the open thoracotomy pleura biopsy obsolete.

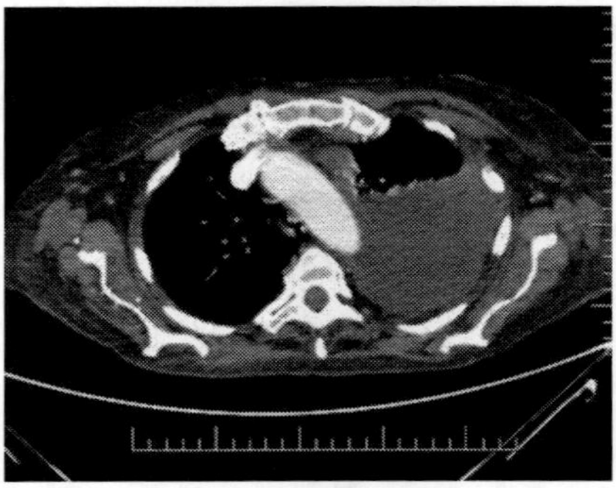

Figure 9. CT of a pleural effusion in the left pleural cavity (axial plane).

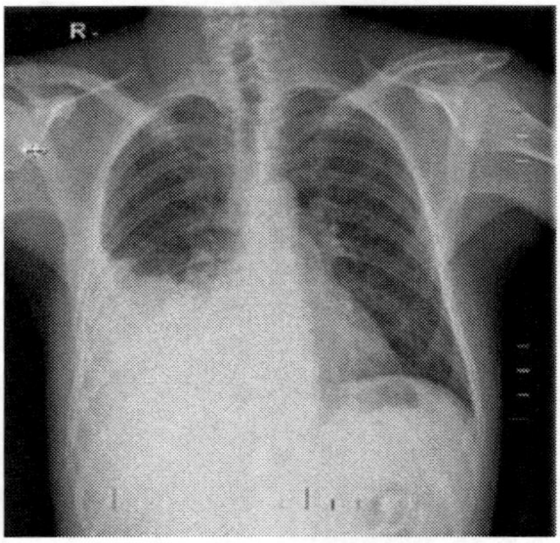

Figure 10. X-ray of a pleural effusion in the right pleural cavity.

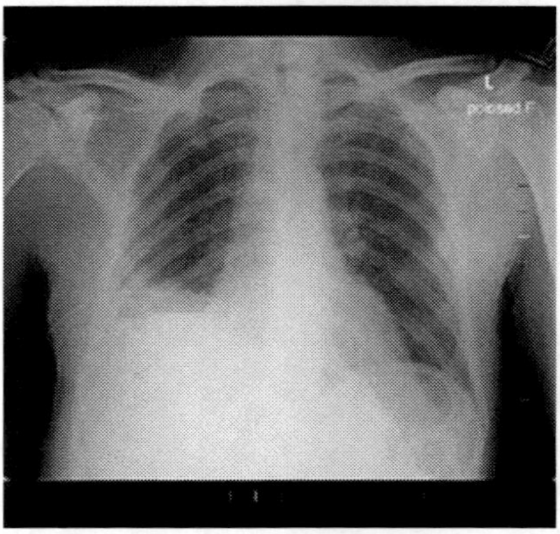

Figure 11. X-ray of a pleural effusion (post-drainage) in the right pleural cavity.

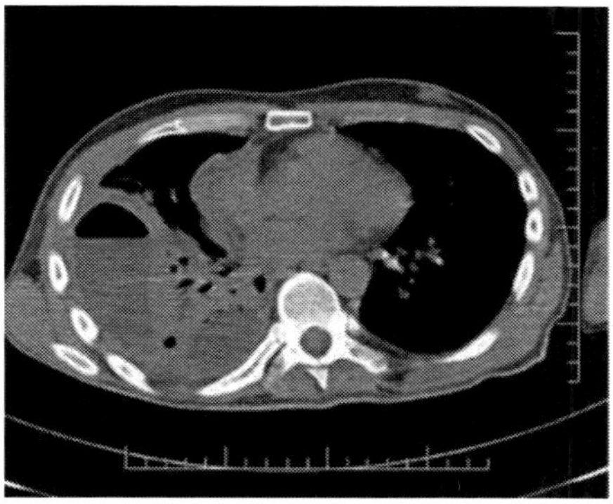

Figure 12. CT of an empyema in the right pleural cavity (axial plane).

The first line of treatment for non-cancerous effusions is the causal treatment of the underlying disease. If the effusion does not subside or is symptomatic, it should be evacuated. The simplest method is pleural tap, but it is also the least effective. Repeated taps carry with them the risk of causing an infection of the pleural cavity. Pleural tap should therefore only be the first step, sometimes done urgently, to make diagnosis easier. However, if fluid continues to accumulate, a more drastic procedure should be used. Inserting a chest tube into the pleural space is a reliable method of solving the most diverse pleural fluid collections (Figures 11, 12). It is an undemanding procedure with high evacuation efficiency, even in the long-term, and it allows pleurodesis to be performed eventually. It is usually the last stage of videothoracoscopic diagnostic surgery. Often, after exudation, severe functional impairment of respiratory mechanics due to lung entrapment in fibrin deposits remains. We must address this condition by removing this cortex on the visceral and often parietal pleura by decortication. For most patients, the most preferred and least burdensome method of treating malignant effusion is tubular chest drainage with instillation of a sclerosing agent. Tetracyclines were used most commonly. Currently, the application of talc is very popular. The success of the procedure should be defined not as the unconditional formation of a complete pleural symphysis, but as the reduction of pleural fluid reaccumulation to such an extent that dyspnea subsides, and no further therapeutic treatment is required.

Chest Empyema

The term empyema means the accumulation of pus within a naturally existing cavity in the body. Chest empyema is a purulent pleural effusion. It can be localized (encapsulated), but it can also affect the entire pleural space. Infection most often enters the normally sterile pleural space from some surrounding intrathoracic structure, but sometimes also from non-thoracic structures or organs. The actual process of empyema formation and development has three stages: exudative, with the formation and increase of pleural membranes, fibrinopurulent with the deposition of large deposits of fibrin, the stage of organization with the growth of fibroblasts and collagen masses. The first stage is characterized by exudation from the increase in permeability of the inflamed edematous pleura. Polymorphonuclear leukocytes are present in small numbers and fibrin begins to deposit on the pleural surface. Initially, the fluid is relatively clear and yellow, but as bacterial invasion progresses, leukocytes increase (more than 500/μl), density is more than 1018, and protein levels rise above 2.5 g/dl. The pH drops below 7.2 and the LDH reaches up to 1000 IU/l. In the further course, large fibrin deposits are formed on both parts of the pleura, although more on the parietal pleura. Fibrin bridges sometimes form between the two parts of the pleura, which later leads to the formation of smaller separate cavities. The bridges divide the empyema of the entire pleural cavity into several cavities. Even the third stage sometimes begins as early as a week after the onset of the infection. It is characterized by the formation of collagen on both parts of the pleura, which binds and immobilizes the lungs beneath it. This process matures for 3 to 4 weeks until the organized collagen forms a hard cortex on the pleural surface. At this stage, the effusion is densely purulent and approximately 75% of its volume is made of a sediment. The chronicity of empyema is characterized by fibrosis, tightening and even confinement of the lungs and chest wall, atelectasis, and prolonged lung infection, to, in the final stage, reduction of the entire hemithorax. Fibrothorax with chest wall invasion and narrowing of the intercostal spaces can be considered the final stage of this process. Despite the advances in medicine, empyema is still a deadly disease with a mortality of between 1-19%, while the mortality of immunocompromised patients can be as high as 40%. The most common causes of empyema are pneumonia and purulent lung disease, thoracic surgery, and injuries. The cause of empyema can also be esophageal perforation, subdiaphragmatic abscess, but also long-lasting pneumothorax with a bronchopleural fistula. The microbiological spectrum of empyema has changed over the years. Although pneumococci and staphylococci continue to be frequent in many series, gram-negative aerobic and anaerobic bacteria (Escherichia coli, Pseudomonas and Enterobacteriaceae) have recently become more than very serious. Fungal mycobacterial infections are now less common. Pleural empyema can occur in the acute form with fever, chills, cough, shortness of breath and tachypnea, or in the chronic form with subfebrile body temperature and weight loss. Sometimes there is weakness, general discomfort, loss of appetite or difficult to define chest pain. Chronic empyema can spontaneously drain into the bronchi, which causes a bronchopleural fistula to develop, which is manifested by a cough with a large expectoration of the purulent sputum. Sometimes chronic empyema is asymptomatic and manifests itself by spontaneous perforation on the outside, through the soft tissues of the chest wall, and possibly also through the skin (empyema necessitans). Chronic purulence is usually accompanied by the formation of nail clubbing. Secondary retraction changes in the chest result in ventilation and respiration disorders. Anemia and leukocytosis are usually present. The diagnosis of empyema is determined on the basis of clinical symptoms, the presence of leukocytosis, a characteristic X-ray picture and the recovery of purulent effusion from the pleural cavity. An X-ray shows pleural opacification. Sometimes gas bubbles appear in the pleural opacification. Today, ultrasonography is an invaluable aid in the detection of pleural lesions. It can be used in the identification of pleural effusions or associated pleural swellings or abnormalities, it helps in the localization of small, confined exudates for puncture, it can be used for possible direction of drainage, can assess possible onset of lung lesions. Chest CT is sometimes an irreplaceable aid in the assessment of pleural diseases (Figures 13, 14). In addition to identifying and localizing pleural effusion, it can assess current pulmonary parenchymal, mediastinal, or even chest wall disorders. It can characterize the nature of the purulent collection and, compared to a conventional X-ray, a CT scan can help distinguish a peripheral lung abscess from an empyema. Especially in cases where surgery is considered, bronchoscopy is important, because it can reveal a foreign body or cancer. A pleural tap is a crucial diagnostic step. The fluid obtained by it should be examined via cytological, biochemical, as well as pH investigations. If clinically suspected, the possibility of mycobacteria and fungal infection should also be investigated.

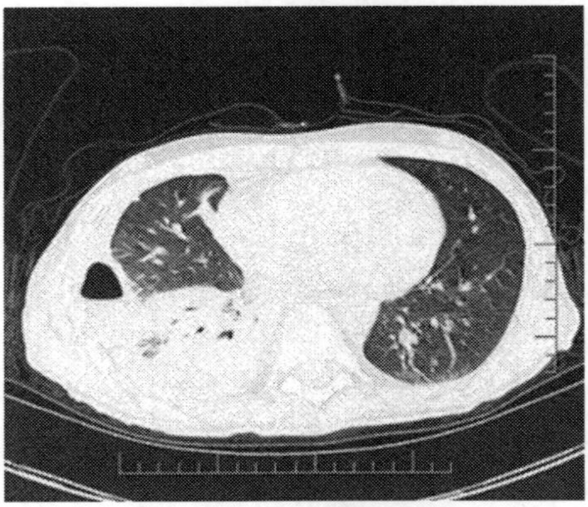

Figure 13. CT of an empyema in the right pleural cavity (axial plane).

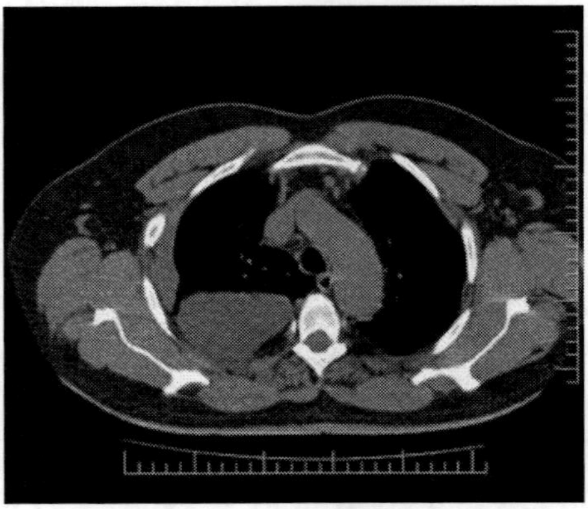

Figure 14. CT of a fibrothorax in the right pleural cavity.

The treatment of empyema depends on its cause, stage of development, the condition of the lungs involved, the possible bronchopleural fistula, the ability to obliterate the empyema cavity, and on the clinical condition of the patient. The pleural cavity is, normally, with well-expanded lungs and with the parietal and visceral pleura touching each other, highly resistant to bacterial invasion. Therapeutic procedures are therefore aimed at maintaining this situation. In most empyemas, the lungs are primarily affected, so treatment should be directed primarily to manage the lung disease. In acute empyema, we use antibiotics to control the infection. An intercostal tubular drainage (chest tube) is the simplest and at the same time very effective method for draining the effusion and obliterating the pleural space. Repeated thoracenteses in conjunction with antibiotics are an unfavorable course of treatment and can only be used if the fluid volume is low and is low in toxicity. Even so, the success of such a method is small, rather it leads to septation of the empyema, the creation of multiple separate cavities. Surgical removal of pus by proper drainage of the pleural space remains the gold standard for dealing with empyema. We will not only evacuate the pus but will also allow the two pleural membranes to be attached to each other, thus achieving obliteration of the space and elimination of the infection. The timing and selection of a suitable type of drainage must be evaluated individually. Connect the chest tube size 28-32F to active suction with a negative pressure of -25cmH_2O. In the optimal situation, in 2-3 weeks, the lungs fully develop, re-expand, and obliterate the pleural space. If drainage does not bring a significant reduction in the volume of aspirated fluid within 48 hours and the septic condition persists despite drainage, we apply rinsing of the empyema cavity with antiseptic agents (0.3% persteril, betadine, chloramine). Intrapleural irrigation can be applied as a permanent rinse or by intermittent rinsing at 6-12-hour intervals. In recent years, video-assisted thoracoscopic surgery (VATS) has been increasingly used as the primary treatment for acute empyema. After marking the exact location of the empyema by ultrasonography or CT, pus is evacuated videothoracoscopically, adhesions that could cause sepsis are broken up, fibrin membranes and deposits are removed from the lung surface, or in some cases, necrotic masses are removed from the pleural sinuses and the drain is introduced into the pleural cavity at the lowest point under visual control. Eventually, the lungs re-expand. As it is a minimally invasive method, VATS is the most suitable procedure for critically ill patients who are high-risk (surgically), not only due to infection, but also overall weakness or weakened immune system. The technique is safe and very effective for the second stage of empyema, but impractical and ineffective for the organizing stage of empyema. Thoracotomy is an alternative to video-assisted thoracoscopic surgery. It is indicated in cases where simple drainage is not effective, usually for a multiloculated empyema, or for inaccessible collections of pus. Under general anesthesia, a small thoracotomy is performed, and we remove the pus through it, break up the adhesions, make the debridement, and eventually peel the fibrin depositions from the surface of the lungs or the chest wall pleura. Insert the chest tube at the lowest point of the cavity. One possibility after unsuccessful closed intercostal drainage is open drainage of the empyema cavity according to Eloesser – the Eloesser flap. Open drainage is maintained better than a chest tube. Suppuration can be managed with regular rinsing using antiseptic solutions and gauze. Lung decortication has proven to be the most appropriate surgical procedure if there remains a large empyema cavity with thick walls that does not tend to regress, or if it is a multi-chamber empyema in which the overall toxic reaction has been managed. The condition for successful decortication is the regression of the inflammatory response and the assumption that the visceral pleura, which the empyema sac pushes onto, is in relatively good condition and will allow lung re-expansion after removal of the sac. The best results are achieved in the early phase of chronic empyema (fifth to sixth week of disease), which developed after pneumonia or post-traumatic hemothorax. Decortication can also be combined with lung resection if the affected lungs are severely damaged. Empyemectomy is another method of treatment that is possible for smaller empyemas in which an uncomplicated separation of the empyema sac is expected. The procedure involves the complete separation of the empyema sac from the lungs and chest wall without opening it. Thoracoplastic procedures are used as a last resort for long-lasting empyema with a firm fixation of the empyema sac to the lungs, but especially for concomitant diseases that do not give hope for re-expansion of lung parenchyma. With thoracoplastic procedures, obliteration of the empyema cavity is achieved by mobilizing the parietal wall of the empyema sac. Primary healing is achieved when the procedure is done successfully. Adverse effects include deformation of the chest wall and restriction of the lung parenchyma.

FIBROTHORAX

Fibrothorax is characterized by the presence of fibrous tissue in the pleural cavity, which is, most commonly, a complication of hemothorax, tuberculosis, or chronic empyema.

As a result of this fibrosis, the lungs are tightened, the hemithorax decreases, contracts, its motility decreases. This then results in a significant reduction in the function of the trapped and collapsed lungs. In the previous century, the most common cause of fibrothorax was tuberculosis. At present, it is mainly chronic empyema, clotted hemothorax, or an untreated pleural effusion. However, in some cases of fibrothorax, neither clinically nor in thoracotomy can we determine the original cause of this condition. In principle, if any pleural fluid is not drained, it causes fibrin to precipitate on the contact pleural surfaces. If the process continues, fibroblasts and angioblasts proliferate, the exudate forms a collagen-rich (but poor in vascular supply, cells, and elastic fibers) raid on the pleura. Gradually, a solid, avascular collagenous matrix is organized. The amount of fibrotic component gradually increases, and the loose membranes almost always form solid adhesions between the lungs, chest wall, pericardium, diaphragm, and mediastinum. The extent of the inflammatory response depends on the nature of the fluid. It can vary from a microscopically thin glossy membrane at the transudate, to a few millimeters thick fibrous deposits from empyema or hemothorax. In doing so, the pleural fluid compresses the lungs and, if there is a large amount of it, causes atelectasis. Compressed lungs affected by atelectasis are trapped by inflammatory tissue that covers the visceral pleura and lung tissue may be destroyed (necrotizing pneumonia may occur). The chest wall and diaphragm are also coated with the same fibrous process, while here this deposit is even thicker, more massive, sometimes it can reach up to 2 cm or more. Calcifications are often on it. Lung constriction and chest wall tightening result in restrictive lung disease and are characterized by a reduction in lung volumes. Pulmonary vasoconstriction occurs as a compensatory mechanism, resulting in a reduction in perfusion in said hypoventilated lungs. Thanks to this mechanism, hypoxia does not occur if the contralateral lungs are normal. However, if more severe bilateral lung involvement is present, hypoxia, hypercapnia, pulmonary hypertension, and cor pulmonale occur. The most characteristic difficulty is shortness of breath on exertion, which gradually worsens and progresses. At rest, oxygen saturation is sufficient, but even with mild exertion, its values decrease. The patient can sometimes experience chest discomfort, from the feeling of a tight chest to chest pain, dry, unproductive cough, loss of appetite and weakness. In extreme cases, cor pulmonale can occur. On physical examination, one-sided fixation of the chest wall with a reduction of respiratory movements and hypotrophy of the relevant musculature is noticeable. The percussion is muted, weakened breathing is detected on auscultation. Careful history and evaluation of the development of the disease, as well as evaluation and comparison of dynamics on conventional X-ray or CT scans, are all extremely important for diagnosis. CT is essential for the assessment and evaluation of the extent and anatomical characteristics of fibrothorax. In addition, it gives the surgeon precise information about the quality of the nearby lung parenchyma. NMR does not offer any major advantages over CT.

Preoperative evaluation also includes conventional examination of lung function (spirometry, diffusing capacity of the lung for CO_2, blood gas analysis, and pulmonary exercise stress test). Avoiding treatment is the best prevention, meaning that any patient with any effusion should be treated with early drainage of the pleural cavity with complete evacuation of its contents. Lung decortication is indicated for patients with symptomatic extraparenchymal restrictive lung disease caused by fibrothorax. Surgery is justified if drainage and suction do not achieve lung expansion and if we can rule out a malignant cause of pleural effusion. Another reason for the operation is the failure of drainage in the treatment of empyema, with the assumption that decortication will achieve the development of the lungs, control of the pleural space, and thus the possibility of eliminating infection. Postoperative improvement in lung function is then evident. Persistent restriction is a sign of incomplete relaxation of the chest wall or diaphragm. It is important to assess the lung parenchyma under the affected pleura, because if a more severe lung disease is present, we will not achieve the expected functional effect in decortication. The timing of the operation is important so that the deposit can be reliably peeled off. Before 3 weeks, the deposit is not yet well organized, it tears, often causing lung injuries with subsequent persistence of air leakage and bleeding. In hemothorax, the optimal time is 5-6 weeks from the onset of bleeding, empyema should be treated in more than 3 months. However, the situation is different in immunosuppressed patients and it is appropriate to solve empyema by surgery in as little as 3 weeks. The operation will be made significantly easier using endobronchial intubation with the technique of separate ventilation of the lungs. The preferred surgical approach is a broad posterolateral thoracotomy in the lateral position through the fifth or sixth intercostal space. Subsequently, the finding is removed from the lungs and chest wall, and the lungs are opened. At the end of the operation, we insert two tubular drains into the pleural space and suction with a negative pressure of -10 cm H_2O to achieve complete evacuation of blood and air from the pleural space. Major postoperative complications include sepsis from residual empyema, or infection in the surgical wound, bronchopleural fistula, and bleeding. The higher incidence of these major complications is in conditions where decortication had to be supplemented by lung resection. The incidence of complications can be reduced by precise surgical technique, achieving optimal lung development, and precise drainage of the pleural space. The improvement in lung function after decortication is evident. Its degree determines the quality of the lung parenchyma under the diseased lung process.

Conclusion

Patients undergoing hemodialysis are often exposed to complications treated by a thoracic surgeon. Following large vein cannulation, pneumothorax as well as hemothorax may occur. In the treatment of the underlying disease, effusions in the pleural cavity are common, requiring repeated pleural taps or chest tube. A complication after pneumonia, but infecting pleural effusion, may be empyema, which requires adequate surgical treatment depending on the stage of the disease. Empyema, pleural effusion, or hemothorax may result in fibrothorax, which also requires surgical treatment.

References

Haruštiak, S. 1993. "Pleura" in: *Špeciálna chirurgia*. Edited by J. Černý. 119-155. Martin: Osveta. ["Pleura" in: *Special surgery*. Edited by J. Černý. 119-155. Martin: Osveta].

Janík, M. 2010. "Pleura" in *Princípy chirurgie II*. Edited by S. Haruštiak et al., 603-629. Bratislava: SAP. ["Pleura" in *Principles of surgery II*. Edited by S. Haruštiak et al., 603-629. Bratislava: SAP.g.

Light, R. W. 2000. "Physiology of pleural fluid production and benign pleural effusion." In: *General Thoracic Surgery. Vol I. 5th ed.* Edited by Thomas W. 687-698. Philadelphia: Lippincott Williams & Wilkins.

Paris, F., Deslauriers, J., Calvo, V. 2002. "Empyema and bronchopleural fistula." In *Thoracic surgery, 2nd ed.* edited by F. G. Pearson et al. 1171-1194. New York: Churchill Livingstone.

Rice, Th. W. 2000. "Fibrothorax and decortication of lung." 2000. "Physiology of pleural fluid production and benign pleural effusion." In: *General Thoracic Surgery. Vol I. 5th ed.* Edited by Thomas W. 729-737. Philadelphia: Lippincott Williams & Wilkins.

Stolz, A., Pafko P. 2010. *Komplikace v plicní chirurgii.* Praha: Grada. [*Complications in lung surgery*. Prague: Grada.].

Vodička J. 2007. *Spontánní pneumotorax*. Praha: Maxdorf. [*Spontaneous pneumothorax*. Prague: Maxdorf.].

In: Surgeon´s Perspective on Dialysis Patient ISBN: 978-1-53619-262-9
Editor: Maria Frankovicova

Chapter 16

SKIN DISEASES ASSOCIATED WITH CHRONIC RENAL FAILURE

J. Baloghová*, MD
Department of Dermatovenerology, Faculty of Medicine,
Pavol Jozef Šafárik University in Košice and University Hospital,
Košice, Slovakia

ABSTRACT

Chronic renal failure, dialysis and renal transplantation are associated with wide range of cutaneous manifestations. Uremia has very important impact on occurrence of dermatological symptoms and skin lesions. Cutaneous changes can be nonspecific – mainly pruritus, disorders of skin appendages, dry skin, dyschromia, or specific – calcinosis, perforating dermatoses, bullous dermatoses. Immunosuppressants have strong impact on occurrence of skin infections and skin cancer. Comorbidities associated with chronic renal failure, more often diabetes, obesity, immunosuppressive therapy and dialysis have also influence on management, diagnosis and treatment of cutaneous disorders.

* Corresponding Author's E-mail: janettebaloghova@gmail.com.

Keywords: skin, pruritus, xerosis, calcinosis, bullous dermatoses, perforating dermatoses, nephrogenic fibrosing dermopathy, skin infections, NMSC

ABBREVIATIONS

CRP	C reactive protein
PCT	Pophyria cutanea tarda
NSF	nephrogenic systemic fibrosis
GBCA	gadolinium-containing contrast agents
VZV	Varicella zoster virus
NMSC	Nonmelanoma skin cancer
SCC	squamous cell carcinoma
BCC	basal cell carcinoma
AVF	arteriovenous fistula
CEAP	Clinical-Etiology-Anatomy - Pathophysiology

INTRODUCTION

More than skin deep, several skin changes reflect internal organs' diseases. Skin examination plays an important role in management of systemic diseases, endocrinological diseases, disorders of the digestive tract, liver, kidneys and other internal organs. Chronic renal failure is more specific, because due to accumulation of catabolites, function of more organs is altered. This leads to numerous disorders - neurological, cardiovascular, hematological, gastrointestinal, endocrinological, pulmonary and dermatological.

Skin changes associated with chronic renal failure represent a wide range of non- specific and specific manifestations. Their occurrence ranges from 50 to 100%, and severity increases with the progression of the chronic renal failure. *Non-specific skin changes* include skin pigmentation, pallor, itching of the skin, prurigo, dry skin, acquired ichthyosis, hair and nail changes. *Specific skin changes* include pseudoporphyriae, perforating dermatoses, calcinosis, calciphylaxis and bullous dermatoses. There are other skin diseases associated with comorbidities and immunosuppressive therapy (Masmoudi et al., 2014, Hu et al., 2019).

NON-SPECIFIC SKIN CHANGES

Pruritus

Uremic pruritus, itching due to uremic toxins, is the most common symptom of chronic renal insufficiency and affects more than 50 percent of the individuals on dialysis. This symptom is not present in acute renal failure (Yonova 2007).

The etiology of pruritus is not well known. There are many factors contributing in the pathophysiology of uremic pruritus: increased levels of serotonin, vitamin A, magnesium, phosphate and aluminium, iron deficiency, peripheral neuropathy, allergic reaction to materials used for dialysis and endogenous opioids. Histamine plasma levels are five times higher in patients with uremia and pruritus than in patients without uremia and without pruritus (Krajnik 2001). Elevated CRP levels and concentrations of chemical mediators in the serum like leukotriene B4, interleukin 6, interleukin 31 and T helper cells also play an important role (Arzhan et al., 2020, Yonova 2007, Krajnik 2001).

Uremic pruritus differs according to type of dialysis. Several studies showed that there are differences. Study in 2007 in Shanghai as well as study during years 2015-2017 in Chongqing had proved, that incidence of pruritus was higher in hemodialysis patients than in peritoneal dialysis patients (Hu et al., 2019). Min et al., in the study during years 2009-2015 showed a higher prevalence of uremic pruritus in peritoneal dialysis patients than in hemodialysis patients (Min et al., 2016). The subjective intensity of itchiness was higher in peritoneal dialysis patients than it was in hemodialysis patients, but without any significant correlation between uremic pruritus and all-cause mortality neither in hemodialysis nor in peritoneal dialysis patients (Arzhan et al., 2020).

During peritoneal dialysis large and medium-sized molecules are removed, while hemodialysis can over time lead to accumulation of these molecules (Hu et al., 2019). Other differences in case of peritoneal dialysis include higher protein intake, longer duration of dialysis, higher blood levels of parathyroid hormone and CRP (Arzhan et al., 2020).

Dry skin, xerosis, plays an important role. Reduced hydratation of stratum corneum, disturbance of epidermal barrier and increased secretion of urea in sweat interfere with the activation of angiotensin converting enzyme leading to impaired function of sweat and sebaceous glands. Defective skin functions together with increased pH of the stratum corneum and increased levels of vitamin A in the epidermis result in xeroderma with pruritus (Hu et al., .2019).

Uremia specific abnormalities include calcium and phosphorus metabolism disorders. Elevated phosphorus blood levels together with blood calcium form calcium phosphate. Calcium phosphate deposits appear in the skin and other tissues to reduce blood calcium. Hypocalcemia can also contribute to secondary hyperparathyroidism leading to a higher secretion of parathyroid hormone which causes renal tubular reabsorption of phosphorus. In the study of Hu et al., (2019) it was found that the levels of urea, creatinine, phosphate, calcium, magnesium and parathyroid hormone in patients with itching were significantly higher than those in people without itching. These biochemical markers can play an important role in the pathogenesis of uremia, although not all uremic patients suffering from pruritus have hyperparathyroidism (Hu et al., 2019, Krajnik 2001).

There are several factors which can influence itching. Air temperature, mostly the heat and humidity may affect skin dryness. High temperatures can cause histamine release provoking itching (Hu et al., 2019).

Pruritus in patients with chronic renal insufficiency and comorbidities can be also induced by drugs as a symptom of allergic reaction or iatrogenic nephrotoxicity. Subclinical sensitivity to any drug may cause pruritus. Pruritus can be induced by analgetics, sulfonamides, chloroquine, angiotensin converting enzyme inhibitors, gold, vitamin A, morphine or contrast media (Yonova 2007).

It is very important to exclude paraneoplastic pruritus which is induced by malignant tumors of breast, stomach, lung, prostate, colon, uterus, nasopharynx and the others. Itching associated with carcinoma can be localized (pretibial areas, inner sites of thighs, upper trunk, shoulders, extensor surface of upper limbs) and generalized. After successful treatment of carcinoma itching disappears (Krajnik 2001).

Pruritus has different clinical features, can be localized or generalized. Can occur daily, or in several patients weekly or monthly, some patients have pruritus during or after the dialysis. Usually uremic itching occurs during 6 months after initiation of dialysis. The severity of pruritus can vary. Pruritus intensity can be mild, moderate or severe leading to psychosomatic consequences with sleep disorders, increased irritability, general stress and disturbance of daily activities (Combs et al., 2015, Yonova 2007).

Treatment of Uremic Pruritus

Chronic pruritus has a strong impact on the quality of life, can be associated with depression, anxiety and lead to worse patient outcomes. For this reason, it is very important to choose the most effective therapeutic approach although in the case of uremic pruritus it is a great challenge.

Dialysis modality can have impact on uremic pruritus as it was mentioned above. High-flux hemodialysis, hemodiafiltration with hemoperfusion and high permeability hemodialysis are alternative methods of hemodialysis which can alleviate uremic pruritus (Arzhan et al., 2020).

Topical and Physical Therapy

Treatment of pruritus, which is mostly combined with xerosis also reflects treatment of dry skin. *Topical emollients and moisturizers* therefore belong to basic daily routine treatment. Moisturizers should be applied once or three times daily to xerotic skin and within 3 minutes of bathing for the most convenient skin hydratation (Elmariah et al., 2011). To keep skin hydrated it is recommended rather to use shower than bathing. Itching can be provoked also by irritative fabrics and too warm clothes leading to more sweating. In one study emollients with high water content such as gamma-linolenic acid had better efficacy than placebo (Blaha et al., 2019).

In case of skin inflammation *topical glucocorticoids* and *ultraviolet phototherapy* can bring relief. Ultraviolet B phototherapy can be effective in treating refractory pruritus in peritoneal dialysis patients and also in eliminating epidermal retinol. Ultraviolet light inhibits the histamine induced pruritus by stabilizing the mast cell membranes at nerve endings. It is important to take to account benefit-risk ratio of phototherapy due to lifetime risk of skin malignancy (Arzhan et al., 2020, Krajnik 2001).

Localized uremic pruritus can be also released by topical treatment with immunomodulators – *tacrolimus and pimecrolimus* and *topical capsaicin* (applied as 0,025% cream). Capsaicin inhibits itch transmission by substance P depletion from the C-nerve endings. Due to burning and redness at site of application capsaicin should be applied only on small areas (Arzhan et al., 2020, Krajnik 2001, Blaha et al., 2019).

Topical anesthetics - lidocaine 5% or the eutectic mixture of lidocaine 2.5% - prilocaine 2.5%, pramoxine 1%, and polidocanol 3% are used with a good efficacy in the treatment of various pruritic conditions (Elmariah et al., 2011). In the randomized, double-blind, controlled comparative trial individuals with moderate to severe uremic pruritus receiving hemodialysis had been treating with topical 1% pramoxine lotion twice daily during 4 weeks. This therapy was well tolerated and significantly reduced itching comparing to control lotion (Young et al., 2009).

Alternative therapy with *acupuncture* and *acupressure* was confirmed as being effective in patients who do not respond to other treatments (Badiee et al., 2018).

Systemic Therapy

Azelastin as an inhibitor of leukotriene B4 receptors has been used as effective therapy of pruritus in hemodialysis patients (Krajnik 2001). As well as montelukast –a leukotriene receptor antagonist, especially on refractory pruritus (Arzhan et al., 2020).

Antidepressant *sertraline* is considered to be a treatment of choice. By modulating inflammatory markers and cytokines can release the itching and moreover there is no need to adjust the dosage in patients with renal failure (Arzhan et al., 2020).

Anticonvulsants *gabapentin* and *pregabalin* had been used in the treatment of chronic pain and diabetic neuropathy. Their therapeutic effect acts through binding to the alpha2-delta subunit of voltage-sensitive calcium channels. A systemic review of 44 randomized control trials with 39 different treatments of uremic pruritus found a statistically significant benefit to treatment with gabapentin and pregabalin (Blaha et al., 2019, Simonsen et al., 2017).

Although increased histamine plasma levels had been revealed in end stage of renal disease, treatment with *antihistamines* has not been shown to alleviate symptoms of uremic pruritus (Blaha et al., 2019, Yonova 2007).

Thalidomide was found to release uremic itching in patients with leprosy. Its effect on pruritus should be based on reduction of tumor necrosis factor synthesis and interference with cytokine production (Krajnik 2001).

Based on hypothesis, that the uremic pruritogen can be part of the intestinal fluid or can be produced by intestinal flora, *oral charcoal* (6g daily) had been the subject of some trials with good results (Krajnik 2001).

Studies suggest that activation of the μ-opioid system can induce pruritus. Consequently, antagonism of μ-opioid receptors and activation of the κ-opioid system receptors relieve the itch. *Nalfurafine,* a kappa-agonist, had showed in one study the antipruritic affect, while in the other one no significant benefit of treatment with nalfurafine was found. Moreover, its side effect insomnia must be taken into account. *Naltrexone* is the μ-opioid antagonist. In two studies naltrexone reached mixed results. One study showed statistically significant benefit over placebo but the other one did not (Krajnik 2001, Jaiswal et al., 2016, Arzhan et al., 2020, Blaha et al., 2019). *Nalbuphine* is a κ-opioid and μ-opioid receptor antagonist. It is a novel therapy for pruritus. In a multicenter, randomized, double blind, placebo-controlled trial of hemodialysis patients nalbuphine significantly reduced intensity of uremic pruritus (Blaha et al., 2019).

Cromolyn sodium, by stabilizing mast cells, can be another possibility for reducing uremic itching (Arzhan et al., 2020). As reported by De Marchi et al., pruritus improved within one week in most *erythropoietin* treated patients probably by decreasing plasma histamine (Marchi et al., 1992).

More intensive pruritus can be managed by *intravenous therapy with lidocaine, heparin and cholestyramine.* Lidocaine seems to be effective in patients with itch due to uremic neuropathy although it is important to concern on its toxicity (Krajnik 2001).

Surgical intervention includes subtotal parathyroidectomy, electric needle stimulation and renal transplantation (Peres et al., 2014).

Subtotal *parathyroidectomy* can release pruritus determined by parathyroid hormone. But there is no correlation between the intensity of pruritus and activity of parathyroid hormone. Parathyroidectomy has poor efficacy in the therapy of uremic itch unless associated with hyperparathyroidism (Hu et al., 2019, Krajnik 2001)

Definite treatment for refractory uremic itching would be *kidney transplantation* (Arzhan et al., 2019).

Skin Discolorations, Dyschromias

There are several pigmentation disorders that have been reported in patients with chronic renal failure.

The most characteristic feature is *hyperpigmentation* referred to elevated levels of melatonin-stimulating hormone in the tissues due to inability of the kidney to excrete it. Increased pigmentation involves especially sites exposed to sun (Van de Velde-Kossmann 2018), can be present also on the lips (Oyetola et al., 2015) and in several cases on the palms and soles (Udayakumar et al., 2006).

Other skin discoloration includes *pallor,* related to anemia of chronic diseases and erythropoietin deficiency. Anemia occurs in patients with renal failure also due to deficiency of iron, folic acid or vitamin B12, blood loss during dialysis and poor erythrocyte survival (Rashpa et al., 2018).

Slate-grey skin discoloration is due to deposits of hemosiderin (Lupi et al., 2011). *Yellow skin* discoloration should be caused by retention of fat-soluble pigments, carotenoids ad urochromes, in the dermis and subcutaneous tissue (Van de Velde-Kossmann 2018, Specchio et al. 2014).

Hyperpigmentation and yellowing of the skin can remain regardless of appropriate dialysis therapy (Van de Velde-Kossmann 2018).

Ecchymosis, purpura and *petechiae* also often occur on the skin of patients with chronic renal failure. These skin discolorations reflect platelet disorders and vascular fragility in hemodialysis patients due to elevated accumulation of guanidinosuccinic acid, which suppresses platelet activity and by this way can account for uremic bleeding (Peres et al., 2014, Rashpa et al., 2018).

Xerosis, Dry Skin

Xerosis is a frequent symptom in patients with chronic renal failure, mainly present in patients who were not dialyzed, but can persists or be worse despite dialysis. This symptom is absent in acute renal failure and does not correspond to the urea plasma levels. Renal transplantation can help to improve the skin dryness (Specchio et al., 2014). It is hypothesized that in renal failure skin integrity is disturbed due to fragmentation of elastic fibers, atrophy of sebaceous and eccrine sweat glands and loss of coherence in the stratum corneum. Dry skin is often associated with uremic itching. Typical clinical manifestation of dry skin is ichtyosiform, thick dry skin with fissures and scaling (Van De Velde-Kossmann 2018).

Prurigo Nodularis

Long lasting itching brings changes to skin structure, which becomes hyperpigmentated, thick, leathery, with lichenificated surface and deep skin creases. Excoriations due to permanent itching lead to skin infection (mostly bacterial) and occurrence of itchy hard papules, nodules or plaques with superficial erosions– *prurigo nodularis*. Skin lesions usually appear and the site of skin irritation or trauma as a sign of Koebner phenomenon and on the sites which are well reachable for scratching – extremities (extensor sites), neck and lower back. Areas which are difficult to reach are clear (Hu et al., 2019, Yonova 2007, Van De Velde-Kossmann 2018, Kestner et al., 2017).

There are several types of prurigo: papular, nodular, plaque and umbilicated type. Lesions in umbilicated prurigo have depressed center covered with eschar –like necrosis. This type of prurigo is more associated with systemic internal diseases. Decreased cell proliferation and angiogenesis together with limited reepithelization of wounds can predispose to formation of ulcerated non healing papules and nodules in patients with chronic renal failure (Kestner et al., 2017).

Hair Disorders

Frequency of occurrence of hair disorders is various. As it was reported in the several studies – Mourad et al., reported more than 70%, Mirza et al., 56,6%, Sultan et al. 47% and Udayakumar et al. 16% of hemodialysis patients with hair changes. The most common reported hair changes are lusterless hairs, sparse scalp and body hairs (Mourad et al., 2014). Alopecia and chronic telogen effluvium also can occur in patients with chronic renal failure, but they had not been studied specifically. These hair alterations can be due to comorbidities like systemic lupus erythematosus and medications (Nunley 2020).

Hair disorders in hemodialysis patients could respond to heparin, hypervitaminosis A, endocrine disorders, accumulation of toxins, anemia due to iron deficiency, disturbed parathormone level, side effect of drugs used during the treatment of chronic renal failure (beta blockers, indomethacin, methyldopa, cimetidine, allopurinol) and also influence of dialysis on quality of life and mental health (Peres et al., 2014, Mourad et al., 2014).

Nail Disorders

The most specific nail change present in 20-40% of patients with chronic renal failure refers to Half-and-Half nails, known also as Lindsay's nails. The nails are named after Lindsay who believed that nail discoloration is induced by constricted venous return (Markova et al., 2012). These changes are probably due to elevated levels of beta-melanocyte stimulating hormone in the tissue or oedema of the nail bed. Typical clinical sign is reddish to brown discoloration of the distal part and white discoloration of the proximal part of the nail. Usually fingernails are involved more often than toenails. This type of nail change should disappear after kidney transplantation (Van de Velde-Kossmann 2019, Blaha et al., 2019).

Other nail changes observed in reported studies included: onycholysis, koilonychia, melanonychia, subungual hyperkeratosis, absence of a lunula, Mee's lines (single white transverse line), Muehrcke's lines (apparent leukonychia, except other reasons also due to nephrotic syndrome in patients with hypoalbuminemia), Beau's lines (transverse deep depressions) and splinter hemorrhages (Udayakumar et al., 2006, Peres et al., 2014, Markova et al., 2012).

Keratotic Disorders

Chronic renal failure can be associated with disturbance of cornification. Typical clinical sign is *follicular hyperkeratosis*, an increased cornification focused on hair follicle. Lesions are manifested as small cone-shaped papules with dry, rough surface. Etiology is unknown but there are several subtypes of follicular hyperkeratosis – familial, postinflammatory, postirradiation or associated with malignancy (Markova et al., 2012). Mourad et al., reported 48,4% hemodialysis patients with follicular hyperkeratosis more often on the lower limbs, mostly in females and Sultan et al. reported 10% hemodialysis patients with follicular hyperkeratosis (Mourad et al., 2014).

SPECIFIC SKIN CHANGES

Bullous Dermatoses

Chronic renal failure is associated with two bullous dermatoses – porphyria cutanea tarda and pseudoporphyria. Prevalence of these disorders is reported 1,2% to 18% in hemodialysis patients, and affects males and females equally (Blaha et al., 2019, Markova et al., 2012).

Pophyria cutanea tarda (PCT) is disease due to congenital or acquired deficiency of enzyme uroporphyrinogen III decarboxylase with clinical findings of vesicles, bullae and erosions at the sites of sun exposure, mostly on the back of the hands also on the face. Healing of these lesions presents with scarring and hyperpigmentation (Blaha et al., 2019, Specchio et al., 2014). Other skin findings include skin fragility, scleroderma-like changes and hypertrichosis, which is often present in women in periorbital areas together with facial hyperpigmentation (Markova et al., 2012). PCT can be manifested in peritoneal dialysis or hemodialysis patients as well as in patients with insufficient kidney function (Markova et al., 2012). Skin manifestations are result of phototoxic reaction of accumulated porphyrins in combination with UV radiation. In case of renal failure PCT can occur despite dialysis if uroporphyrins are not well eliminated by dialysis. Exposure to several factors can deteriorate the condition – alcohol intake, iron deposits, hemochromatosis, estrogens, viral infections – hepatitis B, hepatitis C, HIV. Therapy of PCT includes keeping away from triggers, photoprotection, iron overload decrease, chloroquine, but the most effective therapy is kidney transplantation (Blaha et al., 2019).

Pseudoporphyria is also photodermatosis which clinically also histopathologically looks like PCT, but there are some differences. Occurrence of the disease is 1,2-18% in dialysis patients (more hemodialysis patients). The cause of mechanism of the disease remains unknown, but in the etiology several drugs like nonsteroidal anti-inflammatory drugs, diuretics, antibiotics, antimycotics and retinoids together with exposure to UV light, mainly UVA, can provoke the disease. In case of chronic renal failure decreased antioxidant glutathione plasma levels and erythrocytes due to free-radical injury are supposed to play important role in the pathogenesis of pseudoporphyria. Clinical findings are similar with PCT – skin fragility, vesicles, bullae and erosion with crusts on sun exposed areas (mainly hand and forearms), but hypertrichosis and scleroderma-like changes are missing. Treatment includes drugs withdrawal which can provoke the disease and photoprotection (Markova et al., 2012, Blaha et al., 2019, Specchio et al., 2014).

Calcifications

Soft tissue calcifications are divided into several subtypes: dystrophic, metastatic, idiopathic, tumoral and calciphylaxis (Lorente- Luna et al., 2015). Calcifying skin disorders in patients with chronic renal failure include cutaneous calcinosis, metastatic calcinosis cutis and calciphylaxis (Specchio et al., 2014). Calcification occurs as a result of decreased calcium absorption in hyperphosphataemia which leads to deposits of calcium salts in the skin and other tissues.

Metastatic calcifications occur as a result of secondary hyperparathyroidism due to elevated calcium and phosphorus plasma levels. Deposits of calcium appear in the healthy tissue. *Dystrophic calcinosis cutis* is associated with normal calcium and phosphorus levels and can relate to connective tissue diseases, systemic sclerosis and other diseases, where tissue damage can result in skin calcification. Clinically skin calcifications present with papules, plaques or nodules, of white, yellowish-white color and stone-hard consistency. Skin lesions are usually localized at periarticular sites and also on fingertips, where they are very painful. Other sites of involvement are the superior and lateral shoulder, posterior elbows, lateral hip and buttocks (Jaeger et al., 2017). Calcium deposits can appear except subcutaneous tissue also in kidneys, lung, gastric mucosa and vascular walls (Blaha et al., 2019). Lesions usually disappear after calcium and phosphate plasma levels become normal with dietary measures, phosphate binders, calcium channel blockers, topical, intralesional or systemic calciomimetic sodium thiosulfate, surgical excision, lithotripsy or parathyroidectomy in case of unresponsive metastatic skin calcinosis (Blaha et al., 2019, Markova et al., 2012). Qiblawi et al., had reported apremilast as an adjuvant therapy for calcinosis cutis (Qiblawi et al., 2019).

Calciphylaxis (calcific uremic arteriolopathy) is characterized by calcification of small vessels in the dermis and subcutaneous tissue which leads to thrombosis and cutaneous ischemia. This disease is generally seen in patients with chronic renal failure with 4% frequency, mostly in hemodialysis patients. Risk factors involve hyperparathyroidism, vitamin D exposure, obesity, liver disease, immunosuppression. Elimination of the calcium salts from dermis to the skin surface manifests as a superficial ulceration. Usually there are painful purple reticulated plaques with central non-healing ulceration and skin necrosis, frequently found on the lower legs symmetrically, occasionally on the penis and digits (Markova et al., 2012). High morbidity and mortality of the disease is result of septic complications of ulcerated and necrotic skin lesions. Worse prognosis was reported in the patients with ulcerated lesion, BMI greater than 30 and female gender (Colboc et al., 2019).

Acquired Perforating Dermatoses

Perforating dermatoses are papulonodulars skin disorders with transepidermal elimination of dermal material. They are divided due to the nature of the eliminated material and the type of epidermal disruption (Saray et al., 2006). *Perforating dermatoses* include:

- *Kyrles' disease* firstly described in 1916 by Kyrle, with transepidermal elimination of keratotic material without collagen or elastic fibers. Skin findings resemble dome shaped papules, sized 2-8 mm in diameter, with keratotic plug which can confluent to plaques. Lesions are usually localized on the lower extremities, more often on the calf, tibial and posterior site, on arms, head and neck (Nair et al., 2015),
- *Reactive perforating collagenosis* was firstly described in 1968 by Mehregan and Coskey and in 1994 diagnostic criteria were defined by Faver et.al. Disease is characterized by abnormal collagen fibers elimination through the epidermis. Clinical manifestations include hard skin colored papules with umbilical depressed center covered with crust, healing with scars and hypopigmentation. Lesions are usually localized on the extremities, back, face and neck at the site of superficial trauma or scratching (Kawakami et al., 2020),
- *Perforating serpiginous elastosis* was firstly described in 1927 by Fisher and in 1953 Lutz described its morphology and named it serpiginosa follicular keratosis. Disease is characterized by abnormal elastic fibers secretion through the center of umbilicated papules or plaques. Lesions are usually symmetrical and mostly single, localized on the arms, face and neck (Polanska et al., 2016),
- *Perforating folliculitis,* firstly reported by Mehregan and Coskey in 1968, having overlapping features with Kyrle's disease, is characterized by degenerated follicular units, perforated follicular infundibulum with or without elimination of collagen and elastic fibers through the epidermis. Closely to area of perforation a curled up hair can be seen surrounded by a foreign body granuloma. Disease is characterized by keratotic follicular papules located usually on the extremities and buttocks (Arora et al., 2013, Blaha et al., 2019).

- In 1989 Rapini et al., collectively referred to them as *acquired perforating dermatosis* (Kawakami et al., 2020).

Perforating serpiginous elastosis is associated with Down's syndrome and genetic connective tissue diseases (Marfan syndrome, osteogenesis imperfecta, Ehlers-Danlos syndrome). Diabetes and chronic renal disease suggest to be associated with Kyrles'disease, perforating folliculitis, reactive perforating collagenosis and acquired perforating dermatosis (Kawakami et al., 2020).

Approximately 72% of patients with acquired perforating dermatosis suffer from chronic kidney disease and 2-11% of patients with acquired perforating dermatosis are on dialysis. Chronic pruritus in patients with diabetes and chronic renal failure may lead to the rupture of collagen fibers with consequent elimination. Local inflammation can be associated with diabetic microangiopathy due to substances which are not removed by dialysis (Fernandes et al., 2016, Blaha et al., 2019).

Presence of itching and Koebner phenomenon is helpful for diagnosis, but the skin biopsy should be performed to prove the diagnosis. Lesions can mimic folliculitis, insect bites, dermatofibromas, lichen planus, keratoacanthomas, granuloma annulare, prurigo or psoriasis (Kestner et al., 2017).

Treatment of diabetes and chronic renal disease is important together with controlling itching. Other treatment options include allopurinol, UVB phototherapy, psoralen with UVA phototherapy, corticosteroids (topical, intralesional, systemic), retinoids (topical, systemic), antihistamines, methotrexate, doxycycline, cryotherapy, keratolytics (Markova et al., 2012, Fernandes et al., 2016, Blaha et al., 2019). There are several cases which report perforating folliculitis during therapy with molecular targeted drugs (mainly kinase inhibitors). In such cases it is recommended to stop this therapy (Kawakami et al., 2020).

Nephrogenic Fibrosing Dermopathy

Nephrogenic fibrosing dermopathy is also known as nephrogenic systemic fibrosis or fibrotic uremic nephropathy. Nephrogenic fibrosing dermopathy was firstly reported in 1997 by Cowper et al., as scleromyxedema-like cutaneous disease associated with renal disease. Later fibrosing process was also find in other tissues and organs – myocardium, lungs, muscles, kidneys and testes, for this reason the disease was renamed to nephrogenic systemic fibrosis (Waikhom et al., 2011, Ting et al., 2003).

This disorder is caused by iatrogenic gadolinium administration in patients with acute kidney injury or chronic renal disease, stage 4 or 5 with estimated glomerular filtration rate of less than 30ml/min/1,73 m^2 (Woolen et al., 2019).

Due to increased cases of nephrogenic systemic fibrosis (NSF) reported from 1997 to 2007 the American College of Radiology and European Society of Urogenital Radiology updated guidelines on contrast agents. The lowest-risk gadolinium-containing contrast agents (GBCA) with very low, if any, risk of NSF development, had been termed as group II agents (gadobenate dimeglumine, gadoteridol, gadoterate meglumine, and gadobutrol). The risk of NSF from group II GBCA administration in patients with stage 4 or 5 chronic kidney disease is likely less than 0.07% (Woolen et al., 2019).

Nephrogenic systemic fibrosis has been also reported in patients without receiving GBCAs. Proinflammatory conditions and edema have been reported as additional risk factors (Becker et al., 2016).

Occurrence of the skin lesions varies – from few days to several months. The exact interval between exposure to GBCA and skin symptoms is not well known. Usually immediately after GBCA exposure acute phase appears followed by chronic phase with fibrosis (Waikhom et al., 2011).

Skin induration is a hallmark of nephrogenic systemic fibrosis. At the beginning disease is manifested with erythematous papules and nodules. Later lesions become confluent to form infiltrated red plaques, which can appear slightly edematous with surface similar to orange peel skin. Lesions can be confused with cellulitis or chronic lymphedema. Skin surface is changing over time to have cobblestone appearance with brown hyperpigmentation and woody hard infiltration. Very common symptoms are itching and burning sensation. Lesions are usually localized symmetrically on the extremities, up to the knees and up to the elbows, but may spread proximally or to the trunk. Face and neck is sparing (Waikhom et al., 2011).

Fibrosing process can also involve the joints underlying skin lesions leading to flexion contractures and motion disability – mainly hands, wrists, ankles and knees (Waikhom et al., 2011).

Clinically NSF may resemble sings of systemic sclerosis. But, in systemic sclerosis vascular disease with pulmonary hypertension is cause of death, while in NSF death is due to fibrosis of internal organs (Becker et al., 2016). Visceral involvement include cardiomyopathy, pulmonary fibrosis, esophageal dysmotility and liver fibrosis with esophageal varices, thrombotic events – repeated occlusion of the dialysis graft, peripheral vascular occlusion, transient ischemic attack and brain infarcts. In differential diagnosis it is important to exclude scleromyxedema, toxic oil syndrome, eosinophilia myalgia syndrome, eosinophilic fasciitis and morphoea (Waikhom et al., 2011).

Treatment options involve steroids (topical and systemic), pentoxyfiline, plasmapheresis, PUVA therapy, intravenous immunoglobulins. Skin lesions can resolve also due to improvement of renal disease. In case of chronic renal failure, the best treatment option is renal transplantation as soon as possible because fibrosing process can become permanent and lead to irreversible disability (Waikhom et al., 2011).

Uremic Frost

Uremic frost is a rare skin change that can occur during severe uremia. In the pre-dialysis era, uremic frost was a frequent cutaneous manifestation of chronic renal failure (Udayakumar et al., 2006). This condition occurs due to eccrine deposition of crystals of urea as a consequence of the high urea in the patients' sweat which crystallizes (Specchio et al., 2014).

Skin deposits of urate crystals of white or yellowish discoloration are usually localized on the face mostly on the beard area or on the eyebrows, also on the neck and on the trunk with a frosted appearance (Specchio et al., 2014). Another skin manifestation is erythema papulatum uremicum with large papules and nodules on erythematous base usually localized on the palms, soles, forearms and face (Udayakumar et al., 2006).

Lesions heal with scaling similar to that after a sunburn, sometimes fissures can develop (Udayakumar et al., 2006). Lesions can resemble retention keratosis, atopic dermatitis and postinflammatory desquamation. As for the therapy – hemodialysis should be considered as preventive because during the time before dialysis the incidence of uremic frost was very high (Markova et al., 2012).

OTHER SKIN CHANGES

Skin Infections

Immunodeficiency is responsible for high prevalence of candidial, fungal, viral and bacterial infections in patients with chronic renal failure. Another risk factors for infection are malnutrition, restricted diets, anaemia, diabetes, stress and therapy with immunosuppressive drugs. Increased incidence of skin infections in patients with chronic renal failure has a strong impact on morbidity and mortality of the patients.

Diabetes mellitus is very important risk factor. It is reported that approximately 40% of patients with new onset of renal failure suffer from diabetes. Complications of diabetes involve several systems, skin together with skin infections included. (Van de Velde-Kossmann 2019).

Bacterial skin and soft tissue infections are more common in patients with diabetes and in the other patients. These infections are mainly caused by staphylococcus and streptococcus species, anaerobic or polymicrobial flora. Methicillin-resistant staphylococcal infections are frequent. These bacterial infections involve *erysipelas, cellulitis, infections with follicular and perifollicular involvement and necrotizing fasciitis* (Van de Velde-Kossmann 2019).

Oedema of lower legs which is associated with chronic renal failure together with dry, fissured skin, excoriation or wound and interdigital fungal infection as infection entrance are predisposing factors for erysipelas and cellulitis. Diagnosis and disease management can be complicated in cases of stasis dermatitis with bilateral leg erythema. Appropriate systemic antibiotic therapy is acquired.

Necrotizing fasciitis is a rare soft tissue infection with fast progression. Disease is manifested by necrosis of fascia and subcutaneous tissue, with severe pain, erythema, bullae leading to skin ulcerations with malodorous drainage and crepitus within the tissue. Early diagnosis, antibiotic therapy and surgical intervention are very important to prevent mortality. Alcoholism, advanced age, chronic therapy with steroids and malnutrition are another risk factors in diabetic patient with chronic renal failure (Van de Velde-Kossmann 2019).

Patel et al., reported four cases of *nontuberculous mycobacterial infection* in solid organ transplant recipients. Clinical manifestations included nodular lesion in a heart, in the lung, on the skin and in a liver (Patel et al., 1994).

Fungal and yeast skin infections – superficial and deep one, are also more frequent in patients with diabetes and chronic renal failure.

Candidiasis, usually caused by candida species (*Candida albicans*, *C. glabrata, C. tropicalis*) involves skin folds and mucosal surfaces. Oral mucosa candidiasis is mentioned below. Candidial infection in intertriginous areas – candidial intertrigo, presents with very itchy erythema with satellite vesiculopustules at the periphery and macerated skin surface. Candidial infection involves also urogenital system. Candidial vulvovaginitis and balanoposthitis is commonly recurrent and chronic, characterized by very itchy erythema and edema with discharge, in men complicated with phimosis. Candidial paronychia – painful involvement of the nail fold and nail bed with erythema and pus. The periungual tissue is red, swollen, tender to pressure.

Another superficial yeast infection is *pityriasis versicolor* caused by lipophilic yeast *Pityrosporum ovale*. Circular or oval, yellowish to red and light brown patches with fine scaling on the surface are usually localized on the trunk, on the back and on the neck. After sun exposure non treating lesions become hypopigmented.

Dermatophyte infections involve usually feet, nails, hands, lower legs, scalp and trunk. More common are superficial mycotic infections with erythematous lesions, plaques, often with target like arrangement (ringworm). Surface of the lesions is scaly, often with vesicles on the periphery. Deep, subcutaneous mycotic infection can be focused on hair follicle (beard area, scalp) or can involve tissue at sites where there is a loss of skin integrity (leg ulcers, catheters). Localized superficial mycotic infections can be treated by topical treatment, widespread, erosive and deep mycotic infections require systemic therapy (Van de Velde-Kossmann 2019).

Viral skin infections, mainly caused by human herpes viruses and human papilloma virus, are frequent infections in transplant recipients.

It is reported that viral warts occur in 11-53% of transplant patients. Lesion are multiple and usually are localized at sun-exposed areas. Important is monitoring of patients due to possible cancer. Herpes simplex virus infections involve oral and genital mucocutaneous sites. Immunodeficiency can lead to severe course of the disease with ulcerations at site of vesicles. Varicella zoster virus (VZV) seropositivity is reported in 90% of solid organ transplant patients (Van de Velde-Kossmann 2019). Shingles can progress to very severe course – lesions with grouped vesicles distributed in more than one dermatome, dissemination of the lesions, gangrene at site of vesicles. Dissemination of the infection can lead to extracutaneous complications – hepatitis, pneumonitis, pancreatitis, disseminated intravascular coagulation and involvement of central nervous system (zoster paresis, VZV vasculopathy, meningitis, meningoradiculitis, cerebellitis).

Skin Malignancies

Patients with chronic renal failure have high incidence of malignancies. Uremia in chronic renal failure can induce suppression of the immune status. Carcinogenicity of uremia was firstly explained by Penn in 1970 (Kuddusi 2002).

Nonmelanoma skin cancer (NMSC), predominantly *squamous cell carcinoma* (SCC) and *basal cell carcinoma* (BCC), is one of the most malignancies following renal transplantation (Matinfar et al., 2017). Study reported by Wang et al., confirmed that pre-dialysis patients with chronic renal failure have 1,14-fold higher risk and patients with 5th stage of chronic renal disease have 1,38-fold higher risk of developing nonmelanoma skin cancer (Wang et al., 2017). Cutaneous malignancies mainly SCC and its precursor actinic keratosis occur 5-10 years after kidney transplantation (Ulrich et al., 2006). SCC occurs 50-250 times more frequently in renal transplants than in the general population (Nunley 2020). Actinic keratosis as well as SCC occur more often in younger renal transplants. Some clinical findings are difficult to recognize actinic keratosis, SCC or warts. Actinic keratoses have faster rate and quick progress to SCC (Nunley 2020).

UV light exposure or prolonged UV phototherapy, male sex, older age, fair skin type and immunosuppressive therapy can contribute to occurrence of NMSCs. There is higher prevalence of BCC in general population but in kidney transplants SCC is more frequent with more aggressive phenotype.

Melanoma is 2-9 times more frequent in the transplant population. The melanoma risk may contribute to transmission by the donor (Nunley 2020).

Kaposi's sarcoma associated with immunosuppression and renal transplantation affects up to 5% of patients. Onset is most frequent about 20 months after transplant. (Van de Velde-Kossmann 2019). Kuddusi et al. reported 2 patients with Kaposi's sarcoma with chronic renal disease who were not treated with immunosuppressive therapy and did not undergo renal transplantation (Kuddusi 2002).

Several cases of other malignancies had been reported - cutaneous sarcomas, histiocytomas, atypical fibroxanthomas, dermatofibrosarcoma protuberans and Merkel cell carcinoma (Nunley 2020).

Skin Disorders Associated with Arterio-Venous Fistula

Hemodialysis is considered to be a treatment solution for the patients with end stage renal disease (for those who are and also for those who are not kidney transplant candidates). Well-functioning dialysis access is very important. This access is surgically created as arteriovenous fistula (connection of a vein to artery in an extremity) (Aljouaid et al., 2020).

Erythema and oedema around the arteriovenous fistula (AVF) can be sign of infection, central vein stenosis and allergy (Kaida et al., 2018). It is reported that *infection* accounts for 20% of all AVF complications. The most common is cellulitis. AVF infections respond well to antibiotic therapy. Much more serious is an infection associated with anatomical abnormalities, such as aneurysms, hematomas or abscesses (Stolic 2013).

Arteriovenous shunt dermatitis had been reported in 8% patients on long-term hemodialysis (Udayakumar et al., 2006). Eczema in the area of AVF can be result of contact allergy from exposure to hemodialysis cannulas containing epoxy resin, topical anesthetic creams or patches and polycarbonate urethane hemodialysis venous catheters. Kaida et al reported a case with *allergic contact dermatitis* due to contact with hemodialysis tubing containing di(2-ethylhexyl) phthalate (Kaida et al., 2018). Any other material used during hemodialysis can cause allergic contact dermatitis.

Deguchi et al., reported a case of *stasis dermatitis with ulceration* at the site of AVF due to traffic injury (Deguchi et al., 2010). Stasis dermatitis as a sign of venous insufficiency, can progress from oedema to ulceration. Using Clinical-Etiology-Anatomy - Pathophysiology (CEAP) classification we recognize grade C3-C6, grade C6 of the upper limbs is usually associated as a complication of AVF (Deguchi et al., 2010).

Pseudo-Kaposi's sarcoma had been described closely to arteriovenous fistula. Clinically lesions resemble purple papules and nodules which change to patches covered by crusts and scales. *Septicaemia due to cannulation* had been reported in 8% of the patients (Udayakumar et al., 2006).

Oral Mucosa Changes

Chronic renal failure is associated with a wide spectrum of oral symptoms. Systemic diseases, hematological disorders, disturbance of immunity and infections contribute to manifestation of oral mucosa changes. They had been reported about 90% of patients with chronic renal failure suffer from oral symptoms (Arunkumar et al., 2015).

The most common manifestation is *chronic aphtous stomatitis* with appearance of ulcerative lesions in oral mucosa. Size and number of lesions vary (Oyetola et al., 2015). Maroud et al., reported aphtous stomatitis in 10,7% of patients, may be due to elevated blood urea level and poor oral hygiene, Sultan et al., reported the presence of oral ulcerations in 9% of hemodialysis patients and Udayakumar et al., reported ulcerative stomatitis in 29%. This high incidence was attributed to intake of alcohol, spicy meals, hot food and tobacco smoking (Masmoudi et al., 2014).

Uremic stomatitis due to elevated urea plasma levels and other nitrogenous wastes is usually characterized by white plaques on the buccal mucosa, floor of the mouth and tongue. Four types of uremic stomatitis are recognized – erythemopultaceous, ulcerative, hemorrhagic and hyperkeratotic. Lesions are painful, patients feel burning sensation with unpleasant taste. Lesions can mimic oral hairy leukoplakia (Kuravatti et al., 2016). Except poor hygiene and tobacco smoking also chronic gingivitis, periodontal disease, decayed teeth and xerostomia are believed to aggravate the disease (Arunkumar et al., 2015).

Xerostomia, dry mouth is a frequent sign of oral mucosa involvement in dialysis patients. Uremic involvement of salivary glands, chemical inflammation, dehydratation and mouth breathing contribute to decreased salivary flow (Kuravatti et al., 2016). Xerostomia is also the side effect of antihypertensive drugs and more often occurs in patients with diabetes due to increased thirst and urination (Arunkumar et al., 2015).

Patients suffer from uremic breath (odorous breath). Taste change, dysgeusia, usually *metallic taste* is supposed to be the result of urea content in the saliva and its breakdown to ammonia and carbon dioxide by bacterial urease. It also can occur due to metabolic disturbance, use of medications and zinc deficiency (Kuravatti et al., 2016).

Tongue alterations in patients with chronic renal failure include coated tongue, macroglossia with teeth markings and fissured tongue (Rashpa et al., 2018). Junior et al. reported over 50% patients with tongue alterations with saburral tongues ranking first (Peres et al., 2014).

Pallor of the oral mucosa is due to reduced erythropoietin leading to anemia (Gupta et al., 2015).

Petechiae and ecchymosis which occur on the skin can also occur on mucous membranes of oral cavity. Lesions are usually result of bleeding tendency due to abnormal thrombocyte function and anticoagulant therapy used during hemodialysis (Kuravatti et al., 2016).

Mucosal candidial infections have high prevalence. Oral candidiasis occurs in 20-30% of transplant patients. Clinical signs of oral candidial infection involve angular cheilitis, pseudomembranous or erythematous ulcerations and chronic atrophic infection (Kuravatti et al., 2016). Firmly adherent white plaques are localized on buccal mucosa and on the mucous membrane of the lips. Tongue is swollen, erythematous and painful, can be covered with white plaques. Infection can spread to the oesophagus and trachea. Angles of the mouth are erythematous, swollen, with painful fissures.

Gingival swelling (gingival hyperplasia) is result of the treatment of chronic renal disease with calcium channel blockers and calcineurin inhibitors - cyclosporine and tacrolimus. Gingival overgrowth involves interdental papilla, marginal and attached gingiva (Oyetola et al., 2015, Kuravatti et al., 2016). Condition has impact on the patient's speech, normal oral function and oral hygiene (Gupta et al., 2015).

CONCLUSION

Chronic renal failure is a complex pathophysiological process responsible for a series of complications and involvement of other organs and systems. Skin disorders are very common in patients with chronic renal failure. They can be associated with end-stage renal disease, with dialysis or renal transplantation. Chronic renal failure often becomes a consequence of several diseases – diabetes, hypertension, glomerulonephritis, cystic kidney diseases, vasculitis, rheumatic diseases, connective tissue diseases, cholesterol emboli, systemic amyloidosis and infections. Cutaneous manifestations are very diverse. Dermatological diagnosis depends on cutaneous features and clinical symptoms, in uncertain cases skin biopsy with histopathological examination is recommended. In case of pruritus diagnosis should be done very carefully to exclude other causes of itching. Therapeutic approach to skin diseases depends on several factors and not always is successful. In many cases kidney transplantation is the only one solution.

REFERENCES

Aljuaid, M. M., Alzahrani, N. N., Atalla, A. A. (2020). Complications of arteriovenous fistula in dialysis patients: Incidence and risk factors in Taif city, KSA: *J Family Med Prim Care*, 2020, Jan,9(1), 407-411.

Arora, K., Hajirnis, K. A., Sawant, S. et al., (2013). Perforating disorders of the skin. *Indian J Pathol Microbiol* 2013, 56,355-8.

Arunkumar, S., Annigeri, R. G. (2015). Ulcerative Uremic Stomatitis-Review of the Literature and A Rare Case report. *JKIMSU*, 2015, Jan-Mar, vol 4, No 1. 148-154.

Arzhan, S., Roumelioti, M. E., Unruh, M. L. (2020). Review-Advances in CKD 2020 Itch and Ache on Dialysis: New Approaches to Manage Uremic Pruritus and Restless Legs. *Blood Purif* 2020;49:222–22, doi: 10.1159/000504081.

Badiee, A., Ravanshad, Y., Azarfar, A. et al., (2018). A Systematic Review and Meta-analysis of Using Acupuncture and Acupressure for Uremic Pruritus. *IJKD* 2018; March, Vol 12, N 2:78-83.

Becker, S. et al., (2016). Edema, Hyperpigmentation, Induration: 3 Skin Signs Heralding Danger in Patients on Maintenance Hemodialysis. *Medicine. Observation Study*. 2016, March, Volume 95, Number 12, doi: 10.1097/MD.0000000000003121.

Blaha, T., Nigwekar, S., Combs, S. et al., (2019). Dermatologic manifestations in end stage renal disease *Hemodialysis International* 2019; 23:3–18.

Colboc, H., Moguelet, P., Bazin D. et al., (2019) Localization, Morphologic Features, and Chemical Composition of Calciphylaxis-Related Skin Deposits in Patients with Calcific Uremic Arteriolopathy. *JAMA Dermatol.* 2019;155(7):789-796. doi:10.1001/jamadermatol. 2019.038.

Combs, S. A., Teixeira, J. P., Germain, M. J. (2015). Pruritus in Kidney Disease. *Semin Nephrol.* 2015 July; 35(4): 383–391. doi:10.1016/ j.semnephrol.2015.06.009.

Deguchi, E., Imafuku, S., Nakayama, J. (2010). Ulcerating stasis dermatitis of the forearm due to arteriovenous fistula: A case report and review of the published work. *Journal of Dermatology* 2010, 37, 550-553.

Elmariah, S. B., Lerner, E. A. (2011). Topical Therapies for Pruritus. *Semin Cutan Med Surg.* 2011 June; 30(2): 118–126. doi:10.1016/ j.sder.2011.04.008.

Fernandes, K. A. P., Lima, L. A., Guedes, J. C. R. et al.,(2016). Acquired perforating dermatosis in a patient with chronic renal failure. *An Bras Dermatol.* 2016;91(5 Supl 1): S10-3.

Gupta, M. et al., (2015). Oral conditions in renal disorders and treatment considerations - A review for pediatric dentist. *The Saudi Dental Journal* (2015) 27, 113–119.

Hu, T. et al., (2019). Clinical features and risk factors of pruritus in patients with chronic renal failure. *Experimental and Therapeutic Medicine* 2019, vol. 18, p. 964-971.

Jaeger, V. A., Newman, M. G., Mirkes, C. R. (2017). Metastatic Calcinosis Cutis in End-Stage Renal Disease. *Baylor University Medical Center Proceedings*, 2017, 30:3, 368-369, doi: 10.1080/08998 280.2017.11929652.

Jaiswal, D. et al., (2016). Targeting the Opioid Pathway for Uremic Pruritus: A Systematic Review and Meta-analysis. *Canadian Journal of Kidney Health and Disease.* 2016, Volume 3: 1 –9 doi: 10.1177/2054358116675345.

Kaida, Y., Minami, A., Matsue-Fukuyama, M. et al., (2018). Erythema and Selling Around Arteriovenous Fistula Sites in a Hemodialysis Patient. *Am J Kidney Dis.* 2018;71(5): A10-A11.

Kawakami, T., Akiyama, M., Ishida-Yamamoto, A. (2020). Clinical practice guide for the treatment of perforating dermatosis. *Journal of Dermatology* 2020, 47, 1374-1382.

Kestner, R. I. et al., (2017). Acquired reactive perforating dermatosis is a variant of prurigo nodularis. *Acta Dermato-Venereologica. Medical Journals/Acta D-V*, 2017, 97(2), pp. 249–254. doi: 10.2340/00015555-2492.

Krajnik, M., Zylicz, Z. (2001). Understanding Pruritus in Systemic Disease. *J Pain Symptom Manage* 2001; 21:151–168.

Kuddusi,C. (2002). Increased incidence of neoplasia in chronic renal failure (20-year experience). *International Urology and Nephrology*, 2002, 33, 121-126.

Kuravatti, S., David, M. P., Indira, A. P. (2016). Oral manifestations of chronic kidney disease-an overview. *International Journal of Contemporary Medical Research* 2016;3(4):1149-1152.

Lorente-Luna M, Alfageme Roldán F, González Lois C. (2015). Ultrasound Diagnosis of Calcified Skin Deposits. Depósitos cálcicos cutáneos diagnosticados mediante ecografía. *Actas Dermosifiliogr.* 2015;106 (7):586---588. [Ultrasound Diagnosis of Calcified Skin Deposits. Cutaneous calcium deposits diagnosed by ultrasound.]

Lupi, O. et al., (2011). Cutaneous manifestations in end-stage renal disease. *An Bras Dermatol.* 2011;86(2):319-26.

Marchi, S. De, et al., (1992). Relief of Pruritus and Decreases in Plasma Histamine Concentrations during Erythropoietin Therapy in Patients with Uremia. *New England Journal of Medicine,* 1992, 326 (15): 969-74. https://doi.org/10.1056/nejm 199204093261501.

Markova, A., Lester, J., Wang, J., Robinson-Bostom, L. (2012). Diagnosis of Common Dermopathies in Dialysis Patients: A Review and Update. *Seminars in Dialysis* 2012, July-August, Vol 25, No 4 pp. 408–418.

Masmoudi, A., Darouiche, M. H., Salah, H. B. et al., (2014). Cutaneous abnormalities in patients with end stage renal failure on chronic hemodialysis. A study of 458 patients. *J Dermatol Case Rep.*, 2014; 8(4): 86-94.

Matinfar M, Shahidi S, Feizi A. (2018). Incidence of nonmelanoma skin cancer in renal transplant recipients: A systematic review and meta-analysis. *J Res Med Sci.* 2018 Feb 20;23:14. doi: 10.4103/jrms. JRMS_817_17.

Min, J. W. et al., (2016). Comparison of uremic pruritus between patients undergoing hemodialysis and peritoneal dialysis. *Kidney Res Clin Pract.* 2016 Jun; 35(2): 107–13.

Mourad, B., Hegab, D., Okasha, K. et al., (2014). Prospective study on prevalence of dermatological changes in patients under hemodialysis in hemodialysis units in Tanta University hospitals, Egypt. *Clinical, Cosmetic and Investigational Dermatology* 2014:7 313–319.

Nair, P. A., Jivani, N. B., Diwan, N. G. (2015). Kyrle's disease in a patient of diabetes mellitus and chronic renal failure on dialysis. *J Family Med Prim Care* 2015, 4,284-6.

Nunley, J. R. (2020). *Dermatologic Manifestations of Renal Disease*. Retrieved from https://emedicine.medscape.com/article/1094846-overview.

Oyetola, E. O. et al., (2015). Oral findings in chronic kidney disease: implications for management in developing countries. *BMC Oral Health* (2015) 15:24, 1-8.

Patel, R., Roberts, G. D., Keating, M. R., Paya, C. V. (1994). Infections due to nontuberculous mycobacteria in kidney, heart, and liver transplant recipients. *Clin Infect Dis*. 1994 Aug. 19(2):263-73.

Peres, L. A. B., et al., (2014). Skin lesions in chronic renal dialysis. *J Bras Nefrol* 2014;36(1):42-47.

Polanska, A., Bowszyc-Dmochowska, M., Zaba, R. W. et al., (2016). Elastosis perforans serpiginosa: a review of the literature and our own experience. *Adv Dermatol Allergol* 2016; XXXIII (5): 392–395 DOI: 10.5114/ada.2016.62849.

Rashpa, R. S., Mahajan, V. K., Kumar, P. et al., (2018). Mucocutaneous Manifestations in Patients with Chronic Kidney Disease: A Cross-sectional Study. *Indian Dermatol Online J* 2018, Jan-Feb;9(1):20-26. doi: 10.4103/idoj.IDOJ_160_17.

Qiblawi, S. H., Fivenson, D. P. (2019). Apremilast as an adjuvant therapy for calcinosis cutis. *JAAD Case Reports* 2019, October, vol 5, number 10, 874-6.

Saray, Y., Seckin, D., Bilezikci, B. (2006). Acquired perforating dermatosis: clinicopathological features in twenty-two cases. *JEADV* 2006, 20, 679–688.

Simonsen, E. et al., (2017). Treatment of Uremic Pruritus: A Systemic Review. *Am J Kidney Dis*. 2017, 70(5):638-655.

Specchio, F., Carboni, I., Chimenti, S. et al., (2014). Cutaneous Manifestations in Patients with Chronic Renal Failure on Hemodialysis. *Int. J. Immunopathol. Pharmacol.* 2014, Vol. 27, no. I, 1-4.

Stolic, R. (2013). Most Important Chronic Complications of Arteriovenous Fistulas for Hemodialysis. *Med Princ Pract* 2013; 22:220–228 DOI: 10.1159/000343669.

Ting, W. W., Stone, M. S., Madison K. C., Kurtz,K. (2003). Nephrogenic Fibrosing Dermopathy with Systemic Involvement. *Arch Dermatol.* 2003; 139:903-906.

Udayakumar, P. et al., (2006). Cutanoues manifestations in patients with chronic renal failure on hemodialysis. *Indian J Dermatol Venereol Leprol* 2006, 72:119-25.

Ulrich, C., Busch, J. O., Meyer, T. et al., (2006). Successful treatment of multiple actinic keratoses in organ transplant patients with topical 5% imiquimod: a report of six cases. *Br J Dermatol* 2006, 155(2), 451-4.

Van de Velde-Kossmann, K. M. (2018). Review-advances in CKD 2018 Skin Examination: An Important Diagnostic Tool in Renal Failure Patients. *Blood Prif,* 2018, 45, pp. 187-193.doi:10.1159/000485156.

Van de Velde-Kossmann, K.M. (2019). Review-advances in CKD 2019. Recognizing Common Skin and Soft Tissue Infections in the Nephrology Clinic. *Blood Prif,* 2019, 7, pp.259-264. doi:10.1159/000494594

Waikhom, R., Taraphder, A. et al., (2011). Nephrogenic systemic fibosis: a brief review. *Indian J. Dermatol.* 2011, Jan-feb, 56 (1):54-58.

Wang, Ch. Ch., Tang, C H. H., Huang, S. Y. et al., (2017). Risk of Non-melanoma Skin Cancer in Patients with Chronic Kidney Disease and its Relationship to Uraemic Pruritus. *Acta Derm Venereol* 2017; 97: 1230–1234.

Woolen, S. A., Shankar, P. R., Gagnier, J. J. et al., (2020). Risk of Nephrogenic Systemic Fibrosis in Patients with Stage 4 or 5 Chronic Kidney Disease Receiving a Group II Gadolinium-Based Contrast Agent: A Systematic Review and Meta-analysis. *JAMA Intern Med.* 2020 Feb 1;180(2):223-230.

Yonova, D. (2007). Pruritus in certain internal diseases. *Hippokratia* 2007; 11 (2): 67-71.

Young, T. A. et al., (2009). A pramoxine-based anti-itch lotion is more effective than a control lotion for the treatment of uremic pruritus in adult hemodialysis patients *J Dermatol Treat.* 2009, 20:2, 76-81, DOI: 10.1080/09546630802441218.

About the Editor

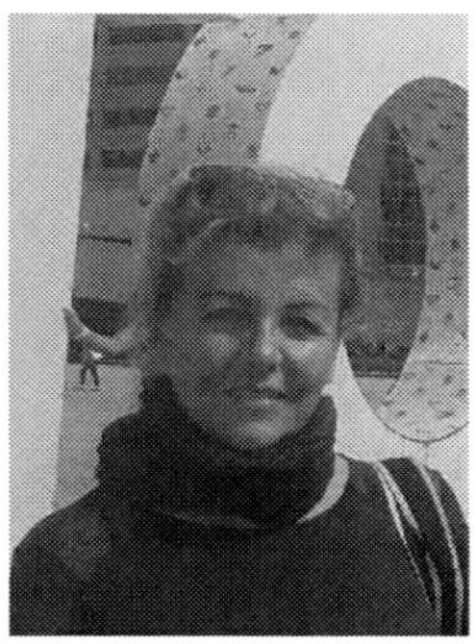

Professor Mária Frankovičová is the first Professor of Surgery in the history of Slovak medicine. She was the head of the Department of Vascular Surgery at the Faculty of Medicine, University of Pavol Jozef Šafárik in Košice, VÚSCH, a.s. (East Slovak Institute of Cardiovascular Disease). At the Faculty of Medicine, she teaches both Slovak and foreign medicine students, and trains future vascular surgeons – specialists.

Prof. MUDr. Mária Frankovičová, PhD worked at respected departments abroad and has significantly contributed to the development of surgery, vascular surgery, microsurgery

(replantation of extremities and their parts) and transplant surgery in Slovakia. Along with a team of co-workers, she was participating on certain priority operations in Slovakia. She was in the role of a regional expert on Vascular Surgery within Košice region and during 2007-2009 held the position as the Chief Expert on Vascular Surgery at the Ministry of Health of the Slovak Republic. She is a member of the European Society for Vascular Surgery as well as the International Society of Surgery (ISS/SIC), where she represented Slovakia as a national delegate of the Slovak Surgical Society for 14 years. She was responsible for the accreditation of the study program Vascular Surgery at the Ministry of Health of the Slovak Republic. She has had plenty of lectures and publications in Slovakia as well as abroad.

Her scientific research activities are directly reflected in her clinical practice in the treatment of cardiovascular diseases. She collaborates with different departments abroad. The Prize of the Mayor of Košice city was awarded to her in 2004 and in 2011, she was announced the laureate of a prestigious award, namely Crystal Wing Award, for the development in the field of medicine in Slovakia. In 2011, she was also appreciated by the Slovak Society of Angiology, and in 2013, the Municipal Executive Board of Košice awarded her with the Košice City Award for exceptional merits in the field of Vascular Surgery in Slovakia and abroad as well as for her special contribution to the development of surgical school.

INDEX

A

B

C

D

E

F

I

K

O

P

Q

R

S

T

U

V

W

X